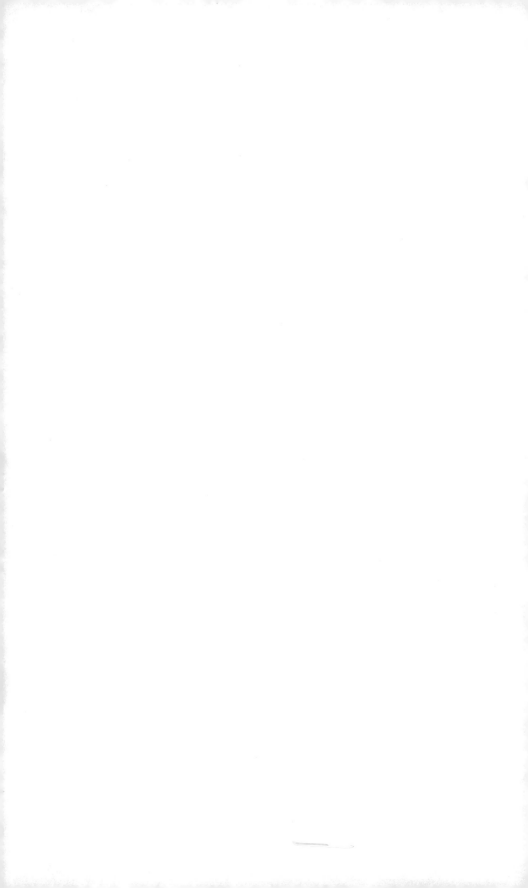

TRAUMA

DR. JAMES COLE

TRAUMA

My Life as an Emergency Surgeon

ST. MARTIN'S PRESS
NEW YORK

www.stmartins.com

Design by Kathryn Parise

Library of Congress Cataloging-in-Publication Data

Cole, James, Dr.
    Trauma : my life as an emergency surgeon / James Cole.—1st ed.
        p. cm.
    ISBN 978-0-312-55222-0 (hardback)
    1. Cole, James, Dr. 2. Surgeons—United States—Biography.
3. Wounds and injuries—Surgery. 4. Traumatology—United
States. 5. Medicine, Military. I. Title.
    RD27.35.C645A3 2011
    617.092—dc23
    [B]

                                                  2011024843

First Edition: October 2011

10 9 8 7 6 5 4 3 2 1

Author's Note

This is not a work of fiction. The case histories I share are all based on real events. However, I have changed the names of all patients and most of my colleagues and military leaders to preserve each one's privacy. Although a few minor details have also been changed, these are case histories of the actual people and experiences that have shaped my life and my professional career as a trauma surgeon. They are the stories of the patients whose lives I have had the God-given privilege of affecting.

To my wife, Michele,
who has supported me in all of my endeavors and adventures
throughout our twenty-four years of marriage.
She has selflessly stood by me during our eight separate moves,
each time establishing a welcoming home within all of the time zones
of the continental United States.
She has been the rock of our family, raising our children during
my conspicuous absences while on deployment over a half dozen times,
as well as during my internship and residency training, at which time
I was too exhausted to function as a parent.

Contents

Acknowledgments

I would like to express my sincere gratitude to my Executive Editor, Marc Resnick, who took a chance with an unknown author's first manuscript.

I would also like to thank all of the staff at St. Martin's Press who took my rough manuscript and made it readable.

I would like to acknowledge my father, Dr. James Cole, who inspired me with dinnertime stories of his patients to pursue medicine as a career. His pearls of wisdom still guide me. And to my mother, Ann Cole, who has always supported me and who was the first to read my rough manuscript.

Finally, I remain grateful to my wife and my four wonderful children, who have supported me during the many hours I was holed up writing this text.

TRAUMA

1

The Trauma Surgeon

Introduction

The stinking man's blood trailed along my arm and torso, and then ran down my leg, soaking through my scrub pants. My foot swam in a pool of the sanguineous fluid, which saturated my sock and was welling up inside my operating room shoe. The shoe—constructed of a lightweight, rubbery material that easily repelled all fluids—was keeping my patient's blood in close contact with my body as I worked. The cool, sticky sensation was terribly unpleasant, but there was nothing I could do to remedy my personal discomfort at the time.

My gloved left hand was pressed deeply into the gaping gash in the left side of my patient's neck. He had only recently been made calm, after an emergency medicine physician accommodated my request to place an endotracheal breathing tube into my patient's mouth after I ordered the senior trauma nurse to administer a hefty dose of an intravenous sedative.

Only minutes prior, I responded to a page summoning me to the trauma room. The anxious paramedics arrived with my patient at the very moment I entered the emergency room trauma area; I had no time to don any protective garments other than a pair of gloves. I had never before seen so much blood. My patient's head, face, neck, and previously white T-shirt were a bright red confluence. His arms, flailing about as paramedics kept him physically restrained to the transport gurney, were saturated with the substance. The paramedic at the head of the moving cart had blood splattered about his face as he struggled to keep the anxious and very agitated victim from rolling off the moving platform. A large pile of crimson gauze was partially secured to my patient's neck with wide swaths of blood-soaked tape, doing very little to control the ongoing exsanguination from the obvious neck injury.

I helped the four attendants move our foul-smelling patient from the paramedic gurney to the trauma cart. I leaned my face as far away as possible from the obviously intoxicated and combative individual, but I could only maintain so much distance from him with my hand firmly pressed into his neck wound. There was too much noise in the trauma room for anyone to hear my orders. Paramedics, nurses, and technicians of every variety were all speaking at anxiously loud levels, completely oblivious to all other conversations. Everyone was speaking above the other—but no one was really doing anything.

"Okay. All eyes on me!" I commanded in a firm, but nonthreatening voice. The room silenced, with the exception of the man whose neck I had in my grasp, who continued to struggle and moan in a most unpleasant manner. The stench of his filthy, inebriated body stung at my nostrils. I took a look about and realized that the volume of blood in the room had been a shocking sight to more than just myself. People all around me looked somewhat frightened. They needed direction, and they needed leadership.

I removed the bulky, ineffective dressing from my patient's neck and dark blood coughed out like water from an old pump of a country well. I placed my index and middle fingers deep within the huge, bloody wound, and I plugged the source of the hemorrhage. I could not move my hand, as it was the only thing preventing my patient from bleeding out on that trauma room table. But with my fingers in the dike, I couldn't do all else that was necessary to manage my trauma patient. I needed help from my team.

As I had done many times before, I ran the ABCs of trauma resuscitation. I ran the mental checklist as I had done repeatedly on past occasions. My patient's airway needed securing. I made eye contact with the nurse and told her to administer the intravenous sedative and paralyzing agents. I told the emergency medicine doctor rubbernecking near the foot of the bed to place the breathing tube. In less than two minutes, the airway was secured. I then asked the respiratory therapist to listen to the lungs. I watched as she nodded affirmatively as she heard breathing sounds on the left side, and then on the right side of my patient's chest. I ordered a second nurse to infuse a one-liter, intravenous bolus of fluid, and told the emergency room technician to get me a set of vitals.

"Eighty-six over fifty-four, sir, with a heart rate of one-twenty," he shouted confidently. I ordered the charge nurse to get me two units of O-negative blood and to run them in as quickly as possible. As she left the resuscitation room, I looked at the nurse who had hung the bag of intravenous (IV) fluid and asked her to call the operating room and prepare for an emergency neck exploration. She pulled a phone from her pocket and she made the call.

About five minutes later, a swarm of trauma personnel was rushing my patient into the operating room. I never left my patient's side; my fingers remained plunged deep within his anatomical defect. Once in the OR, we transferred my casualty onto the operating room table and I told one of our specialty transport paramedics to slide his fingers on top of mine. I guided his two digits into the desired position, losing another several cupfuls of blood in the process. I told him not to move a muscle, and ordered my patient's neck prepped—paramedic fingers and all—as I exited the operating room to scrub my hands.

When I returned, my patient was prepared and ready for me to definitively control the hemorrhage. I shouldered the paramedic holding pressure deep within the neck, and began my procedure. With several swipes of my scalpel and a few bold cuts with my scissors, I exposed the entire length of my patient's internal jugular vein. After instructing the paramedic to slowly move his fingers out of the wound, I witnessed the nearly transected, jagged vein spew blood at me like an erupting volcano. Recognizing the futility of attempting to repair the vein, I decided to sacrifice it. I clamped the vein above and below the devastating laceration, and the bleeding stopped. A few well-placed surgical ligatures stemmed the blood loss indefinitely, and I removed the clamps.

With the hemorrhage definitively controlled, I spent the next thirty minutes performing a thorough neck exploration in full trauma fashion. I examined my patient's carotid artery and all its branches, glad to see that the wounding instrument had narrowly missed the most important of vascular structures in the neck. A man could survive with his jugular tied off, but he could never survive if I had needed to do the same to his carotid. I then examined his trachea and his esophagus, neither of which had any evidence of injury. His thyroid gland was cut and was oozing, but a thorough cooking from careful applications of my electrocautery probe laid that problem to rest.

I concluded my operation by meticulously repairing the layers of damaged muscle my patient's neck had suffered—obviously from the sharp edge of a boldly plunged knife of a vengeful assailant. When my last skin clip had been applied, I neatly dressed the wound with gauze, I thanked the entire operating room staff for their excellent assistance, and I left the room to change out of my bloody scrubs, to cleanse my skin of the filthy patient's bodily fluids, and to seek a family member to brief of the work I had just completed. The blood clinging to the lower half of my body made me a bit nauseated, but I would soon rid myself of the semi-clotted, bloody gel.

I am only human. The other doctors, nurses, and the various health-care technicians who surround me and comprise my trauma team are also human. We are nothing special. But as the trauma surgeon in charge of a team of people, tasked by virtue of my particular job title to take control of otherwise chaotic situations—often horrible situations where death might otherwise seem inevitable—I and the other trauma surgeons who have shared my experiences are often placed in unfair situations.

When gravely injured men, women, girls, and boys are rushed into the trauma room, often by several paramedics panting to catch their breath as they sprint with their limp and bloody casualties toward the trauma beds so as to pass off a responsibility greater than they wish to be in charge of, the multiple members of the trauma team occasionally gasp. They often then take a momentary half step back and close their open, yet silent, hanging jaws, as something terribly shocking overcomes even the most grizzled and well-seasoned of the trauma groupies.

It is in one of these "Holy shit" moments that all eyes glance toward the trauma surgeon, and when the team members quietly look for a momentary sign of confidence—some nonverbal indication or cue that the trauma surgeon will be able to handle the situation in a smooth manner, regardless of whether the patient may live or die. The more seasoned ancillary veterans of the trauma team—often the charge nurse, or a graying, senior X-ray technician—know that the very worst of the worst trauma casualties may not have even the slightest chance of living beyond the confines of the trauma room. But it is often not the amount of blood soaking through the sheets and the mattress of the ambulance cart, the volume of the patient's screams or lack thereof, or even the sight of human bowel billowing out from an open body cavity, that clues those truly in the know as to the likely potential for a badly injured casualty to live another day.

Instead it is that momentary look on the trauma surgeon's face that either says "Okay, bring it on," or "What the hell am I going to do with this?"

All trauma surgeons have thought or have even muttered the latter of the two statements at one time or another. After all, we are human. There is no special place in a trauma surgeon's DNA that gives us immunity to that vile feeling of impending nausea when seeing and smelling the charred flesh of a young man who has been burned to a gruesome char. There is no particular course of surgical instruction that, upon successful completion, imparts absolute fearlessness onto the surgeon's constitution. And there is no special On/Off switch that has been biologically impregnated into a trauma surgeon's soul giving him the unique ability to tune out the blood-curdling screams and the wailing of a mother who has just been given the horrifying news that her teenaged son—whom she gave birth to, whom she nursed for six months, whose diapers she changed, and whom she raised to the best of her abilities with all of the love and hope that she could muster—has just died after an unsuccessful attempt to save him from a stray bullet that tore a hole through his chest while he was mischievously hanging out with his friends.

I can't imagine that there is an honest trauma surgeon out there who has never had his "What the hell am I going to do with this" experience in his career. Fortunately, for the majority of us, we had most of those experiences during our residency training. But despite our thousands of hours of surgical indoctrination, apprenticeship, and well-intentioned brainwashing over the five or more postdoctoral residency years of our early careers, we still continue to experience all of the human emotions.

Yet, it is our responsibility to not allow that component of natural humanism to adversely impact our abilities to critically assess, resuscitate, and manage the most severely injured trauma victims. It is in those very worst of situations, when the trauma team looks at us for direction and guidance, that we must remain the "Captain of the Ship" and do our very best to project strength and confidence to our crew. It is then when it becomes most important that we maintain a quiet calm in a room filled with anxious cacophony, and when we must perform our surgical procedures with precision and smoothness despite the immeasurable levels of adrenaline that surge through our veins.

That is when I have at times felt that I was placed in an unfair situation, as if I was being held to a higher-than-human standard. Attempting to meet that standard has given me challenges which I have accepted yet many of my non-surgeon colleagues have respectfully declined. But it has also been those challenges which have allowed me to excel at my craft, merely and solely by the will and by the grace of God.

Over the course of my twenty-year career as a physician and surgeon, I have cared for thousands of critically wounded and gravely ill individuals. I have treated patients wounded from both common mechanisms of injury, and by every other gruesome cause imaginable. I have treated gunshot wounds, stabbings, slashings, impalement injuries, industrial accidents, farm-equipment mishaps, crush injuries, and war wounds. I have seen the life pass from individuals too numerous to count—men, women, and children—as they died in my presence. And I have on countless occasions borne the unpleasant responsibility of breaking the gut-wrenching news to family members and friends—who just hours prior saw their spouses or loved ones off to work or school—that the person whom they once loved so very dearly in life, had now passed on to the world of the dead. I have heard the wailing and the screaming of grieving mothers, and I have seen the faces of the victims' fathers age before my very eyes. I have often felt that for every family to whom I have given the terrible news, I myself have sacrificed at least a few days of my own life.

Over the years I have crossed paths with presidential cabinet members, admirals and generals, executives of great stature, and the socially elite. I have also crossed paths with drug addicts, gang members and other violent criminals, the mentally unsound, and the homeless. Yet, regardless of whom I have treated as patients, whom I have worked for, and whom I have been directly influenced by, I have somehow been able to retain the understanding that everyone—some of whom present themselves covered in an attractive veneer of success and prosperity, and others literally exuding the stench of poverty and hopelessness—has the same basic wants and needs. All individuals ultimately seek a pain-free existence, compassion and understanding, and the chance to live yet another day.

There were many times in which I could manage my patients' conditions, and other times in which I couldn't. During those times in which I just couldn't resolve my patients' suffering or prolong their mortal existence any longer, I became reminded ever so bluntly that my powers as a physician are limited by something more than the constraints of just science and technology— that other factor being exponentially more powerful and unyielding than all of man's labors, inventions, and medicines combined. It has become clear to me that despite all of our efforts, we mortals are at times powerless in effecting whether one lives or dies.

Yes, I am human. I am nothing special. But my experiences have been nothing short of special, and at times spectacular. It has been those experiences that have made me the bona fide trauma surgeon that I have become.

2

The General Medical Officer

The Early Postgraduate Years

In July 1992, the military sentry guarding the front gate of Camp Pendleton noticed the blue Department of Defense sticker affixed to the windshield of my car, and he saluted me smartly. I drove through the main gate with my father-in-law in the seat next to me, and my pregnant wife in the back, tending to the constant needs of our one-year-old infant boy. We had just driven nearly three thousand miles, from the Atlantic coast to the Pacific coast, and we were exhausted. We had traveled on military orders as I had just one week before completed my internship at the U.S. Naval Hospital in Portsmouth, Virginia. I looked forward to my new adventure on the West Coast. Frankly, looking back, I believe that I could have easily looked forward to any adventure, opportunity, or simple break from the grueling, yearlong, postdoctoral internship I had just endured.

I was exhausted. I had been in academic overdrive for the past nine years— having spent four years earning my premedical degree, four more years earning my medical degree, and the most recent year working as a postdoctoral intern. I knew that I had at least four more years of postgraduate medical education to complete prior to earning my surgeon's wings, but I so looked forward to my next two-year educational break serving as a primary care physician assigned to a United States Marine Corps operational unit.

I spent the last two months of my internship on trauma rotations. In May, I had been assigned to the Orthopedic Trauma Service, and in June, I worked on the Trauma Surgery Service at Norfolk General Hospital—the region's only, major trauma center. I enjoyed my orthopedic trauma rotation, where I became proficient at managing various trauma-related bone and joint disorders, and where I learned the art of reducing fractured bone ends into perfect, anatomic alignment, prior to applying layers of plaster or fiberglass to immobilize the damaged extremities. I assisted on many operations, most of which involved the lower extremity. And I met some very interesting people.

I met a Navy SEAL who was a senior lieutenant attached to one of the East Coast teams. He had previously suffered a terrible injury to his left leg, shattering both his tibia and his fibula—the two bones joining the knee to the ankle. He had become injured months before I had ever met him, and was a regular in our orthopedic trauma clinic. He had been through multiple surgeries, attempting to save his mangled, lower extremity, and by the time we met, his leg was considered almost unsalvageable. I knew that my chief resident had spoken with the lieutenant on many occasions, trying to convince him to consider amputating the useless limb. But being a SEAL, the lieutenant didn't want to do anything that could possibly end his career.

I tried on multiple occasions to have a conversation with the man. I was fascinated by the mystique of the SEAL teams, and I wondered how exactly he had managed to injure his leg so badly. The lieutenant was always coy with me, and I never learned what actually happened to cause him to become so disabled. He repeatedly told me that he had hurt himself on a parachute training accident, but I never believed him. Years later, I would cross paths with the lieutenant again, after he walked into a premission briefing to go over the details of our orders. At some point he had agreed to have his leg amputated and he had learned to walk, run, and swim with a prosthetic limb. I was awed by the comeback he had made, and by the prestigious position he had attained on such an elite SEAL team. Years later still, I would again come to know the man as the commanding officer of the unit leading us into war. I eventually learned that the former lieutenant did not injure himself in a parachute-training accident, but had done so during a real world mission, defending the sovereignty of our nation during the later stages of the cold war.

My most recent month, however, almost broke me. I had been so exhausted after serving that last month of my internship on the Norfolk General Trauma

Surgery Service that I yearned to be done. I worked for a full month pulling continuous thirty-hour periods of duty, followed by eighteen hours of recovery time where I would drive home, sleep, and try my best to fulfill my duties as a husband and father. I was not as successful at my latter endeavors as I was with my former. My wife—a selfless, saint of a woman who dutifully followed me to Virginia, abandoning all other friends and family, just weeks after our first child was born—allowed me to sleep, but there was no such allowance on the trauma service. By the end of my month on trauma, I was a walking zombie. My days as a trauma intern were crammed with chaos, unpredictability, and a never ending load of daily work.

I assisted on trauma resuscitations, surgeries, and endless hours of dressing and invasive line changes. I cared for too-numerous-to-count patients shot during drug trafficking mishaps, stabbed by gang members, and gravely injured in automobile crashes. Every trauma situation had an aspect of newness for me, and adrenaline surged through my body as I was assigned an emergency task during each of the trauma resuscitations. The bursts of energy I experienced with each flood of my body's natural stimulant were always followed by dizzying crashes after the excitement had all been quelled. But after every exciting trauma resuscitation and surgery, I had to move on to completing my daily chores, despite the exhaustive weariness that had become almost too difficult to bear.

I was a young doctor, having just turned twenty-seven, and hadn't yet experienced enough in my career to be comfortable with some of the horrors that working on a trauma service brought to the table. I distinctly remember an eighteen-year-old man who had been distraught over the jilting by his young bride, herself just eighteen years old. I only remember his first name: Jason. As I would later be told, Jason's wife had decided to leave the short-lived marriage for another man. My patient, unable to cope with the humiliation and grief of his wife's infidelity, loaded a shotgun with a single shell, positioned the weapon vertically with the muzzle pressed upward into the under surface of his jaw, and pulled the trigger.

The shotgun blast tore through Jason's mandible, tongue, and facial structures, leaving a tattered mess of human flesh draping from his skull like bits of bloody bunting in a macabre funeral parlor. However, in a bizarre twist of true unfairness, the young man was not killed. He had been severely maimed, but he was still alive. Unfortunately, the shotgun blast had not damaged any part of my patient's brain—all of the weapon's energy was directed away from the cerebral cavity. But Jason was persistent in completing his task: he truly wanted to kill himself. Despite what must have been intolerable pain, exacerbated by the inability to swallow or speak, Jason decided to shoot himself again . . . but he had loaded only one shell into the shotgun. The rest of the rounds were in his car, which was parked outside of his apartment complex.

In his desperate attempt to finally put an end to his life, Jason stumbled down the stairs of his apartment complex, and into his car where he had stored the extra shotgun shells. Somehow, he managed to make it back up into the apartment, where he reloaded the shotgun and prepared to finish the job. But Jason no longer had the courage or the will to take his life. He regretted with all his heart what he had done to himself—and he was scared.

Somehow, paramedics had been called, perhaps by neighbors and they arrived at the apartment just a short while later. After tending to the immediate needs of Jason's wounds, they transported him to Norfolk General Hospital, and the trauma team was alerted.

When I first saw Jason being wheeled in, I was shocked. A wave of extreme unpleasantness sent a cold shiver through my body. What I saw was freakish, twisted, and too unnatural for my mind to handle without forcing myself to rationalize away my instinctive desire to run away from the mutilated figure. But that freakish, twisted figure was a trauma patient. Thankfully, there were several doctors much more senior than I who were able to deal with the gruesomeness of the situation. I would help and do whatever I was tasked with.

He came in sitting up with his back leaning against the upright portion of the paramedic gurney. As I soon realized, there was no way the paramedics could place an endotracheal breathing tube into Jason even if they had wanted or needed to. There was just too much facial trauma. I had never before seen such a sight: he looked absolutely ghoulish. With almost all of his face below the level of his cheek bones completely gone, he resembled an alien creature, with a tiny head perched onto an unnaturally long, bloody neck. There was no mouth per se, but a huge, hanging orifice in the front of the necklike area represented what most certainly had always been directly behind my patient's lower face and jaw, prior to it being blown away. Somehow, despite the massive disfigurement and the dripping remnants of bone and flesh, Jason was somehow able to breathe on his own, and apparently without too much difficulty.

Jason required little more than an urgent tracheostomy, and a fairly extensive debridement procedure—trimming and cutting away the dead tissue—of what was left of his face. The plastic surgery team participated heavily in Jason's care after he had spent about a week on the trauma service. I gradually developed the stomach to change Jason's facial dressings without cringing as I removed the yards of gauze packing from the monstrous cavern in his makeshift face, revealing remnants of sinus cavities, and a portion of his visionless, left orbit. He and I communicated as best as we could. As I unpacked and repacked the man's open wounds, I talked about whatever came to my mind. Jason scribbled a few things in response, obviously frustrated by his inability to freely communicate— not having a tongue, jaw, or mouth to generate any speech.

He did, however, manage to convey to me the details of how he said his wife had devastated him, and how he had been driven to the point of suicide, albeit unsuccessful. The whole story was quite tragic. It made me sad that the young man, hardly yet transitioned out of boyhood, could have felt so hopeless as to shoot himself in the face with a shotgun. According to what Jason later told me, his young bride had been previously married. Apparently, that marriage did not work out too well, either, as Jason penned the details of how the previous husband had also been driven to suicide—the former one having hanged himself. If what Jason told me was true, I couldn't fathom how evil that young wife must have been. Like a black widow spider, she must have lured her men into her web, fostering an environment where self-inflicted death was the most reasonable exit strategy for her prey. She herself was only a teenager!

But Jason and everything else having to do with the East Coast had been put behind me. I eagerly looked forward to my two years away from graduate medical education. Looking back on those years, they were exactly what I needed to recharge both physically and mentally. Unlike most surgical residents, but common in the military at the time, I took a two-year hiatus from my training after I completed my internship, where I worked as a military General Medical Officer (GMO) assigned to an operational Marine Corps unit. There, I was responsible for the routine, general medical care of a large group of marines attached to the 1st Surveillance, Reconnaissance, and Intelligence Group aboard Camp Pendleton, California. Those two years turned out to be very important in my development as a young physician, although I now know that I didn't quite realize it at that time.

Whereas most physicians—after completing their four-year medical school education and thereafter receiving the title of "Doctor"—progress directly into a three-, four-, or five-year postgraduate residency program, where they continue to hone their skills as a physician in the specialty of their choosing, I was ordered to serve as a military general practice physician after completing a one year, post graduate internship. When I began my GMO tour, nearly all of my civilian peers were entering their second postgraduate residency year of continued training, where they would be under the supervision of senior resident physicians and surgeons, as well as seasoned attending staff physicians. The typical residency training model has always provided the physician specialists in training with consultation and supervision from fully trained and seasoned attending specialists, and has long been the typical, postdoctoral, educational pathway for nearly all physicians.

But my case—as was the case for hundreds of other military physicians at the time—was different. Exactly one year after graduating from medical school, I was in charge of, and completely responsible for, all of my medical decisions. I was responsible for the diagnoses I assigned to my patients and for the consequences of the medical treatment plans I prescribed. This is an important distinction that most physicians actively enrolled in postgraduate residency training do not realize at the time. Despite how confident and successful trainees may feel as newly minted, resident physicians, the security of having senior residents and board-certified, attending supervisors always as close as a shout down the hall or an electronic page away provides an invisible source of courage and strength not realized until after it is gone and the independent physician is out practicing medicine on his own. For me, as a General Medical Officer, being responsible for all of my medical decisions matured me at a younger age than most, and made me a more responsible, confident, and experienced physician.

I was never charged with caring for patients with life-threatening medical illnesses or devastating traumatic injuries. However I did treat hundreds of young marines for common medical maladies such as gastrointestinal illness, upper respiratory tract infection, asthma, concussion, various musculoskeletal injuries, and the adverse consequences of poorly thought-out, sexual impropriety. That experience gave me a very valuable two-year, on-the-job immersion course in listening to patients, perfecting the doctor-patient relationship, and learning which routine treatment regimens genuinely helped patients and which did not.

In addition, my two-year general practice experience taught me that outside of the sterile confines of a major medical center—where strange, medicinal odors and crisp, white lab coats on myriads of mysterious, stone-faced individuals can often intimidate patients—patients and physicians are equal partners. One is never superior to the other. As a General Medical Officer, the patients who shared with me their medical secrets and the embarrassing details of their personal lives all worked with me and we all lived in the same military community. I observed my patients on a daily basis, in their places of work, and after hours. I knew which patients were compliant with the care plans I had prescribed, and I knew which ones weren't.

But in turn, the same people whom I had been keeping an eye on were also watching me. If a medication wasn't working, or if a diagnosis I had assigned didn't necessarily seem to be accurate, I heard about it. I heard about it from the individual marines as we would pass by each other in the motor pool, I would hear about it from the company first sergeant who thought that his marine just wasn't cutting the mustard, and I heard it from my wife, who had heard the unhappy rumblings from my patients' wives back in the military housing community. And so I learned at an early stage in my career, the true concept of accountability. I embraced, and cherished the concept. I was accountable to my patients for all of the responsibilities my position and title of "Doctor" bestowed upon me.

Another benefit to that two-year assignment to the Marine Corps was an immersive experience in leadership, which ordinary physicians seldom get offered at such an early time in their immature careers. In addition to providing medical care to the marines of my assigned unit, I was also the senior officer in charge of a detachment of enlisted, navy medical providers. Those young navy corpsmen, some only a few years out of high school, were given the significant responsibility of tending to the wounds and illnesses that the marines suffered during training evolutions.

During times of war and military conflict, the corpsmen would also be tasked with providing life-saving, front-line, emergency medical care—often while under fire on a battlefield—to marines wounded in combat. I was their supervisor and trainer. Our nation was not actively engaged in war when I first assumed my leadership position at Camp Pendleton, but I knew that at any time the marines and the navy medical personnel who supported them could be called into harm's way. And so I actively trained my corpsmen, week after week,

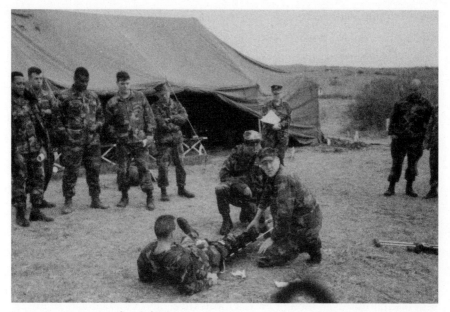

Navy corpsmen assigned to Cole's Marine Corps unit receiving combat casualty training at Camp Pendleton.

to prepare them for the wartime challenges they would hopefully never encounter.

But as fate would have it, in 1993, a large number of marines and corpsmen in my unit were in fact tested, as they were sent off to Somalia to serve during the Battle of Mogadishu. None of our marines were killed, but several of them were badly burned or wounded, and were appropriately cared for by the navy corpsmen I had personally trained. I was proud of their accomplishments. That experience was my first of several, which planted a deep seed into my consciousness reminding me that at any time we could be called upon to be tested with great challenges.

I also came to believe firmly that medical care is not an individual activity but rather a group effort. I couldn't have cared for all of those injured marines in Somalia by myself even if I had been deployed there—which I wasn't. But just like on any piece of machinery, every cog, gear, and valve is as important as the next. Some parts may play a larger role in its overall function, but when a piece of the machinery doesn't work well, the entire mechanism begins to fail. As a result of my realizing this critical aspect of health-care delivery, I became dedicated to the teaching and training of my craft to the ancillary medical providers affiliated with me. I never felt that any one of the nurses, technicians, therapists, paramedics, or military corpsmen and medics with whom I worked were ever any less important as health-care providers than I was. We were a health-care team. And as the saying goes, "there is no 'I' in 'Team.'"

I also learned that personal challenges that may seem daunting, often built great character and confidence in general when successfully completed. While assigned to my marine unit, I participated daily in unit PT—that is, physical training. I ran with the marines, I hiked with the marines, and I swam with the marines. And I kept up.

In 1993, I was offered the unique opportunity to attend the U.S. Army Airborne School. A Marine Corps officer slot at the Airborne School had opened up, and for whatever reason, there was no marine officer at our unit who could attend the course at that particular time. I was offered the opportunity to represent the marines even though I was a navy officer, and I was a doctor. It was an extremely unusual offer. No one that I had spoken to had ever heard of a navy doctor getting sent by the marines to become a paratrooper. The thought of going to jump school—as we typically called it—was quite exciting, and frightening at the same time. I accepted the offer without hesitation. So for the next four weeks, I was subjected to all of the physical training and routine mental abuse young infantry personnel endure at the Army Airborne School aboard Fort Benning, Georgia.

Airborne School was a bit intimidating, but comical at the same time. Every morning at exactly 0500, four platoons of airborne candidates assembled in tight formation on the rocks outside of the first of the 509th Parachute Infantry Regiment command building. The platoons started out with about one hundred eager parachute candidates a piece, but after about three weeks, each platoon dwindled significantly. While assembled, we were not allowed to speak unless spoken to. And despite being spoken to often—make that *screamed at*—we were usually not expected to answer. Airborne instructors did their best to weed out from the group those individuals with the weaker personalities, and those who might freeze when finally faced with having to make their first, several-thousand-foot jump.

We exercised in piles of wood chips and in pits of sawdust. We swung from training equipment and were intentionally dropped onto the hard ground by instructors who wanted to accustom our bodies to difficult parachute landings.

And we ran. We ran at least five miles every morning, and sometimes more. Airborne School was all about getting into both physical as well as mental shape. At the end of each training day, we went back to our barracks to wash our training uniforms and polish our boots. Despite the fact that we rolled in the mud and dirt, we were expected to wear crisp and clean uniforms and black, polished boots every single training day.

My first parachute jump was a nail-biter of an experience. I was genuinely frightened, but I kept my fears to myself. There is nothing normal about jumping out of the open door of an airplane traveling at over one hundred miles per hour. There is nothing normal about being blown backward, thousands of feet above the ground, by the hot exhaust of massive jet engines. And there is nothing normal about floating freely in the sky, completely unattached to any rigid or fixed structure. Yet, by facing and by pushing through my fears, I also learned the thrill of parachuting. Indeed, I became quite good at it. By the end of the course I had completed all of my required parachute jumps, and I was sent back to my marine unit with the distinctive silver parachute wings upon my chest worn by all military paratroopers, as well as my certificate of course completion.

After completing the Airborne course, I was routinely asked to go along with

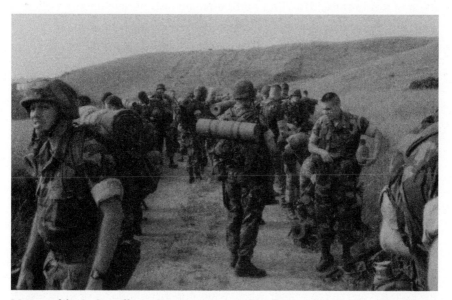

Marines of the 1st Surveillance, Reconnaissance, and Intelligence Group at Camp Pendleton, California on a grueling, fifty-mile hike in 1992. Nearly every member, including Cole, completed the hike within twenty-four hours.

the marines on numerous, parachute training operations. I willingly made many more jumps. I enjoyed the "Hollywood style" parachute activities the most. Jumping "Hollywood style" meant that we jumped out of the airplanes or helicopters wearing only our helmets and our parachutes—uniforms were, of course, a given. Typically, when military paratroopers jumped, we wore a rifle strapped to our leg and a large pack strapped upside down to the waist belt of our parachute harness. Our pack had to fit snugly between our legs, because having our much needed parachute on our back, there really was no other place for our rucksack other than between our legs. With my legs straddling a fully loaded pack, walking the few feet across the smooth metallic, always slippery, airplane deck or helicopter ramp facing the open sky was frighteningly awkward. I always felt that I would one day trip and fall as the aircraft pitched, yawed, or lurched as we traversed a pocket of turbulence. I dreaded sprawling out into the open atmosphere turned upside down and disoriented. But for some reason, I never fell down. Time after time, I was fortunate enough to safely put my "knees into the breeze" and land without much incident.

After having been credited with enough experience to upgrade my status as a parachute jumper, I traded in my silver U.S. Army parachute wings for the gold U.S. Navy and Marine Corps parachute insignia—an elite badge among those in the business. My wings were ceremoniously pinned upon my chest—actually *into* my chest—in front of the entire marine unit, all of whom had assembled in formation to honor my accomplishment. That was an important day for me as a military officer. My gold jump wings afforded me significant street credibility. And on that day, I was so very happy that I hadn't hesitated when I accepted the Airborne School slot, which the marines offered me months back.

I liked the marines, and I guess that they must have liked me as well, because in addition to sending me to Airborne School, they also sent me to military Scuba School. Now, despite Airborne School being somewhat strenuous and stressful, many aspects of the course were quite enjoyable. But there was absolutely nothing enjoyable about military Scuba School. Those ten or so weeks challenged me both physically and mentally, more than anything else I had ever before experienced. The physical challenges included hours of grueling exercises on the hot asphalt, where it was not uncommon for us to do several hundred push-ups, sit-ups, and flutter kicks, then to be followed by a five-mile run in military formation at an extremely rapid pace. Following physical training were several hours of didactic courses that taught us the physics of diving, gas laws, equipment familiarization and troubleshooting, and how to avoid serious medical problems while working under water.

Being a physician, I also learned how to treat—with chamber recompression—those divers who had suffered dive complications, such as "the bends." Scuba School was tough, and oh so exhausting. The goal of the instructors was to get the weak ones to drop out—to quit—before the next phase, which would then get really tough.

Pool Week was something I really couldn't have prepared for. During that phase of our training, the instructors pushed the students to the absolute edge of our human abilities. They took many of us to the brink of drowning. We spent countless periods of time in the deep pool, equipped with a mask, self-inflatable buoyancy vest (which looked as if it must have been held over from the Vietnam War era), two large air tanks, fins, and a weight belt.

We perfected the torturous art of "finning," where we would kick our legs front to back, with large alternating strides, to keep our chests out of the water while we held our hands up over our heads. The instructors knew that every man had a breaking point, and they pushed each of us to that point every day. When the burning and fatigue in our legs prevented us from keeping ourselves above the water any longer, the instructors would jump in and scream at us, stating that we were the weakest group of sorry-assed individuals they had ever seen. They would then often accuse us of cheating—by having air in our buoyancy vests—which, of course, was not true. The instructors would then open the air valves on our vests and push down on us to force out any of the air we had somehow illegally blown in to our buoyancy vests to help keep us afloat. No air ever came out, but by their pushing on our chests, they actually submerged our faces under the water. We often choked and gasped for air. It was very harrowing. They had a method to their madness: they wanted the weak to quit. And I almost did. But I told myself that although I might come very close to drowning, I doubted that the instructors would ever actually allow me to die. So I pushed through my fears and beyond what I thought were my physical limits, and I passed that portion of the arduous course. I was then promoted on to the next phase.

The next iteration of my training started out quiet, calm, and relaxing. Each of the students was adorned in his scuba gear, and we were instructed to crawl along the bottom, outside edge of the pool. We were only allowed to look down—we were warned not to look up or to either side lest we would get kicked out of the program. We would quietly swim at depth for five minutes, ten minutes, or maybe even longer, in complete peace and serenity. And then, *whack!* I would feel a sudden blow to my face and head, my mask would get knocked off, and my regulator—my source of air—would get knocked out of my mouth. I would then feel strong tugging at my scuba tanks as the instructors tried to pull them off my back. I reflexively grabbed hard on to a strap that connected to my air tanks. We were taught to *never* lose control of our air. I would be yanked back and forth by at least a pair of instructors, each of whom wanted my gear. But I wouldn't give it up. I would get short of breath, and oxygen hunger would quickly consume me. And then, as if they knew exactly how many molecules of oxygen I had left in my burning lungs, the instructors would stop fighting me.

As I had been taught, I secured my tanks between my legs and I squeezed them tightly. My mask was far from me, and so I felt with my hands for the air valve on the top of the tanks regulating the flow of air to my regulator hose. Unfortunately for me, the instructors routinely turned off my air valve and tied my hose into tight configurations, which I would have to spend additional precious time—without the benefit of anything to breathe or any functional vision—untangling and untying my life line. Midway through my task, I would routinely experience tunnel vision from the oxygen debt. I would soon pass out if I didn't untangle the Gordian knot. But with hands shaking, I would finally unfoul my hose, open the air valve which the instructors had nefariously closed off, blow whatever air I had left in my lungs through the regulator mouth piece to clear the system, and finally take a life-saving, precious breath. I would then re-don the rest of my gear, clear my mask, and I would then rejoin the rest of the group swimming along the bottom of the pool. Of course it would only be a matter of time until my next "hard hit." But with each successful postassault recovery, I gained more confidence as a military diver, and I got that much closer to course completion.

After completing military Scuba School, I returned to Camp Pendleton. I was now authorized to wear both gold parachute wings, as well as a silver scuba helmet insignia on my military uniform. The marines who greeted me upon my return envied my dual badges. I was told sometime along the way that at that time, there were only two physicians assigned to the Marine Corps who had ever earned both designators. One had previously served in North Carolina aboard Camp Lejeune, and I had been the sole representative in the history of Camp Pendleton. I assume that several doctors have since accomplished what I had, but hearing what I had been told at the time only further boosted my confidence.

During my remaining time at Camp Pendleton, I deployed with the marines on two different missions to Central America, where I provided medical support to the marine engineers and to the intelligence officers engaging in various activities I was not entirely privy to. I provided medical care to the marines, as well as to thousands of locals in each of the jungle regions we had visited. Our living conditions were primitive and quite austere, but we certainly lived no worse than the natives who existed in one-room homes erected from sticks, mud, and ferns. The local people truly lived simple lives and routine medical care was obviously something quite foreign to them.

We spent a few days in each of several different jungle communities, and word quickly spread that an American doctor was in the area. Locals would come up to me and ask to be examined and treated for all sorts of medical problems. Some people walked for days just to see me and my corpsmen. And on a few occasions, I was escorted by our intelligence officers into the local communities via horseback to provide medical consultation and care to the local villagers. Often, people would bring their children to us, but occasionally they would have maladies for which there was no cure, such as Down syndrome, or cerebral palsy. It was heartbreaking to see the last bits of hope in a mother's eyes fade, as the American doctor told them that there were no curative remedies for their children's disorders. My first experiences going to Third World countries were educational adventures, and each one was socially enlightening. Before that time, I never really knew firsthand just how poor some people truly are, and how much they suffer on a daily basis.

As the end of my two-year assignment neared, I knew that what I really needed to do was complete a surgical residency and become a surgeon. I had done many exciting things stationed with the marines at Camp Pendleton, and I had been given a lot of time to decompress from the rigors of my intern year. After those two years, though, I was clearly ready to move on, and ready to begin the next phase of my medical career. I had prepared myself to begin that second year of my residency training at William Beaumont Army Medical Center as well as anyone could have. For months prior to my move to El Paso, I read and reread multiple medical and surgical texts and handbooks. I memorized every page of the most recent *Advanced Trauma Life Support* manual. And I even

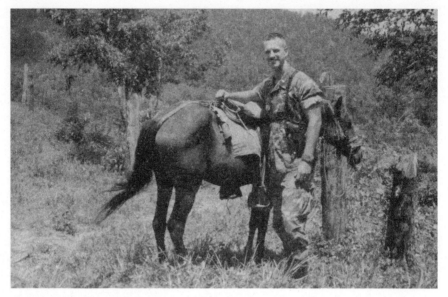

Dr. Cole on deployment to Honduras in 1993, where he occasionally rode into the local communities on horseback to assess sick villagers.

attempted to condition myself to needing fewer hours of sleep, knowing that residency training was notorious for permitting no more than a few hours of rest per night.

I remembered with some disdain and mild anxiety my yearlong internship at the U.S. Naval Hospital in Portsmouth, Virginia, where I would awaken each day no later than 4 A.M. Each day I would work incessantly—often without food or bathroom breaks—until I thought that my work was completed. When I would check out to one of my senior residents, I would almost always receive additional patient care duties taking me well into the dark hours of the night before I was finally able to complete all of my assigned work. I never saw the light of day before being released by my chief resident to go home. When I was not on call, I would usually leave the hospital after 8 P.M., allowing me very little time to go home, spend a few precious moments with my cherished wife, read whatever medical assignment I had been given, and quickly fall asleep knowing that my 4 A.M. alarm call would soon again signal me to start yet another day.

Every third twenty-four-hour period was made even more agonizing by having in-house, on-call responsibilities. That is, my end-of-the-day duties and responsibilities never truly ended as they merely blended into the following day. I would often spend my entire day, night, and the following day rounding on the thirty or more patients admitted to our service, performing inpatient history and physical examinations, assisting senior residents and attending surgeons in the operating rooms or in the clinics, and writing pages and pages of notes documenting the care rendered to our patients. It was the rule rather than the exception for every intern at my training hospital to work forty continuous hours every third day, and over 120 hours in a week's period of time. We were not allowed the luxury of weekends off. If I was fortunate, I would usually be given one entire day off per month—usually a Sunday—toward the end of a monthlong rotation.

That is just how things were back then. That year—as well as during my residency years—was by no means glamorous. Nothing during any portion of my internship or during my residency years mirrored any of the recent television situational comedies or dramas, which inaccurately depict young physicians cavorting with the nurses and the other house staff, enjoying their newly empowered titles as medical doctor. Showering was a luxury, and essentially unheard of when on call. Sleep deprivation was a given, and it was an unrelenting constant. I often thought that sleep deprivation was likely one of the major factors explaining why many physicians become so impersonal, so cold, and so emotionally hard. Going without sufficient sleep for years at a time, in my opinion and experience, alters a person's attitude toward pain and suffering. And when the trainees are in pain and are suffering themselves due to pure, physical exhaustion, there is very little compassion left in the physicians' reservoirs to give to their patients.

But I had been given a two-year break while serving as a General Medical Officer, to rest, to mature, and to develop my skills as a physician. After those two years, I knew with absolute certainty that I wanted to be a surgeon, and I knew that my dream could never be realized without enduring the rigors of a surgical residency. Certainly, there may be scores of physicians—perhaps hundreds, or even thousands—who may have chosen surgery as their profession of choice, only to abandon those dreams and pursue a less-rigorous, less-torturous postgraduate training program in one of the many other medical disciplines. Prior to starting my second year of postgraduate training, I was both physically and mentally prepared for the challenges I would soon face. At least I thought that I was. But nothing really could have prepared me for that first major trauma patient under my care—one which I remember to this day so very well. And I was about to embark on that experience during my very first night of call as a second-year surgical resident.

3

My First Major Trauma

The Junior Surgical Resident

It was early July 1994, and the time was somewhere in the early evening—perhaps 6 P.M. It was my third full day as a second-year surgery resident, and I was already tired. I was working in a very large hospital complex, completely unfamiliar to me. I barely knew the routine of the residency program as I had not even completed one full week. I hadn't yet learned the personalities of all of the other residents and attending surgeons. Yet, despite having been in the surgery program for less than seventy-two hours, I had a complement of over twenty patients of whom I was responsible for knowing every intimate detail. I carried a pocket full of index cards, all of them listing the critical details of each of my patients' medical conditions. The cards included their significant medical history, a list of their current medications and allergies, dates when admitted to the hospital, dates and types of surgical procedures performed, ongoing issues of importance, lab and X-ray data for the past several days, and the treatment plans and directions of each of their attending surgeons ultimately responsible for the patient's well-being.

I carried the monumental responsibility as the first-line respondent to the nurses providing bedside care to each of the patients. There were always questions and concerns, and I just didn't have much experience making critical decisions on matters of that level of importance. My shoulders were tight and my head ached, but that was all part of my new job and it was also all part of my new responsibility as a surgical resident. To make matters worse, however, that evening would be my first night tasked with taking in-house calls. I was not at all looking forward to my added responsibility, but I could not wish it away.

I had barely slept in the previous few days. Even though I was not on call prior to that day, I remained in the hospital well into the night the previous two days learning the hospital's computer system, learning the layout of the facility, and committing whatever details of each patient's hospital record I could to memory, backing up my brain with my stack of note cards. In addition, I reviewed numerous treatment algorithms that spelled out what I would need to do if a patient had a sudden cardiac arrest, how I would treat a life-threatening cardiac arrhythmia, or which doses of which emergency medications and which size endotracheal tube I would choose when establishing an artificial airway in a patient unable to breathe. I also again reviewed the *Advanced Trauma Life Support* manual, otherwise known as the *ATLS* manual. The *ATLS* manual was the guidebook for all physicians caring for trauma patients. The *ATLS* manual had chapters describing appropriate management of every major category of a trauma situation. I knew that William Beaumont Army Medical Center treated many trauma patients and I expected to see at least one during my first night of call.

Despite being a military medical facility, our hospital received about one-third of all of the major trauma patients in the city of El Paso. El Paso, Texas, was an international border community—Juarez, Mexico, being our sister city immediately to our south. I routinely noted the huge Mexican flag flying in the most northern part of Juarez, easily seen from my front yard on the military base aboard Fort Bliss, where I lived. There was good reason why a military hospital would care for as much civilian trauma as we did. Not only were trauma patients an excellent source of great training for members of a surgical residency program, but the civilian county hospital in El Paso just couldn't handle all of the patient volume it received. If our hospital couldn't take care of a portion of the trauma casualties in town, the whole trauma system in El Paso could have potentially failed.

El Paso and Juarez shared more than just an international border. The two cities also shared a more dubious distinction: we were a major international drug region. The drug cartels and their foot soldiers often engaged in small street battles, and at times created havoc in the communities of our neighboring towns. As a result, William Beaumont Army Medical Center cared for numerous U.S. and Mexican citizens who fell victim to the perils of the often heinous drug traders. Fortunately for most El Pasoans, most of the drug dealers kept to themselves and did not terrorize the home owners of the communities in which they lived. However, drug dealers often battled it out with one another, leaving blood and carnage in the streets and barrios.

To feel safe, most home owners had placed heavy bars on their windows to keep out potential criminals. But despite the citizens' fears, significant home burglaries were actually quite rare. Petty theft was common, however, and I think that everyone I knew had at least one bicycle stolen by a cross-border thief who probably sold it for no more than a few dollars or pesos. Cars were stolen fairly often as well, but my family's minivan and our Toyota hatchback were never on the list of preferred vehicles for thieves to steal in Texas and to sell south of the Rio Grande. For the most part, I had no trouble with the crime in El Paso. After all, it often resulted in paramedics bringing me some of the best gunshot trauma I've ever had the pleasure of dealing with.

I was well into my first night of call. It was nearly midnight and I had already awakened myself once from a momentary slumber to walk through the surgical intensive care unit to check up on each of the patients the surgery service was responsible for overseeing. My senior residents had taught me never to sleep for more than two hours at any given time while on call. I needed to have frequent eyes on each of our patients. If I chose to fall prey to my weaknesses and attempt to get some real sleep, a patient could unknowingly begin to decompensate and suffer tragic consequences. If anything adverse was to happen without my knowledge while I was sleeping, I would be forced to explain to an entirely unsympathetic group of staff surgeons the following morning why I was resting when a patient was dying. That was an extremely unpleasant event, which I had witnessed of other residents on two occasions while I was an intern. Both situations eventually resulted in each of the residents being dismissed from the surgery training program. I was absolutely, positively not going to allow such a failure to happen to me.

And so on the sound advice of my senior residents, from that first night of call and on every other night of call for the duration of my additional years as a junior resident, I set my watch alarm to sound every two hours. Each time I heard that terrible beeping sound, I would get up, and I would again walk through the surgical intensive care unit and eyeball each of my patients.

In the late hours of that first call night, despite my youth, I was the senior surgical person in-house, responsible for all of the critically ill patients. Everyone else had gone home. I was responsible for the handling of any problems in the intensive care unit, and for managing any new surgical patients or trauma casualties who should come through the doors of the emergency room. I was only a second-year resident, but for the next two years I would share all of the in-house call responsibilities with two other second-year residents and two third-year residents. In order to survive, we divided our nightly, on-call responsibilities among the five of us. On nights when I wasn't on call, one of the other four junior residents would be in-house and I would be at home trying to get some rest.

On that particular night I was the only surgical resident in the hospital, and I was in charge of everything. It was all quite frightening. The fourth-year surgical residents, the fifth-year chief residents, and the fully trained, board-certified, attending surgeons were all at home in bed, as were all of the subspecialty surgeons. I could call any of them if I had a question or if I needed help. But it had been well ingrained into my consciousness by the other residents that if I were to call for help, I would be demonstrating a sign of weakness, and that would be viewed unfavorably by the others. It was expected of me that I would notify my chief resident if I needed to admit a patient or if a patient needed to be taken to the operating room. In all other circumstances, though, I had best be able to handle every other problem on my own. I wanted to succeed, and I wanted to please my senior residents and my attending surgeons, and so, as unpleasant as my on-call duties would be, I accepted my responsibilities and dealt with every patient problem on my own.

Shortly after midnight the long shrill of the trauma pager sounded. I nearly jumped, as my body was primed with adrenaline and overly filled with caffeine. A trauma patient was being brought into the emergency room, and I was the man in charge. My pulse raced and my chest pounded.

I practically leaped down the stairs, trying to get to the trauma room before the patient arrived. I did get there first, and I was already gloved and gowned by the time the El Paso paramedics brought my trauma casualty into our emergency room. Prior to their arrival, I had again rehearsed the *ATLS* algorithms in my head, but when my casualty was actually wheeled in, my heart sank. It was a child. I had tried so hard to control my destiny by mentally rehearsing over and over how I would manage every trauma scenario imaginable, but I had been preparing to handle adult casualties. When that little boy was wheeled in, my confidence dropped. Kids are just different than adults for so many reasons, and I needed to mentally adjust—quickly.

My first major trauma casualty over which I would have command and control was a very young child, who was the victim of a drive-by shooting. He had been shot through the head. I would later learn that his name was Felix, that he was four years old, and that he was standing with his father out on the front porch of his home as his father argued with men slowly driving by their house. Felix had been shot through the head, from temple to temple. Blood and a scant amount of brain matter oozed through the child's hair and onto the gurney beneath him.

My heart raced. I mustered all of the strength in me to remain calm. I remembered a television commercial I had once seen. It was an underarm antiperspirant commercial where nervous businessmen and women all raised their arms without any physical evidence of wetness. The voice in the commercial stated in a deep and confident tone, "No matter how nervous you are inside, never let them see you sweat." I repeated that phrase to myself, and I vowed to remain calm, to take charge, and to do all that I hoped I could to help that child.

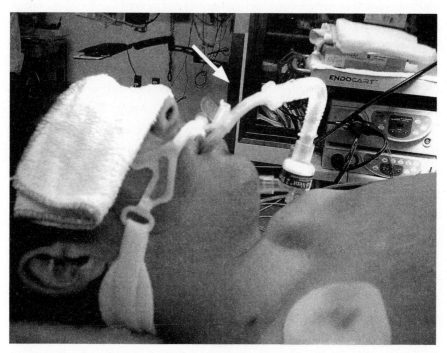

Arrow points to an endotracheal tube inserted into the mouth of an adult casualty.

Felix was not breathing. The paramedics had been bag-ventilating the boy with a mask, but I knew from my *ATLS* manual readings that the child needed a tube placed into his trachea and he needed to be placed on the ventilator. But what size tube would I choose? I had not mentally prepared nearly enough for a child. I then remembered the rule of sixteen plus age divided by four, which would help me choose the appropriately sized device. I estimated that the child was about four years old. Sixteen plus four was twenty, and twenty divided by four was five. So according to the rule, I decided to insert a size 5 endotracheal tube.

I ordered a nurse to administer an intravenous muscle paralytic agent to make my placing the tube easier, without which the child would reflexively bite down as I placed the metal laryngoscope blade into his mouth—a necessary technique that permits visualization of the vocal cords through which the tube must pass. After the medication had taken effect and my patient's little muscles had all become flaccid, I opened his mouth, swept his swollen tongue to the side, and lifted upward on the laryngoscope handle to visualize the little boy's vocal cords. I knew that if I placed the tube into the esophageal opening and not into the tracheal opening, the child would die. This was a crucial moment, and it was my very first pediatric intubation. I saw the cords, I placed the tube, and I breathed a sigh of relief. All was good with step one.

Next, I listened to the child's lungs as I had been taught. I heard breath sounds on both the left and on the right. Everything sounded okay. I connected the child to the breathing machine and I calculated exactly how much air the ventilator should blow into the little boy's lungs, and how often each breath should be administered. Determining those parameters was a matter of simple mathematics, which I was able to calculate in my head after estimating the child's weight in pounds, mentally converting it to kilograms by dividing by a factor of 2.2, and then plugging the resultant number into additional formulas I had memorized.

I then assessed whether or not the boy was in shock. His blood pressure was subnormal and his pulse was fast and thready. The boy's skin color was pale, and he had the generalized look of impending death. I figured that if ever a person had the classic look of shock, my pediatric patient had that look. To counter the shock state, I hastily ordered IV lines to be placed by the ER technicians and nurses, and I ordered an infusion of Lactated Ringer's IV solution, as well as O-negative blood.

I carefully examined the child's head where I saw two abnormally large bullet holes, one on either side of his head. Each hole oozed a dark, gooey substance consisting of blood admixed with brain material. I had seen gunshot wounds before as a medical student and as an intern, but the wounds in that child's head seemed awfully large to me. In retrospect, I realized that what looked abnormal was the unusually small size of my patient wounded by a standard-sized bullet.

The child was not moving even when I pinched the skin of his chest and when I squeezed the nail beds of his fingers. His pupils were widely dilated and they did not constrict in size when I shined a bright light onto them. I felt a terrible sense of doom as I was sure that the child was going to die on me. But he still had a heartbeat, a blood pressure, and a pulse, and I was still very much responsible for keeping that child alive, which I would do to the best of my very novice abilities.

After securing the breathing tube and ensuring that the O-negative blood was running into the child's miniature veins, I pushed the emergency room cart myself into the CT scanner to assess the child's brain and to view the destruction before calling the attending neurosurgeon at his home. After helping lift the child onto the CT scan table, I nearly collapsed from physical exhaustion into a chair in the adjacent CT technician's command room. Remaining vigilant, I viewed my patient at all times through the glass partition and kept my eyes fixated on the portable cardiac and blood pressure monitors. I realized that I was also mentally exhausted, and I did not have a good feeling that the outcome of the shooting would be favorable. At that very moment, I no longer wanted to be a surgical resident. But I also knew that I was into my commitment elbow deep at that point, and there was no reconsidering my choice to become a surgeon at that particular moment in time.

The CT images of Felix's little brain started to pop up on the technician's monitor. Bullet and bone fragments could be seen traversing the brain from side to side. It looked awful! Being so inexperienced, it was the worst brain I had ever seen at that point in my career. I couldn't even imagine how anyone could fix a problem like that. But someone else might know exactly how to deal with the child's injury. I took the opportunity to contact the on-call neurosurgeon to give him a full status report on the child on whom I thought he would almost certainly need to operate. I began to describe the child's injuries to the neurosurgeon including all that I had done to my patient, when suddenly the child took an abrupt turn for the worse. The child began to die. His heart rate precipitously dropped and his oxygen saturation became critically low. I told the neurosurgeon that I needed to hang up immediately and abruptly ended the call.

I ran into the CT room and reassessed my dying child. I started by examining the breathing tube. I had always been taught, and the *ATLS* manual clearly stated, that if there was an unexplainable change in a trauma patient's status, always reassess by starting from the very beginning. So I rechecked the airway tube. I couldn't tell with certainty what I was seeing, and to gain as clear a view of the entire tube as possible, I again placed the metal laryngoscope into his little mouth. I suctioned away the sputum and blood, and I clearly saw that the tube had become dislodged. I threw the useless tube onto the floor in somewhat of a frustrated manner and I began bag-ventilating little Felix. My mind raced as to why the tube could have dislodged, and I shouted for nurses to bring me another size 5, endotracheal tube and the additional medication I again needed.

After bagging the boy for what seemed like an eternity as I awaited the arrival of my new tube and medication, I attempted to intubate the boy once more. After readministering the paralytic drug that I had ordered, I again introduced the laryngoscope into the boy's mouth and again visualized his vocal cords. I passed the tube easily into the correct opening and I once again reassessed his vital signs. The boy's heart rate and blood pressure subsequently normalized, and his oxygen saturation had come up to a perfect 100 percent! Things were again looking acceptable. I securely taped the breathing tube to the boy's face and neck after I connected it back to the ventilator. I then slowed my pace down and I went back into the CT technician's room. I felt that Felix was not yet ready to die. I then called back the neurosurgeon and I gave him the full briefing of all that had transpired.

Lieutenant Colonel Jonathan Rensch was the neurosurgeon on-call that evening—as he always was. Dr. Rensch was the only neurosurgeon the army had assigned to El Paso at the time, and the man worked like a dog. I didn't know Dr. Rensch prior to that first evening, but from that initial night forward, I developed a deep respect and admiration for the man. He was an extremely talented surgeon, an exceptional teacher, and a very pleasant man to be around in general. He was clearly destined for success and greatness as both surgeon as well as military officer. He would one day later get selected for and be promoted to the rank of Brigadier General—a great honor for any officer. I truly was very fortunate to have been taught by such a gifted and talented individual.

During my second phone conversation with the neurosurgeon, I gave my full briefing on the status of my patient. I also explained the temporary setback and the reason for my hanging up on him so abruptly. After listening to my presentation, Dr. Rensch told me to expedite the child to the operating room and to prepare him for emergency surgery. I was both excited and exhausted. But more than anything else, I was relieved. I was finally going to get some real help.

I rushed young Felix to the operating room as instructed and I awaited Dr. Rensch's arrival. In a matter of a few minutes, Dr. Rensch walked into the OR with CT films in hand. He was intensely studying them and mumbling quietly. All I could make out were the words "This is bad . . . this is really bad."

After the anesthesiologist and the operating room nursing staff took over my patient, Dr. Rensch and I went out to the scrub sink where we prepped ourselves for surgery and briefly discussed my encounter with the very first trauma patient over which I had control. We then entered the operating room with hands and arms dripping—his rank and position allowing him to enter the room first—where we each dried off, were ceremoniously gowned by the scrub nurse, and then gloved thereafter. Dr. Rensch then painted the child's head with antiseptic-soaked sponges, and together we applied the surgical drapes exposing nothing but a small window to the child's shaved cranium. Dr. Rensch told me that there wasn't much that could be done for the boy, that his injuries were devastating, and that generally speaking, gunshot wounds that crossed the midline of the brain were almost always lethal injuries. But he also told me that since the child was so young, he had a better chance than most to survive. If our patient had any chance at all for survival, we would have to be very aggressive in our surgical treatment and in our postoperative, critical-care management.

For the next two hours, I assisted Dr. Rensch as he removed both the left and the right sides of the little boy's skull and as we surgically removed the tiny burned and pulverized portions of the irreversibly damaged brain tissue. We irrigated the bullet tract with sterile saline solution, allowing liquid to pour out one side of the cerebrum as we squirted the solution into the hole on the opposite side. It really was quite surreal. The badly damaged brain had become swollen and was bulging in a grotesque manner. There was absolutely no way that we would ever get the removed portions of the child's skull back in place without further damaging the brain, which had expanded like rising bread dough well beyond the confines of its container. We had no other option but to close the skin of the boy's scalp without replacing the skull portions. I asked Dr. Rensch what we would do with the child's two pieces of bone. He then told me that they would go into the freezer for safekeeping. I thought that he was kidding, but he wasn't.

For the next three weeks, I helped care for little Felix in the surgical intensive care unit. The boy had numerous setbacks and complications following surgery. He developed pneumonia on two different occasions, each time receiving an appropriate course of intravenous antibiotics directed specifically at the particular organisms we cultured directly from his lungs. Drains we had placed between Felix's brain and skin had clotted off, and the invasive monitor measuring the internal pressure in his brain stopped working several times requiring replacement on each occasion. On more than one occasion, we were all certain that Felix would soon die, but for some reason that little boy always responded to radical and aggressive interventions.

During the initial postoperative weeks, Felix's head continued to bulge as his swollen brain stretched his young skin to alienlike proportions. We kept him in a deep, chemical coma with the drug pentobarbital—a powerful sedative that slows the brain's activity to a bare minimum allowing for potential, natural healing and recovery. By the end of the third week, we had completely weaned him off all of the pentobarbital and the child was starting to show minimal signs of spontaneous movement. But in no way was he behaving normally, and few of us felt that there was little hope for Felix. All residents, nurses, and staff surgeons dutifully cared for that little boy, hoping for the best, but knowing in our hearts that his chances for meaningful recovery were slim to none.

After another month or so in the surgical intensive care unit, little Felix became more awake, yet remained profoundly dysfunctional. He stared blankly, not even showing an emotional reaction to his own mother's voice. He didn't follow any commands but he reacted appropriately to a painful pinch by moving his hand toward the area stimulated. Felix was by no means cured, but he had become stable and healthy enough to be transferred out of our hospital to a pediatric rehabilitation institution.

Dr. Rensch reattached Felix's skull portions after the brain swelling had normalized. Following that last surgery, the boy's wounds had all eventually healed. His eyes would open but they would roam randomly and without purpose. He could not speak due to the tracheostomy tube we had placed in his neck weeks before, preventing natural speech. He was fed through a tube placed through his abdominal wall and into his stomach. He looked pathetic. None of us was sure if we had done the right thing or not by being so aggressive in attempting to save that child's life. At that point, Felix looked more or less vegetative, and we were sad but relieved when paramedics eventually transported him off to the pediatric rehabilitation facility. We doubted that we would ever see him again, and we weren't sure that we even wanted to. He had consumed every last bit of all of our collective, emotional energies.

Not quite a year had passed since the day Felix was shipped off to the rehabilitation center. By that time I had almost completed a full year of residency training at William Beaumont. I had finally become content. For the most part, I was doing what I wanted to do, and had become more skilled and confident in my trade. I never expected anyone to ever visit me, including my dear wife and children, so I thought that the ICU nurses were mistaken when they paged me and stated that I had a visitor awaiting me. Not being too forthright when I asked who could have possibly come to visit me, they told me to stop asking questions and to head over to the ICU to see for myself.

To say that I was a bit shocked was an understatement. There he was. He walked toward me. Little Felix was smiling and walking, albeit with a limp, but walking nevertheless. He was holding a small, foam baseball and looking pretty much like any other little kid—shy and clinging to his mom. He looked so very much alive, and he certainly seemed to be more than acceptably functional.

Felix had completed many months of inpatient therapy, followed by an even longer period of outpatient rehabilitation. His mother had brought him back for us all to see, and to personally thank each of us for saving her young son's life. I was almost speechless. Despite the choking sensation in my throat, I managed to ask Felix to throw me his ball, which he did a bit awkwardly. But he threw that ball better than I could ever have expected for a boy who had tried to die in my presence more than once, and whose brain I had squirted fluid through months before. I was filled with many emotions: happiness, momentary pride, and more than a little anxiety as I recalled the harrowing days when we first met. He was my first trauma patient, he had been shot through the brain, and I had helped save his life. It was all pretty amazing, yet somewhat surreal as well.

I then realized something very powerful and humbling. While Felix was in our hospital, I never really expected that little child to live, let alone walk and toss me a ball. I also thought that at very best Felix would have had the functional level of a smiling vegetable. That disturbed me greatly remembering all that I had thought when Felix was a patient in our hospital, and how I had felt subsequently on the day he returned to us. It was then that I realized with concrete certainty that humans are not the ultimate authority as to whether a patient lives or dies, or as to their ultimate outcome. Some things—like that young boy's amazing recovery—are just too difficult to explain from a logical, rational perspective.

From that day forward, I allowed the concept of miraculous recovery to enter my realm of possible patient outcomes. And to this very day, I do not discount the possibility that even my most severely traumatized casualties can occasionally recover in a manner that can be classified as nothing other than truly miraculous.

4

Indoctrination, Brainwashing, and Sleep Deprivation

The Training of a Surgeon

After completing my first twelve months in El Paso, I had two years of post-graduate training under my belt—one just completed and the other served immediately after medical school while serving as an intern at Portsmouth Naval Hospital prior to my GMO tour with the Marine Corps. I had adjusted to living the life of a surgical resident as well as could be expected. The year had been difficult—extremely difficult. It was at times demoralizing. I averaged about 120 hours per week in the hospital, and I took a total of twenty-one vacation days that year. Twenty-one days was the maximum amount of leave time our surgical residency program director allowed. By doing the math, I figured that I had put in over 5,800 hours of actual time spent in the hospital during that year. That was about 3,900 more hours than my nonphysician friends back home had worked, each of whom had typical forty-hour workweek jobs. But that didn't bother me much. I felt that despite my suffering, I was probably one of the lucky ones. I had always been certain that I wanted to be a doctor, and by that second postgraduate year of my training, I was still pretty sure that I also wanted to be a surgeon. Even though surgery training was about as close to hell as I could have imagined, I was already two-fifths done with it.

Perhaps my greatest degree of strength and support came not from within, but from my wife, Michele. She and I had been married for close to nine years at that point, and she had been well aware of my desire to become a doctor even long before our wedding. We had dated since high school, and having known my calling to practice medicine even before I had completed college, my wife was nothing less than completely supportive of my endeavors. The support she gave me was certainly at great expense to her, as she bore the complete responsibility of raising our children and managing our home. I was rarely available to her, and when I was, I was usually semicomatose as a result of my chronic sleep deprivation. Although my will to be a better family man was never lacking, the continuous degree of physical exhaustion my internship and residency training programs imposed upon me prevented my accomplishing much outside of the hospital. Without Michele's selfless support and encouragement, I would have never made it through those grueling years of training. She liked me—she loved me—and she made that unquestionably evident by her unwavering support.

I was also fortunate to be well liked by my attending surgeon supervisors. They rarely abused me in a completely unforgivable manner, but they certainly did make life difficult for me at times—as was customary among all surgical residencies at the time—although I don't think that I was tortured as often as many of my residency peers had been. I always did what was asked of me and I didn't try to cut corners in order to garner a few extra hours of precious sleep time.

I would never be critical in any way of the other residents in my program who trained along with me. Each one of us suffered in his own ways throughout our training, and each resident coped with his suffering a little differently. For the most part, all of the residents were very competent and hardworking people. We did have a few stray cats in the mix who I never really understood how they managed to get selected to train in our program in the first place—two of the residents were eventually let go and one guy not in my training year group had a very difficult time as an attending surgeon after completing his residency training. The residents were all well policed by our program director, but our surgery boss didn't have complete authority over everyone, including many of the interns. There certainly were a few less-than-stellar interns who needed what the uniformed services often calls EMI—that is, Extra Military Instruction. In short, assigning someone EMI meant that they were punished with what many would consider to be useless piles of extra shit work.

Reflecting back on the end of my second year of postgraduate training, I remember one particular intern who earned more than his fair share of Extra Military Instruction. I was the junior resident assigned one particular month to the East Team, which was one of the three teams on which we randomly rotated. My senior resident was a short-statured and dry-witted man two years my senior named Jerry Harmack. I really don't remember who served as my chief resident, or which of the numerous attending surgeons we worked for at the time, but I distinctly remember the intern who worked for Dr. Harmack and me. That particular intern's name was Phil.

Now, Phil was actually an intern in a non-surgery specialty, assigned to work on our surgery service for one month so that he could learn some basic surgery and complex patient-management skills. Everyone who had ever trained as an intern knew that he or she would at some time be assigned to the surgery service, and that it would be an extremely long and unpleasant month. Yet, it could also be a very rewarding month because many interesting things happen to surgery patients. As we used to tell people rotating on the surgery service, "Taking in-house call every other night had its distinct disadvantages—you miss half of the great cases when you're not in the hospital." That was the attitude of how things were back then, although I know that residency training has since become much more tame ever since regulatory agencies have enacted the eighty-hour, workweek limitations for all postgraduate trainees.

Most interns made the best of the long and grueling experience, and accepted that they would be working the long and ridiculous hours of a surgery resident, understanding that they would hopefully gain some surgical experience and knowledge along the way. But this did not seem to fit into Phil's plans. In the early morning of the first day on our East Team rotation, Jerry, Phil, and I were scheduled to all meet in the surgical intensive care unit to go over our patients and to discuss our plan for the day. I was ready to discuss my new service, having already made personal rounds on each of the intensive care unit patients by that time. As Jerry—Dr. Harmack—had told us the night before, I was expected to have seen each of the ICU patients and Phil was to have seen each of the less-serious floor patients before 6 A.M. at which time we would present each patient's status to Jerry.

It was customarily expected of us to have checked each patient's vital signs, to have reviewed all fluids administered or consumed by each patient in the preceding twenty-four hours, and to have known exactly how much each patient had voided (that is, urinated). In addition, we were to have checked every lab value that had been ordered, and to have personally spoken with and briefly examined each patient. We knew exactly what was expected of us, and to fulfill our senior resident's requirements and have everything done by six o' clock, I arrived in the intensive care unit at a quarter to five that morning and had completed my tasks by exactly 5:59 A.M. I was right on time and I was ready to begin.

Jerry showed up promptly at 6 A.M. and immediately asked me if there were any patient issues of which he should be made aware. It was his responsibility as our immediate senior to report issues of significance to our chief resident, who might then issue any corrective directives that we hadn't already initiated on our own. It was the chief resident's responsibility to then brief the entire group of attending surgeons at the daily 6:45 A.M., surgical conference. The morning surgical conference was where admissions throughout the night were presented to the group, where critical patient issues were discussed, and where the surgical plan of the day was disseminated. Jerry and I discussed a few patients in particular, but by that late point in my second year of residency I had already been well trained as to how and when to anticipate problems, and how to remedy small issues before they became big problems. Jerry was happy with the report I gave him that day, which was factual and honest. But we did have one very big problem: Phil had not yet shown up.

We paged Phil, who promptly called us back. He told us that he still had a few patients he needed to check on and that he would be down to meet us in about fifteen minutes. I was pretty surprised by what the intern had told us. It was something utterly unheard of in a surgical residency program. First of all, no one ever failed to show up for an assignment, including morning rounds, unless the intern or resident in absentia was actively resuscitating a dying patient. And no one *ever* told a senior resident what he was going to do. Interns and residents were told by their seniors exactly what they were expected to do and when they were expected to do it. Orders were issued by members of an established hierarchy, and all surgeons in training followed them. No one questioned the hierarchy or the orders. It was how things had been done for more than a century, and no person would ever be in a position to change such momentum. As a junior resident, I was pretty much enslaved to all of the third-year, fourth-year, and fifth-year residents, as well as to every attending surgeon. But I accepted my place in the surgical caste system, knowing that things would eventually get better for me as the years passed.

Jerry was not happy with Phil. The stoic senior resident was, however, a hard man to read. I had seen Jerry on his most jubilant of days, and I had also seen him during his most angry and volatile of moments. Unlike most people, during periods of both emotional excitement as well as tranquility, Jerry's facial expressions and voice remained equally calm. Only those of us who really knew the man could tell what his true emotions were. We knew by his laugh. When Jerry was happy he would emit a droning chuckle, ending in a popping sound as his voice cracked from the trailing wind of his breath. But when Jerry was angry, he laughed in a boisterous manner, with plenty of energy and significant volume. Dr. Harmack had been laughing very hard at that particular moment, and I knew that our young intern was going to be in trouble just as soon as he made it down to us from the floor upstairs.

With the phone call still in progress, Jerry told Phil to immediately stop what he was doing and to meet us down in the intensive care unit pronto. While we were waiting for our intern, the cunning senior resident was already planning how he was going to punish Phil for the duration of his rotation with us. I felt somewhat badly for the budding young doctor, suddenly realizing that he couldn't possibly have started off his surgery month on a worse footing. When Phil finally showed up, he was clearly unaware that he had offended his senior resident and was clueless as to his procedural faux pas. Phil seemed surprised that Dr. Harmack had told him to drop what he had been doing, and he seemed entirely unaware that he had already screwed up our morning. The senior man looked sternly at the junior, shook his head, and reminded him of the conversation they had had the previous night regarding what was expected of an intern on morning rounds. Jerry remained calm, as he always did, and he reinforced to Phil that rounds began promptly in the ICU every morning at 6 A.M. sharp.

Then the senior member of our trio asked Phil to present each of the floor patients to him. But before Phil did that which was requested of him, he politely informed Dr. Harmack that he would only be helping us a few days that first week before he would be leaving on a previously approved ten-day vacation. He would, however, be returning to our service for the two or so weeks remaining on the rotation thereafter.

Both of our jaws dropped. That was a painful shocker for both Jerry and me to hear. Phil's vacation meant that I would be responsible for all of the intern's floor work and for pre-rounding on all of his patients every morning. Jerry knew that it would be unreasonable for just one person to pre-round on all of the floor patients as well as all of the intensive care unit patients. Jerry also knew that he would have to pick up the slack and come into the hospital earlier than usual to pre-round on at least some of the ICU patients himself. This was particularly disturbing to him. But a senior resident certainly wouldn't be doing all of my work, which meant that despite Jerry's token assistance, I would have to arrive at the hospital even earlier than my ridiculously early arrival time—now probably no later than four in the morning—and I would have to write all of the floor notes as well as the majority of the ICU notes during the slug's absence.

Jerry was my friend, but he was also my senior resident. I didn't expect him to help me while my assistant was on leave. Jerry felt my pain, but he felt his own pain as well. The fourth-year resident was not pleased, and neither was I. Although I felt that Phil's upcoming absence was completely unacceptable, I also knew that all people needed to take a vacation at some time, and our rotation was theoretically fair game for our intern. However, there was a kind of code among the residents regarding when it was and when it was not socially acceptable to request vacation time. Everyone knew that vacations were only to be taken while assigned to light rotations, such as urology or plastic surgery. But Phil wasn't a surgical resident or even a surgical intern. He aspired to be something not requiring a surgeon's skills. And I guess that it was understandable why he wouldn't choose to spend an entire month on a notoriously difficult service.

But there was more to the problem. Dr. Harmack should have had to approve the intern's vacation request, and if Jerry had been made aware of Phil's temporary absence, we could have distributed the interns among all of us in the residency program a little differently. However, Jerry knew nothing of Phil's vacation plans. Apparently, the sneak took his vacation request slip directly to the Chief of the Medicine department, who approved Phil's absence from our service without anyone in the surgery department ever being made aware of his plans. That was a big no-no. As far as Jerry was concerned, Phil screwed us— either innocently or knowingly—and he was going to pay. I knew it and Jerry knew it, but it was up to the senior resident to decide Phil's fate. Jerry was a fourth year resident and had suffered two more years in the program than I had

at that point. It was not my place to issue punishment. That was Jerry's responsibility, and it was Jerry's privilege. But the Napolean-like leader said nothing
regarding any sort of punitive action at that particular time, and we proceeded
to go on with the tasks of our day.

Near the end of that first day on the East Team service, Dr. Harmack
paged Phil and me, informing us that we would be starting afternoon rounds
at 6:30 P.M., and that we should start checking up on all of our patients. Jerry said
that we would all meet up at our assigned time on the fourth floor where the
majority of our intern's patients were roomed.

Promptly at 6:30 P.M., we all met up on the floor. Jerry decided that he
wanted to do walking rounds, where we would personally visit every patient as a
team and discuss each case. I knew that performing walking rounds would
cause our evening to be long and painful, but it was the senior man's preroga-
tive to decide how and when morning and evening rounds would be conducted.

We stopped outside each patient's room and my senior resident asked our
intern to present the details before we walked in as a team to examine and visit.
Phil did as he was told, but with each presentation Jerry picked up on the subtle
errors in the details of the young doctor's presentations, always making Phil
aware of his mistakes in front of his patients. I thought that Jerry's tactics were
a bit rough, but they did reinforce the concept of paying strict attention to the
details. The routine continued as we rounded on each of the approximately
twenty floor patients. Evening floor rounds that evening were excruciatingly
long, and we finished at approximately 9 P.M. It was at that time that Phil asked
with a look of great anticipation on his face if he could leave and go home.
When Jerry laughed with an enthusiastic guffaw, I knew that was going to be
the moment when the senior man would hand out his punishment to Phil. Dr.
Harmack answered Phil's question through his laughter, stating quite emphati-
cally, "No Phil, now it's time for me to give you your LOS."

Now, I had never heard of an LOS, and I didn't know what Jerry was referring to. Phil looked perplexed and he asked us both just exactly what was an
LOS.

"It's your list of shit, Phil," the senior doctor answered. "And I'm going to
give you so much shit to do that you'll tell every single non-surgery intern who
ever rotates on our service to think wisely how he chooses to request vacation
time in the future."

Phil was completely blindsided. He knew that he had pulled a fast one by having the Medicine department chief approve his vacation request without the senior surgery resident's signature, but he never expected to be punished for doing what he did. There being nothing more to say, Dr. Harmack abruptly turned on his heel and walked away while the intern's jaw hung open. Shortly after our leader left, I talked with Phil on how I perceived Jerry must have felt about everything, and I gave the intern as many tips as I could to help him stay out of any additional trouble. I then took a peek at Phil's list.

Jerry did give Phil an impressive list of work to do—everything from gathering every hard copy X-ray and ultrasound performed on each of the patients, to changing each patient's postoperative dressing. Phil looked dumbfounded, but really, the list contained the same stuff that interns and junior residents had been forced to do for years. Jerry just made Phil's list a little worse than usual by handing it to him so late in the day. I knew that it would take Phil another two to three hours to complete his tasks if he was efficient. But Phil was a non-surgery intern, and they were not well known for being very efficient.

I left the intern, knowing that I had my own additional work to do in the intensive care unit, where I knew that Jerry was likely checking up on the work I had already done that day. Sure enough, I found him checking up on me and the ICU patients. When Jerry saw me, he asked me to present to him any new information, and together we whipped through our final set of rounds in less than an hour. Jerry told me to go home but I had a few more tasks to complete before I could leave the hospital. Once done with my additional chores, I headed off for home. I knew that Phil probably wouldn't be leaving for a while, but I couldn't think about that at the time. I had my own pain and suffering to deal with. After all, it was after 10 P.M., and I had been awake since four that morning. I was exhausted, and I had a full day of work starting in just seven hours.

The following morning, Phil promptly met Dr. Harmack and me in the intensive care unit at 6 A.M. sharp. Phil looked dog-tired. I had no idea how many additional hours it took the intern to complete his tasks the previous night, and I didn't ask. We efficiently went over each of the ICU patients and then discussed each of the floor patients. Morning rounds went by just like clockwork—exactly as it was supposed to happen. We finished in plenty of time for Jerry to present any issues of significance to the chief resident, with time to spare before the 6:45 A.M. staff rounds began. After that we carried out our plan of the day: a full day of surgery for Jerry and me, supervised by our attending surgeons, while Phil the intern took care of the menial matters on the floor.

Later that evening, Dr. Harmack paged us informing us that we were to again meet up on the floor at 6:30 P.M. As tasked, we all met up promptly at the time specified by the leader. Jerry again decided that we would go room to room on floor rounds, having Phil present each patient to us as he had done the day before. I had hoped that our senior resident wouldn't keep us as long as he had the day before. Thankfully, Jerry wasn't as inquisitive as he had been the previous day, and we completed our rounding earlier that evening, by about 7:30 P.M. I figured that Jerry and I would quickly round through the ICU, complete the few additional tasks given to us on our evening rounds, and quietly slither out of the hospital when we knew that we had done absolutely everything asked of us. But the idiot intern had to screw up once again. I was completely blown away by what I would hear next. Not having learned from his mistake made the previous day, Phil again asked Dr. Harmack if he could leave to go home, even though he had a few outstanding assignments and Jerry and I hadn't even been to the ICU. Dumbfounded, Jerry let out another laugh, and I knew that Phil had once again screwed himself.

"No, Phil, you can't," the senior man blurted out. "I have another list of shit for you." Indeed, Jerry did have another list of assignments for Phil to complete, and it was just as punitive as the one prior. The intern sulked as he received his task list, and Jerry and I then went down to the intensive care unit to complete rounds again by ourselves. I said very little to my senior resident. Even though our friendship might have permitted my asking Jerry to lighten up a bit on Phil, I didn't risk angering the man who controlled when I would get to leave the hospital that evening. I was tired, and I thought that saying nothing was better than saying something that I might later regret. Following an additional hour's worth of rounds with Jerry, I completed the few additional tasks he assigned me, and Jerry dismissed me to go home.

The following morning, we again met up as a small team in the intensive care unit at six o'clock. Phil looked worse than ever. We went through our routine of briefings, attended our 6:45 A.M. conference, and again carried out the plan of the day. That particular day was a clinic day, and it was a full one as usual. Now, clinic days at William Beaumont Army Medical Center were unusually painful because in addition to the fifty or so patients that would show up in the morning, another forty or fifty would also show up in the afternoon. Morning clinic routinely carried over into the afternoon, and we were never given a formal lunch break.

I learned after the first few weeks of being a resident to keep a brown grocery bag full of canned spaghetti rings under my desk in the junior resident call room. At some time around midday, I would excuse myself to use the bathroom, and I would sneak off to the call room with lightning-fast speed, grab a can, shake it up, open the lid, and pour the cold spaghetti rings down my throat. There was no time to heat the food, and there was no time to chew. I just swallowed the cold food as fast as I could to give me the boost of energy I badly needed. My body craved the calories, and I needed them as quickly as possible. I estimated that over the course of my residency, I downed well over a thousand cans of those things. Not a very healthy habit for a doctor to practice, but it was a necessity at the time.

On clinic days, the junior resident was also tasked with carrying the SOD pager. SOD stood for Surgical Officer of the Day, or slave dog. I was the junior resident at the time, and as such I carried the SOD pager. As the SOD, I would get paged by any member of the ICU staff, ER staff, or floor staff, for seemingly any emergency, surgical consult, or trauma. I would often run between the surgery clinic, the ICU, and the ER to perform emergency intubations, to resuscitate trauma patients, or to perform minor surgical procedures, only to return to the clinic waiting room packed with displeased patients waiting to be seen. It was not at all a pleasant experience, and I literally learned to triage and personally deal with the sickest and the most complicated patients while simultaneously addressing smaller issues over the phone. The SOD years were not at all enjoyable, but they were a routine part of my—and every other surgical resident's—responsibilities.

As often happened to me throughout the day, my trauma pager went off. I quickly changed the course of my direction to the trauma room, to which I sprinted. I arrived before the paramedics had made it. One of the emergency room nurses informed me that a van had been found about an hour north of us, rolled over alongside the road of one of the expansive two-lane highways spanning the desert southwest. Apparently, an entire family of Spanish-speaking family members had been injured, the worst of whom was the mother. The family members had been taken to various small community hospitals, but the volunteer paramedics had decided to bring the badly injured mother to us.

The news made me a bit nervous, knowing that taking the most badly in-jured victim the greatest distance didn't make a whole lot of sense to me. But I had no way to communicate my thoughts to the paramedics, already en route to our hospital. I waited at least fifteen minutes for the ambulance to arrive. Those fifteen minutes were precious minutes that I could have used to do other things. They were also precious minutes that most critically injured patients could not afford to waste. I hoped that my patient wasn't too badly injured. When the paramedics finally arrived, they rolled in a lady appearing to be of Mexican heritage, groaning in Spanish, and repeatedly mumbling the phrase, "Ay ay ay . . ."

I began my trauma assessment in the usual fashion. Her airway was intact, as she was groaning comprehensibly. Each of her lungs sounded clear, and she breathed in a relatively nonlabored manner. Her blood pressure was low, and her heart rate was fast, the combination of which was troubling. She might have been dehydrated, or more likely, she was in shock. I ordered a one-liter bolus of intravenous fluids, and I continued with my trauma assessment.

I attempted to assess her neurologic status by asking her basic questions and requesting that she follow some basic commands. She did not understand En-glish, but she understood me when I spoke to her in her native language, which I had become pretty good at having lived in El Paso for the past year. She was able to tell me her name: Maria Ortiz. She stated that she was thirty-two years old. She seemed somewhat confused, but I did not suspect that my patient was suffering from brain trauma since I saw no mark or bruise on her head. Her mental status was most likely impaired from a lack of appropriate blood flow to her brain—from a blood pressure too low as a result of uncontrolled bleeding possibly from deep within her abdomen.

As we did with almost every trauma patient back then, I attempted to confirm the presence or absence of intra-abdominal bleeding—which I suspected—by performing a diagnostic peritoneal lavage, or DPL. I had performed the proce-dure hundreds of times before, and knew exactly what I needed to do. I washed my patient's abdomen with antiseptic solution, and with gloved hands, I laid four sterile surgical towels over her so that only a small, square area of skin surround-ing her navel remained exposed.

I liberally injected the skin below her umbilicus with Lidocaine anesthetic, so the skin incision I would soon make would cause her no pain. I made a one-centimeter cut down through skin and fat until I encountered the dense, white layer of heavy tissue known as the fascia. I pierced her fascia with penetrating clamps and I pulled upward, hoping to lift her abdominal wall off any underlying loops of intestine. I then pierced the fascia with a specially designed needle, and using my tactile senses, I determined when the needle had penetrated the innermost lining of her abdominal cavity. I threaded a long, sterile wire through the needle, removed the needle leaving the wire in place, and passed over the wire a rigid, plastic, foot-long catheter deep into her abdominal cavity. I then removed the wire, leaving only the DPL catheter in her abdomen.

Ordinarily at that juncture, I would attach a syringe to the DPL catheter and pull back. If I aspirated back less than ten milliliters of blood, I would then infuse a liter of intravenous solution into her abdomen, and then let the fluid—mixed with any intra-abdominal blood—run back out into the IV bag. If the laboratory technician, to whom I would send the contents of my patient's abdominal washings, would tell me that the fluid contained more than 100,000 red blood cells per microscopic, high power field, I would have sufficient evidence of intra-abdominal bleeding to warrant an emergency, exploratory abdominal operation. But my patient was bleeding a lot. When I pulled back on the plunger which I attached to her abdominal catheter, the syringe filled completely with bright red blood immediately. I knew from having performed numerous diagnostic peritoneal lavages on previous trauma patients that when the syringe filled as it did, I had better not waste any additional, precious time. My patient needed to get straight into the operating room!

I contacted the OR staff and told them to prepare for an emergency, exploratory laparotomy. I paged Dr. Harmack, my senior resident, to let him know that he needed to operate. I fully prepared myself to assist Jerry and the staff surgeon who would certainly supervise the fourth year as he performed the majority of the emergency procedure. But Jerry could not do the surgery. While I had been resuscitating my trauma patient, Jerry had become tied up caring for another patient who was crashing in the intensive care unit. Jerry had planned on emergently taking his patient back to the operating room as well. With the senior resident not able to join us, I would be the one assisting the staff surgeon. The thought of performing a major abdominal operation thrilled me, but it also made me nervous. I was still very junior among the hierarchy of surgical trainees. But I would not refuse a case if it was offered to me. At very least, I would help my boss, and I would function as his first assistant. That option seemed pretty reasonable to me.

As it turned out, the only attending available to take charge of my emergency case was the vascular surgeon. He was a very capable and competent surgeon, but he was a vascular surgeon, and as such, he had less trauma experience than the rest of the staff surgeons. He told me that I would be doing the case—I would be the primary surgeon, and he would assist me!

As I transferred Mrs. Ortiz onto the operating room table, she looked terribly frightened. She had not stopped moaning. As I was about to walk away from her and head out to scrub my hands, she grabbed me just prior to receiving her general anesthetic and pleaded with me in Spanish. She made me promise her that I would not let her die. She told me that she had small children, and that she could not die. I suddenly felt an immense burden thrust upon me. Her eyes said more than her mouth. She had a look of extreme distress and terrible fear. She wanted me to promise that I would not let her die. What else could I do but make her that promise? But I didn't have a good feeling about it. I knew that in good faith, I really couldn't promise her anything. But I did, regardless.

I made my long incision right down the middle of Mrs. Ortiz's abdomen. Immediately upon opening her belly, I encountered a tremendous pool of blood. Having been given the responsibility as primary surgeon, I packed her abdomen tightly with numerous surgical sponges, as I had seen done numerous times while assisting on similar cases. I sucked the bloody contents from my patient's abdomen and I carefully removed each of the saturated sponges one by one, looking for the injury or injuries responsible for all of the bleeding. I initially examined my patient's spleen, as it is typically the most common source of profuse bleeding after abdominal trauma. But my patient's spleen was entirely uninjured. Knowing that the liver had suddenly become the most likely source for the hemorrhage, I pulled out the bloody packs in my patient's right upper quadrant. And there is where I saw the devastation.

Her liver had been cracked nearly in two. As if someone had driven a log splitter through the center of the pulpy organ, it lay splayed apart, with pulsatile bleeding spouting from the depths of the massive gash. I instinctively compressed the hemorrhaging organ between my two hands, hoping to provide temporary control of the deluge of blood loss. But I knew that I could only hold pressure for so long. I needed to do something more definitive than simple hand compression. I looked up at my staff surgeon, who shook his head, and gave me a look of disapproval and extreme dissatisfaction.

"Is that all you're going to do?" he asked disgustedly. "Are you going to do something or are you going to just let her die?" .

I was a bit shocked by his less-than-supportive comments. I had hoped for some real guidance, but wasn't receiving any. I had not even completed my second year of training; I was a mere novice. No one expected someone with my level of training to know how to manage such a devastating problem. I mulled over my staff surgeon's comments for a moment and then came to the sudden realization that he, too, probably didn't know what to do. I then thought about the promise I had made to Mrs. Ortiz—that I wouldn't let her die. I became nauseated.

Not knowing what else to do, I asked the scrub technician for a clip applier. I allowed the liver to again fall apart, exposing the torn central portion of the damaged organ. Blood again quickly spurted up at me, splashing me across my masked face. I quickly applied clip after clip into the depths of the wounded liver, hoping to blindly seal one or more of the small torn vessels. But I wasn't having much success.

"Are you trying to kill her?" my boss stated. "You need to remove her entire right lobe, unless you've got something better to do." He was so condescending and insulting. I needed help—she needed help—but neither I nor my patient were receiving the assistance we needed. I didn't know how to remove the right lobe of a liver. I had never even seen such an operation done before. However, I did know the anatomy of the liver, and I figured that if I wasn't going to get the help I needed, I had no choice but to do that which made sense to me.

I knew that the right lobe of the liver was supplied by one artery, and drained by two large veins. I completed the trauma-induced, incomplete transection through the organ with my gloved fingers, hoping to identify which vessels to tie off. I found the main artery, clamped it, and tied it securely with a heavy, silk ligature. I then divided the tissues on the back of the liver, which were preventing me from seeing the large veins draining the bloody organ. I saw the first vein, and then the second. I clamped both vessels as the entire right lobe fell away from the left. I passed the enormous mass of injured liver to the scrub technician, and worked at securing sutures around the two large liver veins. After several attempts at unsuccessfully suture ligating the large veins, my staff surgeon took over. He carefully passed threaded needles through the veins situated immediately behind my vessel clamps, wrapped them around the vascular tissue, and tied them tightly. He removed my two clamps, and we peered at the mess left behind. The brisk hemorrhage had been controlled, but the oozing was quite overwhelming.

Blood again began to slowly well up in Mrs. Ortiz's abdomen. The countless capillaries exposed on the raw surfaces of the remnant of liver were oozing blood at an alarming rate. I asked for the argon beam coagulator, a device that fires a beam of superheated gas, very useful in cauterizing the raw surfaces of an injured, bloody liver. I had seen it used successfully on minor liver injuries, but I had never before seen any liver injury so bad as the one I was dealing with. I fired the argon beam over all that was oozing, throwing inch-long arcs of fire at the liver, feverishly attempting to cook the organ into submission, but despite the odor of charred tissue, even that wasn't working. Mrs. Ortiz was in a death spiral, and I knew it. My boss knew it, too. Yet, rather than offering any additional suggestions, he just continued to hurl insults at me, asking me mockingly why I wanted her to die.

I looked up at the anesthesia monitors. My patient's blood pressure was too low to support life. It was thirty over zero. I felt my patient's aorta, and not feeling a pulse, I asked my boss if I should start CPR (cardiopulmonary resuscitation). He sneered at me and told me to do whatever I wanted to do.

"It's your patient," he said. "You killed her."

What an ass! I thought. I ripped the surgical drapes off my patient's chest and began performing chest compressions. I beat on her chest with all the strength I could muster. But as five minutes became ten minutes, and then fifteen minutes, I saw no improvement in my patient's blood pressure. I continued pounding on her for another quarter of an hour. After a full thirty minutes of CPR, I stopped. I again felt her aorta and there was no pulse. I looked at the cardiac monitor and saw no evidence of any electrical activity originating from my patient's heart. I knew that she was dead. Backing away from the table, I pronounced her.

I carefully closed her abdomen, no longer bleeding after her heart had stopped. I felt demoralized and terribly saddened. I could not stop replaying the words my deceased patient had said to me before I began my surgery. *"Prométame usted no me dejamá morir!"*—promise you will not let me die! But I *did* allow her to die. I felt sick, and I didn't know how to rid myself of the guilt.

That evening following our disaster of a day, Jerry, Phil, and I all rounded on the East Team patients. I felt very low, and I questioned why I had chosen to become a surgeon in the first place. After the senior resident, the intern, and

I rounded on our floor patients, Phil did not ask if he could leave to go home. I was grateful that the young doctor had finally learned to bite his tongue. I had hoped that the intern's newly found restraint would get Phil and me through with Jerry as soon as possible that evening. I had very little energy left in me, and all I wanted to do was leave the hospital. But I was the in-house resident on call that evening, which always meant extra work would come my way all night long, regardless. I dreaded my night. I hoped to be able to focus on my on-call tasks as soon as possible, rather than have to continue managing my own team's patients.

As matters would have it, Phil was the in-house intern on call that evening, and he knew that he was stuck in the hospital as well. Dr. Harmack said or did very little to ease my personal anguish. Instead, he was still focused on the errant ways of the young intern. We all wasted at least ten precious minutes while the senior resident gave a sarcastic lecture to his intern on how, back in the day when he himself was the low man on the totem pole, he would never have gotten away with the stunt Phil had pulled. In some ways, Jerry focusing on Phil was a blessing for me, as my mind was obsessively preoccupied by my patient's last words. I listened one notch less than passively throughout Jerry's rant.

When the leader had nothing more to say, Phil knew with certainty that he was far from being out of the doghouse. After a series of appropriately timed "Yes, sir" responses, Phil looked at the senior physician with a resigned face and he held out his hand as he politely asked for his "LOS." Dr. Harmack of course obliged, and handed the intern the list he had already written out and had kept in his scrub shirt pocket. Phil accepted the list with dignity and set off to carry out his Extra Military Instruction tasks, which were in addition to his on-call duties.

But Phil knew that he would be going on vacation the following morning, that he had signed leave papers on file, and that nothing could keep him in the hospital after 7 A.M. *Good for Phil*, I thought, as his torture was even starting to bother me.

The next ten days were absolute hell for Jerry and me. Not having an intern on the service meant extra work for both of us and even longer hours of confinement in the hospital than usual. When I was not on call, I typically stayed at work until after 10 P.M. in order to get all of the extra chores done. I became almost sick with exhaustion. When I was afforded a few moments here and there to get some sleep, memories of Mrs. Ortiz came back to haunt me.

After Phil finally returned from his vacation, my workload was lightened by at least several hours each day. I was relieved, but still a little upset that the intern had left us during such a busy rotation, even though technically he had every right to do so. I did everything in my power not to hold a grudge against Phil, because my responsibilities returned to normal when he resumed his duties on our service, and I frankly had no right to be angry with him. I was still preoccupied with Mrs. Ortiz's death and by the way I was treated in the operating room. I wondered at times if I could endure such an experience again. I was in no state of mind to be critical of another surgical trainee, and I decided to let go of all resentment I had toward Phil. But Dr. Harmack wasn't as forgiving. Every evening for the rest of Phil's rotation, Jerry handed him a list of extra work to complete prior to leaving for home. It was pretty horrible for Phil, but like a prisoner resigned to his captivity, he didn't complain.

I must admit that after a while Phil became a rather efficient intern, and he might have even made a good surgical resident if he had just had the guts to make the switch. Near the end of Phil's rotation on our service, he had learned to anticipate surgical problems, to independently address evolving situations of importance, and to complete laborious dressing changes in a fraction of the time it originally took him. I was impressed. But the young doctor would forever be adversely tainted by his surgical experience on our service. I didn't blame him for losing all interest in ever again wanting to work with surgeons for the rest of his medical career.

That seems to be the case with most nonsurgeons who have rotated on a surgery service during some portion of their training. Everyone who rotates on a surgical service gets treated poorly at one time or another. Some trainees handle the harsh treatment well, but most don't.

Phil made a terribly unfortunate, critical error in judgment on that first day by telling his senior resident that he would be going on vacation, and by asking to go home. He set himself up for failure from the very beginning. I wish I could have known Phil's plans ahead of time and perhaps convinced him to go on vacation during a different period. But I didn't. I know that Dr. Harmack treated Phil harshly, but in the end Phil became a good intern. So perhaps the end justifies the means. But who really knows? Surgical training has always been a grueling and painful process, with longer work hours than perhaps any other discipline in the world. Teaching surgery and care of the surgical patient can at times require punitive teaching methods. Perhaps the staff surgeon who berated me in the operating room as my patient died in front of me was conditioning me in the very manner that Jerry had been conditioning Phil. Personally, I don't know if the way our intern was treated, or if the manner in which I was treated during that fateful case, was either right or fair. I surely didn't think so. But if I was going to complete my residency and become a surgeon, I knew that I would have to develop a thicker skin and deal with loss and bad outcomes, regardless of the punitive nature of the lessons learned.

Losing my patient was a very personal and painful experience for me, and I knew that it would certainly happen again. I hoped that I could muster the courage to move beyond the memory of Mrs. Ortiz. I hoped that I would be able to bounce back. I was more than a bit demoralized. My complete, physical exhaustion further exacerbated my low feelings. I had hoped to God that I could become a good resident, and I prayed earnestly that I might one day become a good surgeon. But I was no longer certain that I would be able to accomplish that goal.

5

Baptism by Fire

The County Hospital

In August 1995, I began a three-month, trauma surgery rotation at R. E. Thomason Hospital in downtown El Paso, Texas. I was one month into my third year of residency training and I was starting to regain confidence in my abilities and with my skills. As was customary at my residency program, each of the third-year surgical residents spent a three-month period of time at the county hospital in order to broaden our fund of knowledge and to experience patient management from a different perspective. I had heard great stories from senior residents who shared their past memories of the Thomason General Hospital experience with me. I had heard that Thomason was very busy, that the hospital staff treated a lot of gang members, and that the surgery residents were given a lot more autonomy than we were typically given at William Beaumont.

I was definitely looking forward to that rotation. I was excited that I would be treating more *penetrating* trauma patients, as opposed to blunt trauma victims. Nearly every trauma surgeon I know agrees that blunt trauma patients (such as those injured by motor vehicle crashes and high altitude falls) are often more complicated, more difficult to work up, and often don't require any emergency surgery. On the other hand, penetrating trauma patients (including those wounded by gunshots or stabbings) almost telegraph their injuries by virtue of the holes in their body, usually making the workup extremely straight-forward and simple. The other benefit of penetrating trauma is that the very nature of the injuries often necessitates the urgent intervention of a trauma surgeon and his scalpel. And, thus, most trauma surgeons receive their greatest pleasures when managing penetrating trauma patients as opposed to blunt.

I was excited at the thought of having more freedom and independence in the operating room. Now, don't get me wrong. My chief residents and attending surgeons at William Beaumont gave me plenty of freedom and autonomy, but for the most part that all took place outside the operating room. If a patient was crashing in the intensive care unit and he or she needed the attention of a doc-tor at the bedside—to push medications, to squeeze bags of blood into a shocky patient's circulatory system, to emergently place central venous catheter lines for greater IV access, or for just about any other time-consuming bedside proce-dure or activity—we were given complete freedom and autonomy. But once we were actually performing major surgery in the operating room on a patient un-der general anesthesia, we were under the continuous, close supervision of someone very senior to us who was scrubbed in either across from or immedi-ately next to the surgical resident.

Wise people have told me on several occasions to be careful of what I wished for. That advice rang true for me on one particular evening while I was working in-house and on call at the county hospital, a specific evening that typified my overall Thomason experience. It was well after dark, but also before midnight in the late summertime. Now, recall that I was in El Paso, Texas, where summer days often peaked at 115 degrees. But that particular time was during the evening hours and I believe that it was around 80 degrees and dry outside. As was the case at William Beaumont, after typical working hours while on call, I was the senior surgery member in the hospital. I had one intern work-ing for me, a chief resident at home sleeping but available if needed, and an at-tending trauma surgeon, also at home. I had been pretty busy that day and was beginning to experience that subtle ill feeling—as my body's natural adrenaline secretion was fighting the waves of exhaustion—which usually occurred when my body knew that it needed some rest, but wouldn't be allowed to lie down.

I met up with my intern, Rafael. Rafael was a very soft-spoken family prac-tice resident from Laredo, Texas, and was spending a one-month surgery rota-tion on the trauma service. He was Mexican by birth, but came to America during his school years and had intended on opening up a family medicine clinic somewhere along the Texas-Mexico border to serve the international community. Rafael was a good and noble man, but he did not have the tenacity of a surgeon. That is not a criticism, but it is an honest observation. Rafael was kind and gentle. Surgeons, on the other hand, were often aggressive and sometimes rough. Rafael probably demonstrated more true doctorlike qualities than I did, but I didn't realize it at that particular time. All I knew was that Rafael was slow.

He had been busy addressing a plethora of minor problems patients were having in the hospital. Nothing of what Rafael told me about the patient problems he was managing seemed too concerning to me, but Rafael was a family practice resident and I wasn't sure that I could trust his assessments of our surgical patients. I debated whether or not to check up on the patients Rafael had seen. But as the circumstances of that night unfolded, I did not have any free time to follow up on the problems Rafael had managed. As had happened several times throughout the day, the trauma alert had again sounded.

I arrived at the entrance of the emergency room just as the paramedics rolled our patient in. He was lying calmly on the cart, gazing upward with a peaceful, almost happy stare, while covered in blood from his waist to his knees.

"A bunch of kids were mixing it up near the auto show out in town," the paramedic stated. "Two got shot. This one took a round in the groin, but the other guy looks much worse—he took multiple rounds to the belly. He should be here pretty soon," he concluded.

Suddenly, I felt a bit nervous when I realized that at any minute I would be in charge of two simultaneous major trauma casualties. I decided to assess the first victim as quickly as possible so as to have a handle on the matter before the second patient arrived. My first patient appeared to be about twenty years old, and he was dressed in a bloody, white T-shirt and jeans. I quickly assessed the airway: good. I then checked his breathing: also good. And then I checked his pulse and his blood pressure. I really couldn't find much of a pulse but I thought that I felt one in the foot opposite where he had been shot. It was very fast and very weak. But to be honest with you, I couldn't really tell if the pulse that I was feeling was my own.

The technician was having a tough time getting me a blood pressure, and so I wasn't yet sure if my patient was in shock and if so, how badly. But he had lost a lot of blood. That was obvious from the good soaking his pants had taken. There was a pile of gauze taped down over the open area cut through

my patient's jeans overlying the left groin. It was absolutely saturated with
blood. I untaped and removed the bloody dressing. It must have weighed several pounds from all of the blood that saturated the bandage. As soon as I removed the compressive material, blood began spurting up at me. I quickly
grabbed another handful of dry gauze and firmly applied direct pressure over
the pumping vessel. My patient had an obvious arterial injury. I tried to assess
the patient's neurological status. His eyes remained open spontaneously but he
wouldn't answer any of my questions or follow any of my commands. He just
kept staring blankly up toward the ceiling.

"Classic shock," said the deep voice behind me. I glanced back to see an
emergency medicine physician, about fifty years of age, with a long, gray pony-
tail calmly looking over my shoulder.

Of course, I thought. *This guy is in class-four shock.* It hadn't sunk into my
head until that very moment that my trauma patient would die if he didn't get
blood as soon as possible and into an operating room quickly. I ordered four
units of O-negative blood stat and began infusing IV fluid as quickly as possible
until the blood I ordered had arrived. I told a nurse to continue holding pressure on the wound as firmly as possible. And then the second guy rolled in.

While I wasn't feeling comfortable abandoning my first patient, I had no
choice other than to assess the second casualty. He, too, was a young guy, perhaps twenty or twenty-five years of age, a bit portly, and with gang tattoos covering his unclothed chest. As in every trauma assessment, I assessed my second
patient's airway, his breathing, his circulatory status, and his neurologic function. I established an IV line and ordered the nurses to administer a liter of
Lactated Ringer's, an intravenous solution. I also ordered that labs be drawn
and that several units of blood be typed and cross-matched, anticipating that
my patient would need blood transfusions soon enough.

As opposed to the other casualty I had just assessed, my second patient was
not at all calm. He was cussing, groaning with agony, and he appeared to be in
significant distress. He told me that he had been shot multiple times in the gut,
and he acted in a manner I considered to be appropriate for the injuries he had
received. I assessed his wounds. I counted four holes in the front of his abdomen, and one on the back of each of his flanks. Six holes likely meant that two
of the bullets had gone completely through his body, but that two of the bullets
probably remained within him.

I ordered stat abdominal and chest X-rays, where I found one of the bullets

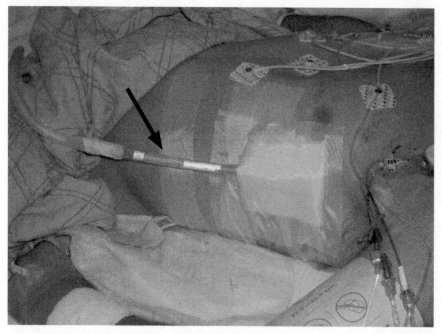

Arrow points to a chest tube inserted into the patient's left thoracic cavity. Chest tubes are often placed to drain blood from the chest and to reexpand collapsed lungs.

in his lower abdomen and the other in the left side of his chest, obscured by a thick shadow of what I presumed indicated that a layer of blood was collecting within his chest. One of the bullets had to have passed through his abdomen, through his diaphragm, and into the chest where it remained lodged. I could see on the X-ray that his left lung had partially collapsed, and I knew that I needed to place a large diameter chest tube to drain his bloody, left hemithorax and reexpand the partially collapsed lung. It was also quite obvious that the guy also needed to go to the operating room.

I asked the trauma crew to set up for the placement of a chest tube, and I asked that my chief resident be paged.

After several minutes, all of my supplies had been gathered for me to perform my bedside trauma procedure and insert the chest tube, but my chief had not yet called back. I sterilely gloved and gowned, prepped my patient's left chest with antiseptic solution, and began injecting a local anesthetic into the skin of my patient's left chest, just below the nipple. He screamed and writhed as I stuck him with the needle, which caused me to jump back so as not to stick myself. I ordered an intravenous sedative and some morphine to calm my patient. After both drugs had been administered, I then continued with my procedure. After infiltrating his skin with the anesthetic, I cut deeply into his chest. I cut boldly down to the rib with one quick stroke. My incision was less than an inch long. That was all that I needed. I then inserted a curved, metal Kelly clamp—similar to a large hemostat—into the wound down onto the rib and rolled the Kelly up and over the rib into the soft, muscular tissue. I remained keenly aware of the fact that if I pierced *below* the bone, that I could potentially tear into one of the vessels that hugs the undersurface of each rib. I needed to remain as close as possible to the *top* of the rib so as to avoid a bloody catastrophe.

As I had done by that point in my young surgical career many times before, I leaned into the Kelly clamp with a significant, but appropriate amount of force, and I punched a hole through the deep, dense tissue layer lining the inner surface of his chest cavity. He squirmed and wailed through his drugged haze as I spread the clamp, enlarging the hole just enough to permit my finger to probe the wound. Blood was already draining out from his chest and onto the floor. I examined the wound with my gloved index finger, gently palpated his beating heart, and brushed away the lung tissue from the chest wall adjacent to my incision. I then inserted the clear, plastic, multiholed tube, directing it upward toward the top of his chest. Blood quickly filled the tubing and began to pour out onto the floor where people were stepping, creating scores of blood-streaked, shoe prints all around the trauma cart. I connected the chest tube to the suction apparatus and secured the tube to my patient's chest with heavy sutures passed through his skin and wrapped tightly around the half-inch thick, clear piece of plastic. I then taped a gauze dressing over the wound completing my minor, surgical procedure.

Strangely enough, my chief resident still had not yet called me back. I asked that he again be paged. Knowing that both of my patients needed surgery urgently, I contacted the operating room myself and told the OR nurses to prepare for two emergency cases—one abdominal operation, and one groin operation. They asked me which surgeons would be performing which procedures. Since I had not yet received a call back from my chief, I really didn't know how to answer them. I assumed that I would be doing one of the cases with either the attending surgeon or with the chief resident, and that one of the two would be doing the other case. But I wasn't sure who exactly would supervise me and on which patient. The senior operating room nurse told me that two rooms would in fact be set up, but that someone needed to inform them before we actually brought our patients back to them. She wanted to know exactly who would be doing which case.

After I hung up the phone I went back to check on my first victim—the one with the hole in his groin. He was not doing well. His blood pressure had only transiently responded to the four-unit blood transfusion, and much of that which had been transfused was now on the bed and floor adjacent to the patient's cart. I ordered four more units of blood and decided to call the attending surgeon directly. That was against protocol by all accounts, but I had patients in my charge who were dying, and I needed someone in there to help me sooner rather than later. I asked that the attending be paged immediately.

After just a few short minutes I received a call back from the attending. We had never before met. I apologized for calling him directly, but explained the urgency of my situation. We discussed the two patient cases for what seemed to be more time than I thought was necessary, but then again, I had been at the patients' bedsides for the past twenty minutes or so, and the attending had been at home completely unaware of the events that had taken place. A thorough briefing was appropriate considering the situation however I wished he would stop talking and come in to help me. The attending surgeon told me that he would get in touch with Joe, the chief resident, and that both of them would be at the hospital shortly.

About five minutes later, Joe called me from what was at the time a novelty item: his cell phone. He was driving into the hospital to meet me. He asked why he hadn't been paged first, which of course I had done—twice! After I explained that fact to him, he told me that his pager must not have been working correctly or something. But I didn't really care. I just knew that my patients needed surgery. Whatever Joe had been doing to prevent him from answering his pager was of little concern or interest to me.

Both the chief resident and the attending surgeon arrived almost simultaneously. I had already explained the details of both patients to each of them, and we walked together to the bedsides of the victims. Each of the surgeons senior to me briefly examined the patients, and they walked away from me and discussed the situations together, leaving me out of the loop. I wondered which patient I would be operating on, and I wondered which of the two surgeons I would be operating with. I just hoped that whichever of the two I was assigned to assist would let me do at least a part of the operation. After all, I was a third-year, and I had assisted on many trauma operations by that time. I definitely had been hoping for a little more autonomy.

As it turned out, I received exactly what I had wished for—more autonomy, that is. The attending surgeon walked back my way and informed me that he would be operating on the groin patient with the chief resident, and that I would be operating on the abdomen-chest guy by myself. He then walked away and prepared to do his surgery. An entirely familiar wave of anxiety once again came over me. I was being given a new challenge, an arduous one. I had been an assistant on similar cases many times before, and I had performed various parts of many operations under direct supervision on countless occasions, but I had never yet flied solo on such a major endeavor. I told myself those words that I had repeated on many occasions while in similar, prior circumstances: "Never let them see you sweat."

I quickly rehearsed in my mind all of the steps necessary to perform an emergency abdominal operation—the exploratory laparotomy. I operated pretty well as I rehearsed the operation in my mind, but I had a few uncertainties and questions, which I just could not answer.

"How do I free up the colon attached to the lateral side wall again?" I asked myself. "Which tissue plane do I cut through to see the buried portion of the pancreas?" I knew that I had very little time to find the answers to those questions in a book. The two trauma patients were getting wheeled off to the OR as I was contemplating my thoughts. But I knew of a good source of immediate information . . . Jerry! Yes, I would call Jerry, my former senior resident and current chief resident at William Beaumont. And that is what I did.

I had Jerry's phone number, as well as all of the other surgeons' phone numbers, written on a card in my wallet. I grabbed one of the hospital phones and dialed Jerry's number. Thankfully, Jerry answered.

"Hey, Jerry, it's Jim," I stated in a very cool voice. After we cordially chatted for a very long minute I told him that I really hadn't called to socialize at such an unusually late hour, but that in fact I needed his help. I explained my imminent challenge and asked him the few questions I couldn't answer regarding my impending trauma operation. Jerry happily acquiesced and helped me, quickly explaining each of the steps of an exploratory laparotomy. I envisioned each step as he explained them to me. When he addressed the two areas I had questioned, it was as if I had been filming a V8 juice commercial. I struck my forehead realizing that I had already known what Jerry had just told me, but I guess that with all of the excitement, and with essentially no time to prepare, I had simply drawn a blank on the details of those few steps. After completing my tutorial, Jerry wished me luck in his usual, calm, emotionless fashion, and off I went to the operating room—now much more confident, and now very excited!

As I stood over my patient—all scrubbed, gowned, gloved, and ready to go—I quickly went over a mental, preoperative check list. I wanted to perform that operation correctly from the get go. Never before had I just had a scrub technician assisting me. Never before was I the senior surgeon in the room, entirely responsible for the results of a major surgical operation. I could think of nothing else that I needed to do at that time other than cut. I asked the anesthesiologist if he was ready for me to begin, and he gave me an affirmative, "Go for it."

I placed a surgical lap pad on either side of the midline of my patient's abdomen, asked for the scalpel, and cut right down the middle. I knew that if I stayed perfectly midline I should have little if any blood loss from the abdominal wall because I knew that the abdominal midline was one of the many "bloodless planes" of surgical anatomy. I cut through skin and fat until I saw the white, glistening, gristle layer known as fascia. I handed over my scalpel to the scrub technician and, grabbing the handheld electrocautery probe, I proceeded to simultaneously cut and cauterize as the electrical energy of the probe melted through the midline fascia. Once I was through the dense layer of tissue, I could see the bulging, blue hue of blood under the final, thin layers of tissue in need of opening before I was actually in the true abdominal cavity. I grasped the two thin adherent layers of tissue with a forceps, gently pulled upward, and cut through, entering my temple of surprises.

As I had done many times before as an assistant, I rapidly grabbed lap pad after lap pad and I quickly packed all quadrants of my patient's abdominal cavity, hoping to blindly compress any areas of active bleeding. Next, I grabbed a large handheld abdominal wall retractor, placed it against the edge of the incised abdominal wall opposite me, and told the scrub technician to pull as hard as he could. It was a maneuver that every medical student, intern, and junior resident was quite familiar with—a maneuver known among the surgically anointed as "holding hook." But that was, in fact, the first time I had ever given orders to hold hook. While my assistant retracted away the abdominal wall, I removed the lap pads one by one, carefully suctioning away the blood, allowing me to inspect the underlying organs to determine what was and what

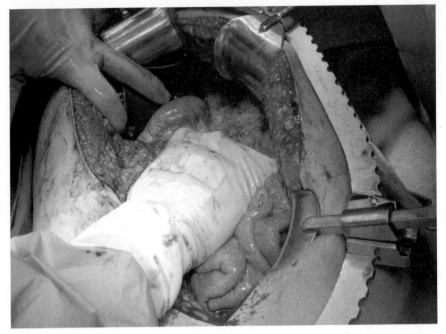

The typical exploratory laparotomy exposure. A metal retractor is pulling the incision open as the surgeon's hands explore the insides of the abdomen.

was not injured. I methodically examined all areas of my casualty's insides, moving from the patient's right upper quadrant, to the right lateral abdominal sidewall, to the right lower quadrant, and eventually all around the entire abdomen. I didn't identify any solid organ injuries—that is, the liver, spleen, and kidneys were all uninjured. But I had yet to carefully examine the bowel.

I ran the bowel with my fingers, inspecting every inch of the small intestine, from its origin where it emerged at the ligament of Trietz just below the middle aspect of the transverse colon, all the way to where it joined the right side of the large intestine. As I moved my hands along the bowel, pulling up eight- to ten-inch segments at a time, I inspected both the front and the back of each loop. As I identified the many holes where the bullets had perforated the intestine, easily recognized by the spillage of liquid stool, I placed a Babcock bowel clamp over the orifice, both to remind me where the various injuries were, as well as to minimize further spillage of the highly contaminated material into the abdominal cavity. I placed twelve clamps on the small bowel, as each of the bullets had pierced through the matted mass of small intestine in multiple areas.

Next, I ran the large bowel. I carefully examined each segment, carefully mobilizing portions of the left and right colon off the lateral, abdominal sidewalls via the techniques I had reviewed in my phone conversation with Jerry just minutes earlier. I examined the stomach and the pancreas—also via the technique of Jerry. I completed my exploration by examining the huge, vascular structures running vertically down the deepest portions of my patient's abdominal cavity—the aorta and the vena cava—relieved to find that they had not been injured. However, I did find a surprise. Hidden underneath the numerous piles of intestine, lying freely in the depths of the abdominal cavity, in the recess alongside the large midline vascular structures was a single bullet. Thrilled to have the opportunity to do next what I had dreamed of doing for many years, I grasped the bullet with a long forceps and plunked the projectile down into a silver, surgical basin, creating the metal-on-metal clinking sound I had heard so many times before while watching the TV show *M*A*S*H.*

Feeling rather energetic and relieved knowing that none of my patient's injuries were anything more complex than I could handle, I began to repair the bullet holes in the bowel. One by one I removed each of the Babcock clamps, and I sewed closed each of the holes in two layers. After I finished, I reran the entire small bowel, making sure that each of my repairs was done to my satisfaction, and making sure that I had not missed anything.

I then remembered the chest tube I had placed in the emergency room. I realized that somewhere in the left hemi-diaphragm was a hole that needed fixing, and somewhere in my patient's left thorax was a bullet. I checked the collection bottles attached to the chest tube I had placed earlier. A total of 500 milliliters of blood had drained from my patient's wounded chest, through the chest tube, and into the bottles. The anesthesiologist told me that he had been watching the collection tubing and that very little had bled during the course of the operation. I knew that 500 milliliters was really nothing to worry about. I knew that my chest tube would be all that my patient needed, as eight out of ten penetrating lung injuries, appropriately drained with a well-placed chest tube, stop hemorrhaging on their own.

Unlike the rest of the body, the blood pressure in the lungs normally runs low—comparable to the pressure in most veins. Bleeding from the low pressure organs usually clots off, eliminating the need for any major surgical treatment. Because opening my patient's chest was unnecessary, there was no need for me to dig for the bullet likely embedded deep within one of his lungs.

Thus, my patient would get to keep his bullet as a souvenir because removing it could cause him more potential harm than leaving it in. It seemed that all I needed to do at that point was look for and repair the bullet hole that had traversed my patient's diaphragm. Fortunately for me, it was in a very accessible area, and I easily sewed it closed with two, heavy sutures.

I then washed out my patient's abdominal cavity with multiple liters of warm saline solution, and I sucked out the fluid until it all ran clear in the collection bottles. For all practical purposes I was done. All I needed to do at that point was to close the abdomen. Although I was feeling jubilant after having had such an awesome experience, I was a little reticent to close without having one of the senior surgeons inspect my work.

Fortunately, as if someone had been reading my mind, one of the OR nurses had already informed the other two surgeons in the next room of my imminent closing. The attending surgeon walked into my room a few moments later to check on me and to inspect my work. He asked me how things had gone, and I informed him of my findings and of the work I had completed. He then asked me if he could scrub in and take a look for himself. Of course, I obliged—as if I could have really said anything to the contrary anyway.

The boss scrubbed, gowned, and gloved, and he ran his hands through the belly like an old pro. He rechecked everything I had already examined, and he inspected my intestinal repairs. He was pleased with everything I had done, but he did remove a few of my outer-layer bowel sutures and replaced them with his own, stating that I may have tied the two sutures a little too tight, potentially making the passage channel through the injured bowel a bit too narrow. I was fine with that. My ego wasn't bruised. If that was all that he could find wrong with my work, I would be thrilled.

He stayed with me and we closed the abdomen together, as if I had become his true apprentice. He chatted with me about the other case, telling me that the other guy had suffered a complex vascular injury to the high femoral artery. Now, I didn't realize it at the time, but a high femoral artery injury is one of those extremely difficult injuries to repair. In hindsight, I became doubly glad that I had been picked to do the belly case by myself. I may have done very little if I had been assigned the other patient.

I really can't remember if I treated any additional trauma patients that particular night, and I don't remember if I had a chance to catch any sleep that evening. But I am certain that it didn't matter one bit. I had been given a great opportunity—a great challenge—and I felt like I had succeeded. I knew that I did well, despite the fact that I had handled the much easier of the two cases presented to me that evening. From that night forward I craved additional opportunities to take on bigger challenges, to do more complicated surgical procedures, and to operate independently again. I knew that I would have very little opportunity for the remainder of my residency to be the true cowboy that I was that night—operating solo without a senior resident or attending surgeon even in the room. I was so grateful to have been on call that night, and I subsequently viewed every long night spent away from home, sequestered in a hospital, not as a duty or punishment, but as a potential opportunity to excel.

6

The University Experience

The World's Greatest Trauma Surgeon

During the course of my fourth year of surgical residency, I spent a total of seven months far from home: two months each in New Mexico, Colorado, and Washington, and one month in San Antonio, Texas. The months the surgery residents spent away from our home base of William Beaumont Army Medical Center had been arranged years before I had been admitted to the program. Each of the away rotations offered the residents unique opportunities to experience concentrated periods of training in areas of surgery not well represented at William Beaumont. The away rotations were clearly important to my overall, well-rounded development as a surgeon. I learned tricks of the surgical trade from renowned university professors and private-practice physicians alike. I operated alongside highly compartmentalized subspecialists who limited their surgical adventures to one or two organs. Plus, I also operated with true general surgeons, capable of performing surgery on everything from the thyroid gland to the uterus.

The additional training I received while away from home was superb. My away rotations offered me refreshing, new perspectives on managing common surgical problems. They also afforded me a set of in-depth experiences at managing surgical disorders perhaps seen only a few times yearly by most general surgeons. But there certainly was a downside to that great opportunity, and it was a true sacrifice which I was forced to make. In those seven months, I rarely saw my family. While I was away from home my wife continued with the daily rituals of all that is necessary to keep an elementary school–aged boy, a pre-school girl, and a toddler all safely occupied, appropriately disciplined, and well loved. Not that she had much, if any, assistance from me when I wasn't hundreds of miles away—as spending nearly all available hours of the week in the hospital just a few minutes' drive from our home often made her feel like a "residency widow." When I was away on those rotations, my wife and I were completely out of touch. Therefore, a most unfortunate consequence of my training obligations was the sad fact that I missed almost every aspect of my third child's first year of life.

In the fall of 1996, I served for two months as the acting chief resident on the Burn-Trauma Surgery Service at the University of New Mexico in Albuquerque. UNM was a very large facility, with five separate intensive care units each delegated to care for a different category of critically ill patients. I spent most of this time in the Burn-Trauma Intensive Care Unit—or the BTICU, as we called it—where my patients resided after I excised hundreds of square feet of cooked flesh from the bodies of numerous badly burned casualties. After I removed the burned tissue, I grafted what seemed like miles of healthy skin harvested from often unusual areas, such as their backs, buttocks, and occasionally from my patients' unburned scrotums. When most of the body had been burned and I needed to cover the postexcisional, bloody flesh with living skin, sometimes the only healthy tissue I could find was in these most sensitive of areas.

I became quite the burn aficionado, relishing the opportunity to spend hour after hour in the superheated operating rooms configured especially for the treatment of burn patients. Sweat soaked through my scrubs and dripped down the inside of my liquid-impermeable, surgical gown, as room temperatures were often as hot as 90 degrees—intentionally kept warm so as to prevent hypothermia in the patients on whom nearly all of their thermoregulatory skin I had excised. Large, bizarre traction pulley systems attached to the operating room ceilings tugged upward on mottled arms and legs, which resembled sides of beef or giant hams hanging at a butcher shop. The suspension devices looked somewhat barbaric, but they were critically necessary to keep large, burned limbs off the operating room tables, allowing several surgeons at one time to excise and graft skin on both sides of the extremities—a technique that facilitated quicker operations, and subjected each burn patient to less anesthesia exposure.

I reveled in my ability to be able to excise burned flesh to the perfect depth within the tissues below. I took great care not to cut too shallow, which would have resulted in the subsequently placed grafted skin to not take. I also took care to avoiding cutting too deeply, which potentially would have caused excessive blood loss as extensive networks of veins within the fatty tissues below the outer layer of skin could have become inadvertently sliced during the tangential cutting process. I carefully arranged my long, narrow sheets of freshly harvested skin—often no thicker than ten-thousandths of an inch—in careful patterns, gently stretching the meshed skin grafts and then securing them to the body with surgical staples. My desire was not only to appropriately treat my badly burned patients; I also challenged myself to give them cosmetic results comparable to the work of a plastic surgeon. Burn patients carry horrible scars both inside and out for the rest of their lives. If I could make the scars on the outside just a little less noticeable, perhaps the emotional ones within could be a bit less painful.

One night while I was in-house and on call, after spending an entire day excising and grafting skin in the operating room, I chatted with the chief of surgery at UNM, Dr. David Berger. Dr. Berger was a technically outstanding surgeon as well as a true gentleman. I was honored to not only have had the opportunity to meet him, but also to have been able to work with and be taught by this very talented educator.

For whatever reason, Dr. Berger looked out for me. On one occasion, my car had been booted by the university police for parking in what I later learned was a lot not intended for surgical house staff. I was angry to have had my car booted, especially when I found my surprise after working for thirty or so straight hours. Both my energy level and my patience were low, but I had no choice other than to pay the substantial fine to get the steel trap off my car. When Dr. Berger heard what had happened, he somehow felt responsible for not having informed his out-of-town resident about the university parking regulations. To my complete surprise, Dr. Berger reimbursed me for my fine from his personal checking account. To this day I am grateful for that entirely unsolicited act of generosity and true kindness.

While I was chatting with Dr. Berger that evening, the trauma alert sounded. Dr. Berger was my attending surgeon on-call that night. He and I went down to the trauma room together. When we arrived at the emergency room, the triage nurse informed us both that a teenaged boy was being flown in by helicopter from one of the rural New Mexico communities. According to the report, he had shot himself in the chest with a rifle of unknown caliber, and he was last reported as being unresponsive. With a concerned look, Dr. Berger informed me that we had better meet our incoming patient up on the helicopter landing pad.

Before the engines turning the helicopter blades had even shut down, the crew frantically waved for us to approach the bird. We kept our heads low and moved quickly to the passenger compartment where we found one of the crew members performing CPR on our gunshot patient. We were told that immediately prior to landing, the boy had a detectable pulse, but as soon as they had touched down, it could no longer be felt. This was a crucial moment in that kid's life. He had a penetrating wound to the chest, possibly wounding his heart, and he had just lost his pulse. I knew that the boy had a chance of surviving if we could just get his chest opened within the next few minutes. I planned on taking him immediately to the emergency room's trauma bay, where I would crack his chest and hopefully stop the hemorrhaging. But Dr. Berger had other plans. He said that we would be taking that boy directly to the operating room!

Dr. Berger was the boss, and as ordered by him, we whisked our patient directly to the OR. One of the flight medics continued to perform CPR along the way, while the other one bag-ventilated our young casualty via the orally inserted endotracheal tube. I pushed my patient's cart at a fast walking pace. Perhaps, I was actually running at a moderate jog. When we arrived in the OR, we transferred our boy onto the operating room table, and the anesthesiologist began connecting our patient to monitor circuits and to other lines and tubes, all necessary to keep a trauma patient both anesthetized and resuscitated. Blood was hung right away, and I was told by the boss to gown and to glove up. I motioned toward the operating room door, indicating I would quickly wash at the scrub sink. Instead I was ordered to abandon scrub and to gown and glove immediately. We had no time to wash.

The operating room nurse literally threw a bottle of antiseptic solution all over the chest and upper abdomen of our patient as the flight medic stopped his chest compressions just long enough to get out of the way of the splashing fluid. Dr. Berger and I hastily threw some surgical drapes over the sides of our guy, and I was handed the scalpel. I had never before performed a median sternotomy—the midline cut through the skin and breastbone used by cardiac surgeons as the preferred incision when performing coronary bypass procedures—but I had seen it performed several times before, and I was eager to act and not ask questions. I sliced with confidence through skin and underlying fat from the top of the breastbone down to the upper abdomen. I didn't bother to cauterize the little vessels that were oozing as a result of my sharp slice. I needed to get into that chest. Those little vessels would wait.

I reached over and grabbed the oscillating saw used to split the sternum, and I positioned it so that the cutting blade faced toward me. Dr. Berger briefly stopped me and asked if I had ever cut through the breastbone before. I told him that I had, but in fact I had not. That was not the time to discuss whether or not I had enough experience to do what needed to be done. I knew that if I had hesitated and told him the truth, I would not have been allowed to perform that procedure. With my own heart pounding, knowing that every nanosecond wasted was a potential for life to be lost, I hooked the upper part of the patient's breastbone with the guard of my power saw. I squeezed the trigger activating the saw blade, and I pulled firmly downward as I had seen the heart surgeons and several of my chief residents do many times before. One thing I clearly remember was that I didn't expect the saw to cut as easily as it did through the bone. It truly felt like a hot knife cutting through butter. I was glad that I somehow managed to stay exactly in the midline. Veering off course would have created a complicated wound, which I would have had difficulty repairing.

I handed the saw to the operating room technician as Dr. Berger placed the sternum retractor into our young man's chest. He cranked the retractor handle as fast as he could, further opening the chest with each turn. Dr. Berger was fully aware that if he opened the chest too quickly that he would likely crack a few ribs, but that was of no concern to either of us. We needed to expose our patient's heart, and we needed to do it damn fast!

Once the chest was widely opened, we could see the dark, bluish fluid within the sac surrounding our patient's heart. I quickly grabbed a pair of surgical scissors and I incised the pericardial sac right down the middle. That was when we best witnessed the bullet tract, skiving through the heart sac, but for some amazing reason, missing the ventricular and atrial cavities entirely. The bullet did, however, catch the main left pulmonary artery within about one centimeter of its origin on the heart. This was a difficult injury, and visualization was suboptimal due to the ongoing blood loss. Our patient's blood pressure was extremely low, despite the anesthesiologist literally pouring in multiple units of blood.

Dr. Berger made a few snips with his scissors, trimming away tissues obscuring our view, so that the large vessel with the bleeding side hole could then be well visualized. Dr. Berger grabbed the injured vessel with two surgical clamps, pulling together the open edges. He then told me to sew, and I carefully repaired the injured pulmonary artery with the fine, vascular suture that the operating room technician handed me. I didn't even have to ask for it. The OR technician carefully placed a surgical instrument into my hand, which held a tiny needle attached to a hairlike stitch. The OR technician had more experience repairing pulmonary artery injuries than I did, and similar to the way a smart golfer trusts his caddie, I trusted that whatever she handed me must have been a good choice.

The sewing went well, but Dr. Berger elected to tie the knot. I later learned that sewing the pulmonary artery can be a harrowing and occasionally catastrophic experience because its substance is not tough and durable like most arteries, but thin, causing it to tear easily. I was fortunate to have used the right amount of tension to repair that injury, and likely even more fortunate that Dr. Berger did the knot tying.

I looked up at the anesthesiologist and asked him how our guy was doing. He told me that he was looking better, but that we were not yet out of the woods. My repair looked secure and tight, but blood was still oozing at a moderate rate from below the outer edge of our wound cavity. Our patient was obviously still bleeding from another unknown source, somewhere in the chest that I could not visualize. We needed to find this other source of bleeding, and the only way in which we would be able to find it would be to extend our excision. I needed to cut laterally into my patient's left lung cavity. To do this, I needed to breach one major limiting barrier—the left portion of the divided sternum. I discussed my plan with Dr. Berger, and after agreeing on what we needed to do, I regrasped the oscillating saw, and I cut left through the remaining inch of bone, converting my patient's linear gash into a T-shaped wound— not optimal for healing, but necessary in that particular case.

I incised the skin of my patient's chest from the midline on down to where the left side of his body met the table. With a pair of heavy surgical scissors, I then cut through the muscular tissue between ribs four and five, creating a massive exposure. I opened his chest cavity similar to the way mechanic opened the hood of a car to expose the engine, and cranked open the ribs with a second chest spreader, enabling me to see everything. Looking at all of God's glorious creation, I saw the area where the bullet had tangentially skived into the lung tissue, and identified our source of the continuous ooze.

I knew immediately that the bleeding would not stop spontaneously, and that an additional procedure was required to definitively stabilize our young man. I knew that he had more than enough lung tissue, which allowed me to sacrifice a portion of it without causing him any long-term harm. I applied a large, clamplike, linear-cutter-stapler device across the lung tissue between the damaged bleeding area and his heart. I closed the device tightly and I saw that my maneuver had caused the bleeding to cease. With an affirmative nod from my boss, I fired the surgical device, sealing the large, feeder vessel, and removing the damaged segment of injured lung tissue in one fell swoop. The patient bled no more.

I placed a chest tube into the young man; I would later it use to inflate his remaining lung and collect the residual blood well after I had tightly closed his chest. I also placed a second tube through the skin of his upper abdomen and laid the centimeter-thick, clear tubing directly over my patient's heart. I removed both chest spreaders, allowing the thoracic wounds to reapproximate under their own power, and cinched closed the large wound between the ribs with multiple sutures the diameter of heavy twine. I repaired the breastbone with heavy wires, passed directly through the sternum, and then tightly twisted with a pair of what resembled surgical pliers. I closed the skin with conventional sutures. I knew I was almost finished: my final requirements were to secure bulky dressings atop my patient's fresh wounds, and then to help get him wheeled over to the intensive care unit.

After getting my patient settled, I wrote a full set of postoperative orders. I chronicled the events of the operating room in written format on several sheets of paper, adding them to the patient's chart. I then breathed a sigh of relief, and went looking for some liquid sustenance since I hadn't had any food or drink for a very long time.

I found a soda machine, and filled the largest cup I could find with an overly sweetened, highly caffeinated beverage. It was very late at night, and I was enjoying a few moments of peace and solitude as I walked down one of the dark hospital corridors, replaying the white-knuckled, yet exhilarating, life-saving encounter I had just experienced. I prayed momentarily, giving thanks for the skills passed through my hands, and for the overall well-being of my patient whose chest I had just violated. I then realized that I didn't even know my patient's name.

I knew him only as "Yankee Doe." He would have been known as "John Doe" in most other hospitals—an unknown brought in emergently from the field—there being no time to look for identification prior to aggressively engaging him in advanced trauma life support activities. But at the University of New Mexico, all unknown trauma victims were assigned a unique alias. The unknown's last name was always "Doe," but the first name was a sequentially assigned, phonetic representation of one of the letters of the alphabet. Patients were assigned names such as "Alpha Doe," "Bravo Doe," "Charlie Doe," and so on. Our casualty, being the twenty-fifth unknown patient brought in, was appropriately assigned the alias of "Yankee Doe."

About midway down the long corridor, a middle-aged woman approached me at a frantic and unsteady pace. I assumed that she would walk past me, and I politely nodded in her direction as we came within a close distance of each other. She quickly crossed into my path and asked me with a quivering voice if I knew where patients were taken after emergency surgery. My curiosity was piqued, and I asked the lady what type of surgery the particular patient in question had had. She told me that her son had been brought in by helicopter after being shot in the chest. She said that she heard her son was still alive, and she wanted to see him with her own eyes.

A cold shiver moved down my spine as I realized that the boy on whom I had just performed surgery was this woman's son. I introduced myself, and I asked her son's name. I then learned that Yankee Doe was actually named Michael.

I slowly briefed Michael's mother of the events that had taken place. I described in slow, methodical detail, basic components of what I did to her son in the operating room. I also told her that I was fairly confident her son would live. The frantic mother wobbled backward and excused herself as she collapsed slowly to the ground. I helped her down, and I held her hand. I continued to give her words of reassurance and encouragement, but I also didn't want to be overly optimistic, as at that time, any one of a number of potential complications could still occur. The woman understood more than I knew as she eventually disclosed to me that she was a nurse, and that she had worked in a rural emergency room into which patients with gunshot wounds had occasionally been brought.

She then began to open up to me, describing with great pain the details of what had happened to her son at home. She told me that her son had been acting despondently for the previous several weeks and that he had been contemplating suicide on occasion. The two lived in a small, one-level home in a very remote part of the New Mexico desert. Michael had been in his bedroom while Mom had been working in the kitchen.

She paused. Choking back tears, she told me that she had heard the sound of a gunshot, and knew full well what had just happened. She described her mad dash into her son's room, only to find him almost lifeless on the floor, with his rifle by his side. She described a huge splash of smeared blood on the back wall, from where he had slid down while collapsing into a crumpled, limp mass. It sounded like a horrible experience for her, which at the time I could not fully appreciate. I was thirty-one years old, and my oldest child was only six at the time—I could not even begin to imagine the horrors of having a teenaged child inflict such great harm to himself.

I escorted Michael's mother to the Burn-Trauma ICU, and I informed the nursing staff of Yankee Doe's new identification. The woman, whose son I knew better on the inside than on the outside, thanked me profusely. She hugged me while still sobbing. She then turned toward her son and began to cry openly.

Just a few hours before, an unknown trauma casualty had been flown in to me most unexpectedly. He had been one of my most challenging trauma cases up to that point in time. But after meeting his mother, he became something so much more to me than just a "case." After that powerful interaction with his mom, Michael became my very personal patient. More importantly, he became the living, breathing son—the flesh and blood—of a very despondent mother whose heart I saw was broken. My whole perspective on everything had changed. Michael's well-being became personal to me. I wanted my patient to do well, not only for my own sake, but for my patient's mother's sake.

Michael's recovery went better than I could have been expected. After less than a week, in a most amazing fashion, he had recovered well enough to be discharged from the hospital. But because Michael had attempted suicide, he needed to spend the next several weeks in the psychiatric unit, where he worked at overcoming the demons that had taken him to such a dark and dangerous place.

Several weeks passed, and my time spent with Yankee Doe—Michael, that is—became just one of my several new and powerful memorable experiences.

I received a page to the trauma administrator's office. I dialed the number and was told to stop by and pick something up that had been dropped off addressed to me. When I arrived, the trauma administrator handed me a card and a small wrapped package. She had tears in her eyes, and I wondered what this was all about. I opened the card. The card was a thank-you note, hand-delivered to the trauma office by Michael's mother. Handwritten on the top of the card were the words, "To Dr. James Cole—World's Greatest Trauma Surgeon." Also included was an open invitation. I was invited by Michael's mom to stop by their home at any time should I ever find myself in their area. I was profoundly humbled.

I opened the little wrapped box. Inside was a small bolo tie, obviously hand-crafted by a local artisan. I was speechless. I knew that Michael's mom had purchased the tie for me as a token of her appreciation for my saving her son. I cherished the gift, and I do to this very day. After all these years, I still keep both the card and the bolo tie—still in the box—in my top dresser drawer. I look at them often, and I occasionally remind myself of that day when I made a significant impact on not just one, but two lives. And on that one day, so very long ago—to at least one person—I was known as The World's Greatest Trauma Surgeon.

7

A Tragic Ending

Albuquerque

I found Albuquerque to be a unique city. Its climate was hot and dry, much like the other communities I had been through in the desert southwest. I was surprised to meet what I considered to be more than the usual share of aging hippies: long-haired, free-spirited individuals. Most had a calm, mellow demeanor, and were unusually parochial regarding their opinions of the various varieties of hot peppers. I found that particular topic most peculiar, and most interesting. I had never before met such a large group of people who could describe in such great detail all the nuances of green chilies and red chilies.

Fully integrated within all parts of Albuquerque were the regional gangs. Their members were typical street thugs, prone to violence, who often populated our trauma rooms after engaging in intergang activities. A robust representation from the Native American population resided both in Albuquerque, and on the numerous reservations all within the regional trauma network's catchment area. The combination of excessive alcohol consumption and socialization around fire pits often led to numerous visits to the University of New Mexico emergency room and to our burn-trauma service. Our intensive care unit was overrepresented by members of the Native American communities.

I had the distinct pleasure of working for some truly great surgical attendings. Dr. Vince Janus was certainly one of them. Dr. Janus was a forty-something, laid-back, and mustachioed cowboy of a man with a thick, Southern drawl. He never became too excited during any of our trauma resuscitations or surgical engagements, no matter how heinous the trauma, and no matter how dire the situation. He was an interesting individual. He was unmarried at the time, and he lived in a basement with about eight hundred square feet of living space. I knew this fact because one day, after completing my postcall responsibilities, Dr. Janus asked me to help him move from his old dwelling into a new home—a real house. At first, I was a little reticent to commit myself to moving someone's entire home after being awake all of the previous day and night. However, when I saw that all of his worldly possessions consisted of a twin bed, a few coffee tables, a dresser, and a makeshift desk configured from a sheet of plywood balanced atop several piles of boxes, I knew that my job would not be too taxing. In fact, we made the entire move in two trips, using Dr. Janus's pickup truck to transport everything.

Dr. Janus led a simple life, but he had a complex series of accomplishments that made him anything but simple. I understood his employment contract with the hospital to be unique. Agreed upon by Dr. Janus and the hospital administration, was a carefully written leave-of-absence clause exercised each summer for a period of three months. During that time, the good surgeon traveled to the most godforsaken parts of the world, operating on the people who needed him most. He had been to Rwanda, Somalia, and many other, war-torn areas. He lived among the natives, and he performed any and all necessary surgery on locals who had been wounded by land mines, gunfire, and by the many machete-wielding marauders. He often described operating day and night for weeks at a time, on scores of wounded, while under the constant threat of imminent risk of his own life. Dr. Janus did not travel as a representative of the U.S. military, nor did he officially represent the U.S. government. He traveled as an individual citizen of goodwill to unstable nations that needed him more than we did.

Dr. Janus had exceptionally diverse surgical skills and a plethora of experience. Unlike most trauma surgeons—where operating on the chest and abdomen were commonplace—he was additionally skilled at surgically fixing long-bone fractures, and at performing complex, urologic procedures. He passed along his expertise to surgical residents such as me, with the patience of Job, and with the skill set of a true master surgeon.

Strangely enough, whereas I had absolute respect and reverence for Dr. Janus, for some reason, he admired people like *me*. He admired members of the military who dedicated their young careers to caring for military service members. He and I spoke often of the military, and of my personal past experiences with the U.S. marines while on deployment. He was always looking for a new avenue to seek excitement. As I would later learn, Dr. Janus eventually joined the drilling, Army Reserves, and he served our nation at war in Iraq.

Working for instructors like Dr. Janus, Dr. Berger, and the many other stellar trauma surgeons was a distinct pleasure, and provided me with an outstanding learning experience. I developed significantly in the areas of burn surgery, vascular surgery, and trauma surgery in general. During those two months, I padded greatly my surgical case log, but by working at such a busy facility, being far from home, and missing my family enormously, I grew tired of my experience at UNM. As I approached the end of my two-month rotation, despite knowing that I would miss my new friends, colleagues, and mentors, I again was ready to move on.

On my last night of service at the University of New Mexico, I was the man tasked to carry the trauma beeper. I was in-house, on call, and I was tired. As I had done so many times before, I worked all day and nearly all night. It was around 4 A.M., and I knew that in just a few short hours, my period of obligation with that facility would be complete. Nothing would have pleased me more than a few hours of horizontal time in the call room, studying the backs of my eyelids before the sun rose. But because there was yet one more life-altering experience awaiting me at the university, sleep was not in the cards.

As had occurred so many times before, the shrill of my trauma pager pierced the quiet of the night. I dragged my weary body to the trauma bay of the emergency room and waited for my briefing as to what was coming in. I was told that we were getting a patient with a stab wound to the chest. Whereas during the previous weeks I might have become excessively anxious, by that juncture in my training, I just couldn't get too excited. I had already managed dozens of victims stabbed in the chest, and virtually hundreds of additional trauma patients in general. If I didn't know how to handle a stab wound by then, I was in trouble.

"Paramedics are doing CPR," the telemetry-radio nurse informed me. My antennas went up a little, but only a little. I knew that I would be opening the guy's chest right there in the trauma room just as soon as he had arrived. Patients stabbed in the chest who had lost their pulse en route to the hospital had the best chance of surviving if an emergency thoracotomy—that is, surgical opening of the chest with rapid closure of the bleeding wound—was performed immediately upon arrival into the emergency department. The critical component needed to potentially save those patients' lives was the immediate availability of a well-trained and skilled trauma surgeon. I had performed that very procedure many times before. I was ready, I was able, and I was confident.

I wondered if the victim was just another Albuquerque gang banger, a drug dealer, or perhaps an abusive husband, stabbed in his sleep by the woman he had manhandled so many times before. Whatever the reason, I didn't care. I was so tired, and I just wanted to get the whole ordeal over with. I ordered the adult chest trauma tray to be opened, and I gowned and gloved awaiting my patient. In the last few moments before my mystery patient's imminent arrival, I mentally rehearsed my anticipated procedure. I was well prepared for my man's arrival, and eager to complete my last procedure at the University of New Mexico.

But despite having previously treated numerous trauma victims, and having learned over and over to expect the unexpected, what rolled in that door was certainly *not* what I had expected. And to this very day, I still have vivid images emblazoned into my memories of what I was about to see. My stabbing victim was not a gang member, a criminal, or even an adult for that matter. To my great angst, who the paramedics rushed into the trauma room was a very young boy! He was a child, for God's sake! He was no bigger than my own son—kindergarten aged at best. My own heart beat frantically because I knew that he was in the throes of death. One paramedic pumped his tiny little chest in a frantic effort to give the boy every chance for survival that he could. As the transferring crew moved the boy from the paramedic gurney onto the trauma cart, I could see the source of that child's critical state. An industrial-size screwdriver handle, at least six inches in length, emerged from the center of his chest, the remainder obviously buried deep within his little body's organs.

This was definitely one of my "Holy Shit" moments. I was momentarily paralyzed—frozen at the sight of that helpless little kid. My mind conjured images of the horror he must have felt as the monster with the screwdriver committed his heinous act. My senses were blunted. I could hear the shouting of anxious nurses and technicians, but as if my eardrums had been blown, my brain perceived the volume of the sounds around me at a bare minimum. All activity seemed to take place in slow motion, as if I were a member of the movie *The Matrix*. I recognized that I was impaired at that moment, but I also knew that I needed to overcome it immediately and do everything possible to help that small, helpless child. If that boy had any chance at all for survival, it would be me. I could not afford to waste one more moment.

I physically shook my head and cleared my dulled sense of reality. Everything became as clear as day, and it all looked so very bad. The boy's color was ashen, but he was already being bag-ventilated—manually breathed for—by the respiratory technician at the head of the bed through the pediatric-size endotracheal tube, which had obviously been placed by paramedics in the field. As I had decided even before my patient arrived—despite the fact that my patient was a child and not an adult—the kid needed his chest cracked. He needed a thoracotomy, and he needed one ASAP!

A nurse instinctively poured the brown antiseptic liquid over the boy's chest. Because he was so small, his entire chest, shoulders, abdomen, and thighs turned the color of the dark liquid. I instructed that CPR continue as I began my bedside surgical procedure. I held the scalpel in my hand, and I had one more hallucination: I saw my son on that table. A squeezing sensation gripped my chest, and my vision grew momentarily dark. But in a flash of a moment, that horrible image went away, and I proceeded with what I needed to do.

I boldly cut down the left side of his chest, starting where the ribs and the breastbone joined, running my scalpel all the way down to the table's edge. Everything on my patient was smaller than I was accustomed to. All of the muscles and tissues in that tiny body were thinner than those of an adult. I didn't even need the surgical scissors to cut the layers between the ribs; I simply poked through them with my gloved finger and stripped the flesh off the bone in one rapid movement. I widely opened his chest and I grabbed the rib spreaders to maintain my area of exposure. I looked up at the medic still performing cardiac compressions and he looked at me. His face was grim as he was feeling pains similar to mine. Momentary anger overcame me as I wanted to do nothing more than replace the defenseless little child on my table with the killer who had perpetrated this crime. But I could not allow anger to distract me. There would be plenty of time for that later. I needed to keep working.

With the boy's chest now widely opened, I ordered that CPR stop. I peered

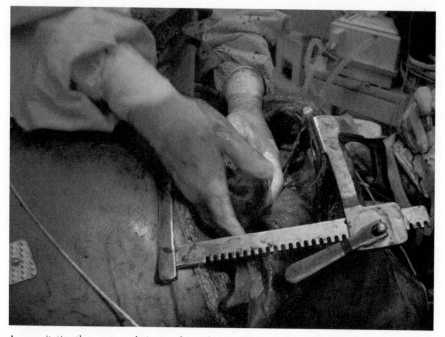

A resuscitative thoracotomy being performed on an adult patient. The metal retractor is spreading the ribs of the left side of the patient's chest and the author is holding the heart.

into the open cavity and I saw the long blade of the screwdriver piercing his small lung. I placed my hand on his still-beating heart after opening the sac surrounding it. It was beating at the rate of a hummingbird's, too fast to possibly measure, and too fast to effectively pump oxygenated blood to his brain. I lifted his left lung upward and I swept the blood that was pooled in the lowest portion of his chest directly onto the floor below my feet. I suctioned whatever blood remained, but a source of bleeding persisted.

I reached back to the tray of surgical tools and grabbed a vascular instrument, intending to clamp the aorta—the largest of the body's arteries—high up in the chest, anticipating that all blood flow below the level of my clamp would be interrupted and the bleeding would cease. Clamping the aorta is a common maneuver used in emergency resuscitations of the sort. I easily identified the aorta, but it was badly damaged. The tool of impending death had torn through the child's largest artery. In fact, the screwdriver had not only pierced the aorta, it had lacerated an approximately six-inch segment of the vessel along nearly its entire length within the chest. The evil monster who had wanted that child dead obviously plunged the screwdriver into his victim and then rocked the handle up and down, creating the tear that I was seeing—a tear which I knew was likely not repairable. My spirits sank as the sad futility of the horrible situation became apparent to me.

But I drove on regardless. After all, if anyone deserved a heroic salvage effort, it was that kid. I placed the vascular clamp across the badly damaged aorta as high in the chest as I could, nearly at the level of his shoulder. Blood flow to everything but his brain, heart, and upper extremities was arrested. I directed my attention to the little boy's heart, which was nearly fibrillating by that point. I grasped a corner of the right atrial chamber and rapidly placed sutures in a circular arrangement through the thin, beating muscle. Within the center of my circular arrangement of sutures I made a small nick, through which I passed a rubber tube. I tightened and tied the sutures, creating a tight seal. I then connected the heart tube directly to an intravenous blood line and transfused a unit of blood directly into the child's body by way of his heart. His heart filled almost immediately, but he subsequently went into full cardiac arrest. I ordered a dose of epinephrine and I grabbed the pediatric paddles, preparing to deliver a series of defibrillating shocks. After three consecutive deliveries of energy directly to the heart muscle, nothing changed and the heart was still fibrillating. The situation had become about as bleak as possible, and I had pretty much run out of options.

I knew that I needed to stop, but I needed confirmation to assure myself that it was indeed an appropriate time to abort any additional efforts. I stepped up to the head of the bed, and I opened his eyelids. I couldn't help but be overcome with sadness as I looked at his cherub of a face—so young, so innocent, and so undeserving of such a fateful outcome. His pupils were blown and they had absolutely no evidence of a functional light reflex. I knew that the poor little child was almost certainly brain dead and already beyond saving. I finally felt comfortable ending the resuscitation, but not at all comfortable with my newly gained experience. I had just performed my first pediatric resuscitative thoracotomy, and my efforts were unsuccessful. I was pretty sure that no one else could have had any different of an outcome, but I still took that death personally. I was certain that I hadn't made any mistakes and that I did all that I could have done. But the fact still remained that the kid was dead, and it was all quite saddening.

I informed the rest of the team that I was declaring the child dead. Everyone became silent, and there was little movement in the room. Several nurses and technicians were quietly crying, and I, too, did everything in my power to prevent the heavy moisture in my eyes from gaining momentum. I breathed a heavy sigh and looked over toward the police officers standing post in the corner of the room, themselves looking somber. I asked them if they had known any details of what had happened to the boy. They motioned for me to walk out of the room with them, and they started talking.

Allegedly, the child had been living with his father and he was starting his first year of kindergarten. Apparently, the child had gone to bed prior to his very first day of school and he was scared. The father—a known felon in the community—was apparently flying high on an all-day, cocaine binge, revealed by his own admission and evidenced by the numerous incriminating items found by police at the home. According to what the dad had told the police, the boy woke up in the middle of the night after wetting his bed, throwing his father into a psychotic, drug-enhanced rage. In a fit of uncontrollable anger, the father grabbed a screwdriver and plunged the blade deep into the boy's chest. Then, coming to his senses, the dad recognized the horror of what he had just done and dialed 911, routing paramedics to his home. When police and paramedics arrived, the father had shrouded the boy with his own body, preventing initial care to the child. Several police officers wrestled the man off the child and placed the man into custody as paramedics worked on the boy, and then transported him to me.

I was shocked by the tragic story I had just been told. All I could think of was my own child, and how much I cherished his precious little life. If I was that father I would have killed myself. There was absolutely no way that I would have been able to live with the circumstances of what I had just done. All I wanted to do at that moment was hug my own son, tell him just how much I loved him, and hold him tight. But I was far from home and it was too late at night—or too early in the morning—to call home. I excused myself from the police, and I slumped away with thoughts of sadness and horror still streaming through my head.

That was not how I had wanted my tenure at the University of New Mexico to come to a close. That was not the last memory of the place, which I wanted to retain. But nothing could have changed what had happened, and nothing would ever erase the memories of that day from my consciousness. To this day,

I still think of the events of that fateful night, and I still imagine what could have come of that boy if he would have lived. As I have watched my own son grow up—now over six feet tall and successfully enrolled in college—I have often thought of how two very similar people, living such very different lives, had such very, very different outcomes.

8

Pure Hell

Cardiovascular Surgery

On New Year's Day of 1997, I sojourned up to the state of Washington to begin a sixty-day rotation on the cardiovascular surgery service at Madigan Army Medical Center in Tacoma. That was a particularly bad weather day, and a foot of snow blanketed the area within a twenty-four-hour period, making roads nearly impassable. The Seattle area was more rugged than usual and highways were littered with numerous wreckages and spinouts. Driving was hazardous, but weather had never been an acceptable excuse for the tardiness of a surgical resident, and I was not going to start off my new rotation on the wrong foot. As I navigated the treacherous roads of the Sea-Tac region, I could see the majestic peak of Mount Rainier off in the distance. I would later learn that an entire group of psychiatry residents from one of the area's teaching hospitals had all tragically fallen to their untimely deaths while on a group-bonding expedition.

I was about a thousand miles from home in El Paso, but that was of little importance as even if my family had been right there with me during that two-month period, I would not have had any time to spend with them. Little did I know that my next sixty days would be spent in Dante's most inner circle of hell, and only my own death could have given me rest.

Throughout the two-month course of instruction, residents specializing in surgery are exposed to a wealth of educational opportunities while serving on their residency rotations. Although infrequently called upon to perform surgery outside the usual and customary limitations of a general surgeon, after success-ful completion of all training, surgeons could conceivably be tasked—usually in the most critical and urgent of situations—with handling surgical problems of any variety. To prepare young surgeons for such possible occurrences, surgical residents spend considerable time learning aspects of every surgical trade, often away from their parent institution.

In my case, I spent many months at William Beaumont learning surgery's core components of abdominal surgery, breast surgery, chest surgery, vascular surgery, neck surgery, and trauma surgery. In addition, I learned key aspects of neurosurgery, orthopedic surgery, plastic surgery, urologic surgery, obstetrical-gynecologic surgery, and critical care. But I also spent months far from home receiving additional concentrated blocks of training in trauma surgery, burn surgery, pediatric surgery, transplant surgery, and cardiovascular surgery.

I had great hopes and expectations for my upcoming two months of cardio-vascular surgery training. I held glamorous visions of performing harrowing open-heart procedures—the signature operation being the coronary artery by-pass graft procedure, commonly referred to by those in the trade as a CABG (pronounced *cabbage*)—and learning the nuances of the cardiopulmonary by-pass pump machine. But my cardiovascular surgery rotation was nothing glam-orous. I was the one and only resident on the service, and I was subordinate to three attending cardiovascular surgeons, each of whom had graduated from prestigious cardiac surgery programs; the Cleveland Clinic, the George Wash-ington University, and the University of Massachusetts. I worked for each of the surgeons and, in the great tradition of cardiovascular surgery training, each at-tending surgeon considered me his personal slave and whipping boy. I had only one intern assisting me. He was an exceptionally strong first-year surgery resi-dent who primarily attended to the patients on the cardiology floor who were well into their recovery. But he was just one person and he, too, was overtaxed. He could do little to relieve me of my extensive burdens. I truly believe that I had never worked as hard as I did on that rotation as compared to any other time in my entire life.

My typical day would begin (assuming that the previous day had, in fact, ended) at 5 A.M., when I arrived at the hospital and checked on my three or four intensive care unit patients on our small but painful service. Every one of my patients was either preop or postop—which meant that they were either really sick awaiting surgery, or really sick because he or she had just had surgery. I reviewed all of the past day's lab values and other ancillary tests. I examined the whole slew of invasive monitoring data trends—right heart pressures, left heart pressures, pulmonary artery pressures, cardiac outputs, and so on—and queried the volumes of bloody fluid draining from the various tubes we had placed into our patients' chests. I also checked to be sure that all patients requiring intra-aortic balloon pump (IABP) treatment were, infact, surviving. An IABP is a gargantuan-size tube threaded through a groin artery up to a level just below the heart, where intermittent mechanical inflation and deflation, carefully synchronized to the continuous electrocardiogram monitor, provided just enough additional assistance to the weakest of the weak hearts to live a little longer. After prescribing fine-tuning treatments or occasionally providing hands-on, aggressive resuscitative care on morning rounds, I reviewed all of the day's patients' preoperative, cardiac catheterization films, which were basically the radiographic road maps indicating which vessels needed bypassing, and to where.

At approximately 6:30 A.M., I would meet up with the cardiac surgeon with whom I would be operating that day. Again we would go over our pregame films, and set our plan for the day. Immediately following our brief discussions, we would head off to the operating room where our first patient would already be asleep on the table in the care of the attending anesthesiologist. The following is how a typical CABG procedure would go from beginning to completion.

An extensive set of monitors would be placed by the anesthesiologist, through neck veins and through arteries in the wrist, to measure all major and minor changes in our patient's cardiovascular status, prior to us even washing our hands. Once the anesthesia boss declared that he was ready, we would scrub up, gown up, and glove up. Cardiovascular surgeons get unusually pampered by surgical assistants, and that was the case for us on every occasion. By the time our gloves were secured onto our hands, our patient's body was already prepped and draped.

As was the rule, I would stand next to the patient's right side, because I was right-handed. That position afforded a right-handed surgeon the greatest comfort and flexibility when operating on the midline of the chest. After receiving the go-ahead from the anesthesiologist behind the drape, I would hold out my hand without uttering a word, into which a scalpel would be placed in such a manner that I did not have to manipulate it even one millimeter. The cardiac scrub technicians were consummate professionals, and they prided themselves on every aspect of surgical assistance, including anticipating which surgical instruments were needed and when, and then perfectly placing them into the surgeon's hand, ready for use. The boss and I would then exchange nods, and I would cut directly down atop the tissues over the center of the sternum from top to bottom. After appropriate applications of the electrocautery probe, the sternal oscillating saw, and the bone spreader, the heart would be exposed. I would then open the pericardial sac surrounding the heart, tack it out of the way with several sutures, and prepare to place the patient on cardiopulmonary bypass.

For me, that was the most harrowing part of cardiac surgery. At that stage, if we really needed to, or for some reason wanted to, we could close the patient's chest, reverse the anesthesia, and call it a day. Very little life-altering harm was done to the patient by that point. But in the next fifteen minutes, we would place large tubes into our patient's frail heart and aorta—suturing them into place with common, sterile sutures—diverting all of our patient's blood from the beating, muscular organ to the cardiopulmonary bypass machine. Blood would then flow through the numerous yards of clear, plastic, three-quarter-inch tubing, from the patient to the machine. I would watch as the trail of red would leave my patient and arrive at the complex box of roller pumps, oxygenator, and valves. We would then give the go-ahead for the perfusionist—the man running the pump—to administer the drugs that would chemically arrest the beating heart. The cardiac contractions would become weaker and weaker, and within a few minutes, the heart would become completely flaccid. We would then apply a large clamp across the body's largest artery immediately at its emergence from the heart, and the patient would as a result be completely dependent on the big machine and our hands.

Many things could go wrong during those few, critical procedures, and any one of them could result in either massive blood loss or a premature, fatal, cardiac arrest. To place the aortic cannula—the main hose returning blood from the machine back to the body under relatively high pressure—I would carefully place two series of circular-arranged sutures, plunged deeply into the thick tubular artery, and leave them long and untied. I would then hold both ends of the inner, circular, suture arrangement and wait for my attending to pierce deeply within the center of my sutures, and insert the aortic tube into the arterial wound before too much blood had poured out, while I *calmly* and slowly tightened the inner suture.

Remaining calm was an essential part of the technique. If I was to be just a little too anxious, speedy, or aggressive, I could pull just a little too hard and break the suture or tear through the aorta, either of which would result in a bloodbath, and the possible death of our patient. Sutures did indeed break on occasion, which was why I always placed an outer, second row of circular-arranged suture. That was my safety valve, which I would rapidly turn to and cinch down in case I broke that first stitch. But I only had one safety valve—only one additional row of sutures—and if that broke, we were all in trouble. Fortunately, I personally broke a suture only once—repeat, only *once*—and that never, ever, happened again.

Placing the second cannula was not nearly as harrowing. The second cannula was actually a pair of tubes that collected all blood returning from the body to the heart by way of the superior vena cava and the inferior vena cava. Both tubes were placed through snipped corners of the right, thin-walled, atrial chamber. We fed one tube into one of the large feeder veins, and the other into the second of the two. Ordinarily, those tubes were fairly easy to place, and because the blood pressure in the chambers of the right side of the heart was seldom greater than that of any ordinary vein, the amount of blood lost while performing that portion of the procedure was quite limited. Nevertheless, however, the sutures used to secure all tubes to the heart have to be placed with great care because pulling too hard could easily tear the thin-walled muscle of the atrial chamber. Once both of the tubes were in place, all blood ordinarily returning to the heart was bypassed entirely to the machine where it was mixed with the powerful blood thinner, heparin, to prevent clot from forming in the bypass machine circuitry. At that point, the heart became nearly bloodless.

My next task was to move down to our patient's legs, where I would begin removing a long segment of saphenous vein to be used for portions of the bypass procedure. This was a fairly simple process of making a very long cut into the inner aspect of the lower leg, just above the ankle and dissecting out the long, wormlike, blue tube. We would usually bypass four or five heart vessels during the same procedure, and so I always dissected out plenty of vein. Often, I would have to remove the entire vein from the ankle up to the patient's groin to be sure that we had enough plumbing to work with. The vein harvest left a huge wound the entire length of the leg, which we would not close until after the entire bypass procedure was complete. When harvesting the saphenous vein, numerous tiny side vessels would routinely have to be tied off and separated from the rest of the leg. It had to be done rather meticulously, as failing to recognize the presence of a tiny feeder vein, and accidentally pulling it away from the rest of the leg tissues could tear a tiny hole in the future heart bypass vessel. And if not recognized until after the bypass procedure was complete, there could be a lot of bleeding in the chest when the heart again began beating. If that happened, it would inevitably be followed by much yelling and screaming from my attending cardiac surgeon. None of that was desirable, as all of it placed our patient in jeopardy.

Opening the chest, placing the patient on cardiopulmonary bypass, and harvesting the saphenous leg vein would take me about thirty minutes to complete. At that point, I would break scrub—that is, I moved away from the operating room table and removed my gloves and gown—and leave the OR. It was a time of critical importance to me as it may be my only true break for the day. I would leave as the attending cardiac surgeon began performing meticulous dissection of a narrow artery off the undersurface of the patient's chest wall, also to be used as a bypass channel. His procedure usually took about twenty or so minutes. And I knew that in that precious amount of time I had to find some fast food, wolf it down, and rush back to the OR to be scrubbed back in before the next phase of the operation began.

I cannot overemphasize just how important that food break was to me. After that point in my morning, I would usually be so busy that I had not a moment of time to get any real food into me. Other than a bag or two of chips from the vending machine, or perhaps a small candy bar, that morning snack was about my only guaranteed period of nutrition. Sadly enough, my food break usually consisted of a slice of calorie-dense, meat-lover's pizza, which I purchased on an almost ritualistic basis from the hospital snack shop in the front lobby.

Once back in the operating room—again scrubbed, gowned, and gloved—my job was to assist the attending heart surgeon in performing the ultrafine process of suturing narrow little tubes to other narrow little tubes. One end of saphenous vein actually would get sewn to small holes punched into the aorta, but the far end would get sewn directly to the tiny coronary arteries. To see it done is a wondrous sight, but to actively participate in the process is even more impressive.

Coronary artery bypass is really a microsurgical procedure. Often, heart vessels as narrow as two millimeters in diameter need bypassing. Suture as fine as a strand of human hair attached to a curved needle an eighth of an inch long is used to circumferentially sew a paper-thin vein to a small nick made in a diseased coronary artery. Sewing under such conditions requires an extremely steady hand and exceptional vision. Nearly every surgeon I know, including me, needs special magnification glasses not only to see the suture, but also to place each stitch with the precision and accuracy needed for a perfect outcome. Meticulous sewing is critical, but tying the knot in a microscopic piece of thread without breaking it can be even more crucial. You can imagine the pain felt if, after spending ten minutes working on an area the size of a grain of rice, you break the stitch trying to tie the knot, which resulted in your having to remove everything, and starting all over again.

Once all bypass sewing had been completed, the second-most nerve-racking part of the entire procedure would take place: taking the patient off the bypass pump. It was usually not a difficult process, as in most cases the heart would again start pumping once the perfusionist running the bypass machine normalized the concentration of the potassium circulating through the tubing back into the body. Occasionally, though, the heart would require a little electrical motivation to again get started. A few quick jolts with the paddles usually jump-started the human engine, but bleeding, from the sutured bypass sites, was not out of the ordinary. Performing microscopic surgery on an arrested, nonbeating heart is a truly difficult feat, but having to throw a stitch to close a spurting pinhole on a now-moving target is an extremely difficult, technical adventure. Accurately placing just one or two additional sutures once the heart had been restarted was absolutely critical and it sometimes took us as much time as sewing an entire vessel prior to coming off pump. Placing those last, critical sutures just a fraction of a millimeter too deep could result in closing off the entire coronary artery and making the patient worse off than he had been even before the operation began.

Next, we removed the bypass tubes. It was a two-man process. One surgeon pulled out the tubes while the other one tightened and tied the circumferential sutures placed around the cannulas at the initial stage of the bypass process. Once the sutures were tied, there could be no leaking. If there was even a trickle of blood, or if there was any chance that one of the cannula stitches might loosen, the result could cause catastrophic bleeding well after the patient arrived back to the intensive care unit after surgery and after the normalized blood pressure pounded away at the tenuous closure areas. That might necessitate a painful take-back procedure for all of us, and when that occurred, it *always* seemed to happen in the middle of the night.

Placing a few drainage tubes and closing the bony sternum, in addition to closing the chest and leg wounds, concluded the final phase of the operative procedure. Prior to our closing all wounds, the anesthesiologist administered just enough medication to reverse the effect of the blood thinner, but not so much as to cause our tiny bypass grafts to clot off. Once all dressings were in place, we stepped back from the table and took a few deep breaths. The OR crew escorted our postop patient to the ICU, and I followed just as soon as I completed the obligatory postoperative orders and procedure note.

This entire operation from beginning to end lasted no fewer than three hours. I was both physically and mentally exhausted after every case, and we typically repeated that entire process one to two additional times each and every day. By the completion of all surgeries, I was thoroughly wiped out. But caring for cardiac patients involves much more than just the operative procedures themselves, and even though we had completed all of the surgeries, my workday was far from complete.

The cardiac surgeons at Madigan Army Medical Center had established a policy that every patient be fully awakened and removed from the ventilator on the same day of his heart surgery. On paper, it was a great policy. Patients had shorter recovery times, had fewer complications, and had shorter hospital stays. It was all good for both the patient as well as the hospital. But it was, in fact, not good for me. Having that early extubation policy meant that long after the surgery was completed, I spent many hours at the patients' bedsides trying to determine when it was an appropriate time to remove the breathing tubes. Unlike the case in many other types of surgery, the anesthesia used on heart patients is a little deeper than most, and has a longer, postoperative, anesthetic effect.

During the immediate postoperative period, heart bypass patients can be very unstable with wild variations in blood pressure and heart function, severe heart rhythm disturbances, and excessive postoperative bleeding. As a result, I spent plenty of personal time at my patients' bedsides, and it was fairly typical for me to not be able to consider taking patients off their breathing machine for perhaps four to six hours after the surgery was completed. If we rolled our final patient out of the OR at around 4 P.M., it would be common for me to not be able to finally extubate him until after about 10 P.M. or later, if a particular patient was not doing as well as we had hoped. If we were just *starting* our last case at four, I would usually end up spending most, if not all, of the night right there in the intensive care unit. The patient would sleep, but I wouldn't.

Now, that's not entirely true. I would fall asleep at times, but it wasn't officially approved of, and it certainly wasn't encouraged. The cardiovascular surgery resident didn't even have a call room, so I couldn't lie down even if I had wanted to or if I had the time to. But every person does have his physical limits, and on occasion, after spending countless late nights in the hospital, perhaps averaging two to three hours of sleep per night for weeks at a time, I couldn't help but fall asleep in a chair next to the bed of a postoperative patient I was watching. For the most part, the nurses were kind to me, and didn't wake me if I had fallen asleep unless they really needed to tell me something important. Ordinarily, the nurses understood that the surgical residents were treated like caged mice in some bizarre, real-world experiment, which studied torture, sleep deprivation, and human behavior.

If I was lucky, and if everything had gone perfectly well that day, I would have the luxury of leaving the hospital sometime after 10 P.M. By that time, I was inevitably exhausted, dehydrated, hypoglycemic, and starving. I lived in a one-room motel approximately one mile from the military hospital. I often debated with myself as I was departing the hospital what was more important to me at that very moment: sleep or food? Usually, I would end up stopping at the gas station along the way to my motel and pick up a bag of jumbo gumdrops, or perhaps some corn chips, and consume them by the time my car had reached the motel parking lot. At that moment in my life I was focused on survival: sleep, water, and food were my priorities in order of greatest importance. I craved sleep. I yearned for it with every one of my muscle fibers and nerve cells. I needed it so badly that I might have given just about anything for a handful of hours of pure, restful, uninterrupted sleep.

But that was never the situation. I was always on call. I was on call continuously, day and night, for the entire duration of my time on the cardiovascular surgery service—sixty continuous days. I would always get paged at night after leaving the hospital. If I made it back to my motel by midnight and I knew that I had just four and a half hours before I needed to again awaken, I would usually sleep for only about half of that time. The rest of the time, I spent answering pages from the intensive care unit nurses and cardiology nurses. On a good night, I wouldn't have to drag myself back into the hospital at zero dark thirty to eyes-on assess a problem I had been called about. But as my luck would have it, I did go back to that hellhole at least every other night on average. I was more exhausted than I had ever been in my entire life, I was becoming physically ill, and I was starting to mentally unravel.

Amassing a huge sleep debt does take a physical toll on the body. I felt sharp pains in my upper abdomen—in the pit of my stomach—on a nightly basis. The source of my pain could have been from the excesses of coffee and caffeinated soda I drank to overcome my zombielike condition. It could have been from malnutrition, as a daily diet of one slice of pizza and a bag of jelly candy surely must have lacked something of nutritional importance. Or, it could have been due to the massive amount of stress I was experiencing. I took my responsibilities as the sole resident on the cardiovascular surgery service very seriously and I wanted to impress my attending staff members by being a good, diligent, and hardworking resident. As a result, I thought about my patients constantly. I was consumed by cardiovascular surgery, but at the same time I was torn between providing hands-on care to my patients, and surviving myself. I was truly starting to think that I might actually die on that rotation.

The pain in my upper abdomen worsened on a daily basis. There were times when I was in so much agony that I would go off into a remote part of the hospital where I would pull my knees up to my chest to blunt the knifelike pain grinding through my insides like live beetles consuming me from within. I always carried a bottle of liquid antacid in my hospital coat's pocket and I sipped it several times per hour, just to keep me going. One late night when I finally made it back to the motel room some time after midnight, I was nearly writhing in pain. I was so incredibly uncomfortable that I just could not ignore it any longer; at the same time I was so exhausted that I just couldn't physically do anything about it. I needed to sleep, but I couldn't sleep because of the pain. I couldn't get up to address my discomfort because I was just too darn tired. I was in the Catch-22 of my lifetime, and in my desperate condition, I could not find a solution to my problem. All I could do was pray. I prayed that the ulcer, which I assumed was the source of my pain and was torturing me, would penetrate my stomach entirely, and that I would develop an emergency surgical condition—one that would necessitate my calling paramedics, one that would give me rest while under anesthesia as some other surgical resident fixed the hole, and most important, one that would give me a legitimate excuse for taking a few days off from the cardiovascular surgery service. My irrational prayer request was all that I could do to give me peace. I had no other options. That night, I did somehow fall asleep, and I don't remember getting any pages from the hospital staff waking me. By early morning, I had felt a bit more rested, and my stomach did not hurt as much. None of that which I had prayed for ever materialized, but I do believe that my requests were heard.

At the end of my period of indentured servitude, the chief of cardiovascular surgery called me into his office. I remember him well, as we had spent so much time together in the operating room. He was an emotionless man. He never smiled, and he never cracked a joke. To him, nothing was funny; everything was serious. Cardiac surgery was serious, and cardiac surgery was his life. He congratulated me on a job well done, and he reached out and shook my hand in what I think was the first evidence revealed to me that he was, in fact, human. He then sat me down and started to recruit me into his chosen specialty. He continued, saying that he thought that I had the work ethic, the drive, and the fortitude to make it through a cardiovascular surgery fellowship. He continued, saying that he had connections at the Cleveland Clinic, and that he would write me a favorable letter of recommendation on my behalf to his former mentor at the clinic, Dr. Delos Cosgrove, an absolute giant in the field of heart surgery. It was all incredibly flattering to me, and for a moment I actually considered taking him up on his offer.

But then my senses returned to me and I remembered just how much I had suffered, and was still suffering in fact. No, I would not be considering cardiovascular surgery any longer. I would never again wish that I had chosen heart surgery as a career. In fact, never again would I think that heart surgeons live glamorous lives. To this day, I feel a little sorry for those surgeons who sold their souls to the devil in order to become what many people in our society consider to be at the pinnacle of the surgical specialties. And I am also grateful for that grueling experience I received at Madigan Army Medical Center. One of my residency instructors used to often tell me, "That which doesn't kill you, makes you stronger." Well, I didn't die, so I guess I must have been made at least a bit stronger by that whole painful ordeal. But most important, my experience at Madigan convinced me not to choose to become a cardiac surgeon. And for that, I am most certainly grateful.

9

Good Fortune

The Chief Surgical Resident

I spent my entire final year of residency—my chief resident year—back in El Paso at William Beaumont Army Medical Center. As residents progress throughout their months and years of surgical training, increasing amounts of independence, and increasing levels of responsibility are entrusted to them. Once into the latter half of the chief year, most residents have attained all of the necessary surgical skills and decision-making abilities to go out into the communities and establish a surgical practice. At that stage of my educational career, I, too, felt confident and competent. I had endured years working all day and all night, juggling the responsibilities of simultaneous emergency room, intensive care unit, and clinic disasters, and operating on routine, difficult, and horribly complicated, surgical patients. I had made it into the final stretch, and I was finally beginning to see the light at the end of my residency tunnel.

Although I knew my residency would soon come to an end, very little changed throughout the year to ease the burden of my work. One afternoon, while both residents junior to me on my service were occupied performing gallbladder and hernia surgeries, I found myself having to respond to the emergency room to manage an incoming trauma patient. According to the report that came across the paramedic radio, a man had been pulled from a house fire, unresponsive and not breathing. He was said to have been badly burned.

Preparing myself for whatever was to roll through the trauma room doors, I threw on a pair of gloves and a protective overgarment. The smell of burned hair and charred flesh arrived before my casualty did.

Paramedics were busily performing chest compressions on the pulseless, badly burned body of what appeared to be a middle-aged black male. His hair had been completely burned off and his skin was cooked. It was deep brown in color. I then realized that the person whose skin appeared to be that of an African-American man was actually that of a Caucasian male, bronzed by prolonged exposure to an intense heat.

My patient had already been intubated by the paramedics in the field. He was being ventilated by the man squeezing the bag attached to the breathing tube, whom I noticed was using both hands to force air into my patient's lungs. I ran my hands over the casualty's chest as I quickly assessed the entirety of his completely nude body. He had been badly burned from head to toe. Not one area of his skin had escaped the flames that had caused his moribund condition. His skin was thick, leathery, and tight. I imagined one of the many well-done turkeys I had pulled out of the oven, having allowed it to bake longer than was optimal. I noted the similarity in my patient's tissues to my memories of the overcooked birds, with skin crisp and shrunken, and form-fitted to the underlying carcass. My patient's skin had indeed been cooked, and his leathery flesh was making it nearly impossible for the paramedic to expand his thoracic cavity and allow for good ventilation of his lungs. As if a straitjacket had been tightly cinched down onto him, I knew that the only chance at saving my patient would be to relieve him of the confining grip of the flesh that bound him.

Knowing that all nerve endings had been irreversibly burned from his skin, I requested a scalpel, and began carving away. I sliced the right side of my patient's chest, starting from the tissue just below his collarbone, and ran my blade all the way to his groin. I carefully avoided the hands of the technician who had taken over the paramedic's role of performing chest compressions. As I sliced through the thick gauntlet of flesh, the cut edges quickly retracted away from my knife as the underlying fat and unburned tissues bulged into the crevice created by my blade's cutting edge. As my scalpel reached my patient's groin, his right chest expanded with a new easiness, as if I had split a biological cast binding his torso. I then repeated my procedure on the opposite side, witnessing a similar bulge of fat billowing between the released edges of the crispy tissue. I completed my bedside escharotomy procedure by connecting both vertical slices with a horizontal gash positioned just below my patient's nipples. The resultant H-shaped series of cuts allowed unencumbered respirations, albeit all mechanical, from the ventilator on which our burn victim had been placed.

I knew that if I was going to take things to the ultimate end point, I would have to perform numerous, extensive skin incisions to release nearly all of the burned tissue, which was undoubtedly preventing adequate circulation to my patient's four limbs and to all of his digits. But before I would subject him to what would be a mutilation, I decided to check to see if he was even salvageable. Being unable to breathe for what must have been a very long time, there was a distinct possibility that my patient had long since been brain dead. Doing any more than I had already done in such an instance would be of no benefit to anyone, and would certainly be unnecessarily morbid, considering his already unfortunate situation.

I checked my casualty's pupils. Indeed, they were fixed and dilated. They showed absolutely no signs of constriction when I passed a bright light before

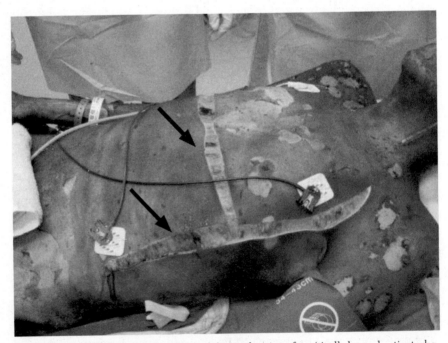

Escharotomies performed on the thoraco-abdominal region of a critically burned patient who succumbed to his injuries. The arrows point to the incisions made.

them. Undoubtedly, my patient's brain had suffered the irreversible effects of prolonged hypoxia, either from a lack of oxygen in the burning building, or from the inability to breathe due to the restrictive forces of his excessively tight skin. I ordered the technician to stop CPR. I peered at the cardiac monitor and saw what I had suspected: a flat line. There was nothing resembling any signs of life. My patient had died, perhaps even before he had arrived at my hands. But I did what was expected of me, and I gave him every opportunity to live. He was dead. And I pronounced him as such.

I sought out the chaplain, who directed me to the grieving room where a sole family member awaited my briefing. She was a portly, white woman of about thirty-five years. Her hair was disheveled and she was missing most of her teeth. She wore an oversized, dirty T-shirt bearing the inappropriate image of two animals engaging in a sexual act. She looked confused and bewildered, and her mouth moved as if she could not stop chewing at her lips.

I broke the bad news slowly to her, and she wailed. It was clear to me during our very brief discussion that the woman was not well from a mental health perspective. She had apparently been living for some time with my much older patient, who had just expired. She repeatedly stated that she would have no place to live because she had no money, and the home in which she once stayed had been burned to the ground. Ironically, she spoke little of the man who just died. Clearly, he was her source of stability, but I suspected that she actually cared little about him.

I offered my most sincere condolences, but I don't think that any of my words were heard. Realizing that there was absolutely nothing more that I could do, I politely entrusted the lady to the chaplain, who would have her hands full trying to accommodate the homeless woman. I excused myself after showing the lady one last sincere gesture, and I left the room. Unfortunately, I may not have done my best at consoling the mentally handicapped friend, as my mind was heavily preoccupied. I could not stop thinking about Mr. Breckenridge.

I was exhausted and I had very little patience left in me. I had to leave my dead, burned patient's friend behind me. Less than twenty-four hours before, I had spent the entire day and night operating on Stanley Breckenridge. It was the longest and most painful surgical endeavor I had ever undertaken. I loathed the thought of going back to the OR with Stanley. I had already checked on him that morning, and he was doing reasonably well. But I needed further reassurance to convince me that I could relax and not worry that my twenty-six-hour operation was not all for naught.

Mr. Breckenridge was a cantankerous old coot who refused to quit smoking despite being a horrendous vasculopath. That is a term we use to describe patients whose entire circulatory system has degenerated into a disheveled tangle of blocked arteries from years of smoking, high cholesterol, and poorly controlled, high blood pressure. They are often diabetics who don't feel the need to adhere to a strict diet, and they often undergo multiple operations over the years to salvage limbs and prevent strokes. Vasculopaths are a surgeon's nightmare.

Mr. Breckenridge had been admitted to our trauma service ten days previously after falling. His right foot had become wedged between pieces of furniture in his home, and the resultant application of forces applied to his lower limb as he fell caused his ankle bone to break through the skin as it snapped off the long length of tibia to which it had been previously attached. Orthopedic surgeons realigned his fracture and secured its position with a carefully applied plate and screws. The jagged wound created by the shard of bone piercing his flesh was trimmed and closed with surgical precision. Mr. Breckenridge was hardly what I would have ever called a typical trauma patient. He had not been shot, stabbed, or the victim of a major car crash. But because his list of medical problems was longer than nearly every other patients' in the hospital, he was admitted to our trauma service for us to manage his medical co-morbidities.

Unfortunately, ten days postop, Mr. Breckenridge's wound began to fall apart. Ordinarily, the body's natural healing factors and oxygenated blood, which circulate through our large and small vessels, gradually provide the building blocks necessary to allow the body to heal itself. But when a vasculopath suffers even trivial injuries—especially on the foot and ankle region—they often don't heal without performing a complicated, revascularization surgery.

The staff vascular surgeon and I studied Mr. Breckenridge's angiogram performed several days after his orthopedic procedure. We had already suspected that his wounds might not heal and that Stanley might need a revascularization procedure to improve the blood flow to his ankle. We didn't want to operate on Stanley, but if we needed to, we needed a preoperative "road map" to guide us as to which area of diseased vessels might need bypassing.

Stanley's vessels were a complete disaster. The angiogram revealed partially obstructed vessels in nearly every vascular conduit from his mid-abdomen on down. The main arteries of each of his thighs were diseased throughout, although wisps of blood could be seen trickling down to areas behind both knees, where the vessels divided into three, smaller arteries. With his injury clearly not healing properly, we planned the simplest of procedures that would help Stanley's situation yet not subject him to any of the risks ordinarily associated with major surgery. We vowed to perform our surgery under regional anesthesia—that is, anesthesia where the patient is not put to sleep, yet all feeling is deadened with a spinal anesthetic. Such anesthesia is often used when pregnant women undergo caesarean sections, allowing them to remain awake as the baby is surgically delivered by the obstetrician from the mother's womb.

At 7 A.M. of the previous morning, Mr. Breckenridge was positioned on the operating room table, fully prepped, and with a heavy dose of anesthesia bathing the nerves of his spinal cord. He was not under general anesthesia, but he was not fully awake, either. To allow Stanley some emotional comfort, the anesthesiologist had given our patient a mild sedative, allowing us to cut on our patient while he rested in a pain-free state. We planned on performing a femoral-femoral bypass procedure, in which we would divert blood flow from Stanley's less diseased left femoral artery to his nearly occluded right femoral artery. Increasing blood flow to an area just beyond the level of greatest vascular blockage would hopefully allow just enough increased blood flow to allow his injured ankle wound to heal.

The operation started off well. I made incisions over both groin areas, and I dissected out both right and left femoral arteries. I created a tunnel in the fatty compartment below the skin of Stanley's pubic region through which I passed a synthetic vascular tube constructed of polytetrafluoroethylene, which we usually just refer to as PTFE. I clamped both femoral vessels, incised into each of the vascular structures, and meticulously sewed the synthetic tube from one vessel to the other.

Using my high-powered, loupe magnification glasses, I had a perfect, enlarged view of the ten-millimeter incisions created in both Stanley's femoral artery and the PTFE graft. I sewed carefully. Even one poorly placed throw of the fine, vascular suture could result in failure of the entire revascularization procedure. With my Castroviejo needle holder in my right hand and my delicate Gerald forceps in my left, I passed the tiny needle attached to the ultrathin suture through Stanley's artery, then through the PTFE. I repeated my technique numerous times, taking great care to be sure that each stitch was spaced exactly one millimeter from the next, and creating a running, water tight connection between the two tubular structures.

After throwing the last pass of the suture with a gentle twist of my fingers, I tied the hairlike material with just the right amount of tension. The scrub technician squirted water onto my gloved hands before I tied. The water created just enough slippage between the suture and my gloves to help prevent me from breaking the suture—a potential faux pas, which could earn me a vicious head butt from the vascular surgeon standing less than one foot across from me. After successfully sewing together the right-sided vascular structures, I repeated the procedure on the opposite side. When done, a brand-new bypass channel had been created, intended to divert the flow of blood from the left femoral artery to the right. In all, the whole painstaking process took me about two hours to complete. But when I released my vascular clamps hoping to identify a healthy rush of blood down the vessels of Stanley's previously injured leg, I was disappointed. The flow was inadequate. We needed to do more.

The next step was for us to perform a femoral-popliteal bypass. Our decision was an audible, made at the line. Like a quarterback standing behind the center, when he sees a defense that bothers him, he changes the play. We didn't previously discuss what we would do should our femoral-femoral bypass fail, but we couldn't leave the operating room without having the desired result of our planned procedure. I shifted gears mentally, and I planned on connecting a second piece of synthetic vascular tubing from the right-sided portion of the femoral-femoral hook-up site, to a piece of Stanley's large artery behind his knee. I repositioned my patient's leg with his knee flexed. I incised through his already cleaned skin and I dissected away the tissues, allowing me exposure of his popliteal artery. As I had done on my patient's pubic area, I created a tunnel down his thigh from groin to knee, and I passed a second, precut length of the white, rubbery, PTFE tubing. I strategically placed my clamps, made my cuts into the vascular conduits, and placed my sutures. I sewed and sewed, eventually creating a second vascular bypass.

But to my chagrin and moderate frustration, that, too, was inadequate. Despite having just spent a total of almost five hours in the operating room, there still was not enough blood flowing down to Stanley's ankle. Again, studying the angiograms we had attached to the X-ray viewbox in the operating room, we surmised that there was just too much vascular disease in Stanley's abdominal aorta to allow for adequate blood pressure to infuse into my pristinely placed bypass channels. We had a few options, one of which was to open Mr. Breckenridge's abdomen and perform an aorto-femoral bypass—attaching a synthetic, Y-shaped graft to the largest of all vascular structures in the body and connecting it to the synthetic tubing in his groins. But we had vowed to minimize significant risk to Stanley, and we didn't want to have to open his belly. That would certainly require a general anesthetic, and we really didn't want to take that risk.

A better option would be to perform an axillary-femoral bypass, where we would obtain our much needed pressure head of blood flow from an artery just below Stanley's collarbone, and bypass it yet again to the tubing in his groin. That is exactly what we decided to do.

To facilitate our procedure, we needed more anesthesia. I drew up a large syringe of numbing agent and liberally injected it into the skin and fatty tissues of Mr. Breckenridge's upper chest and clavicle area. I made my incision and dissected out the desired vessel. I then injected more of the local anesthetic agent below the skin of my patient's chest and abdomen along a route I planned on passing a much longer portion of artificial blood vessel.

I passed a blunt-tipped, hollowed-out, aluminum tube through the incision below my patient's clavicle, and I directed it along the path of my recently injected local anesthetic. I passed it below Stanley's skin, exiting the incision I originally made in his right groin. I uncapped the top of the hollow tube and passed yet another piece of synthetic tubing through the aluminum pipe. With portions of the artificial vessel exposed on both ends of the metal tube, I carefully withdrew the aluminum structure leaving the bypass tubing situated under Stanley's skin. I clamped, incised, and sewed. And nearly three hours after deciding to perform the third bypass procedure, I released all clamps. But to my extreme dissatisfaction, and growing frustration, that too had not adequately restored flow to Stanley's ankle.

Too-numerous-to-count procedures followed. The staff surgeon leading me throughout the painful process had become angry with me. Despite doing all that was asked of me and all at a reasonable pace, he needed someone to blame for keeping him tied up far longer than he had desired or anticipated. I was the resident, and thus, I was the appropriate scapegoat.

Over the next ten hours, we performed numerous additional bypasses and procedures to remove clot from the grafts we had already sewn in place. Despite all of our efforts, we still didn't have the inflow to Stanley's ankle that we desired. I had been operating for eighteen straight hours! I was tired, my legs and back were aching, and I desperately needed to use the restroom. My boss had already left the room on several occasions to sneak some juice and to use the facilities, but I had not been permitted yet to do the same. I wanted to abandon the operation entirely and suggested that we do so. The wrath of the attending surgeon who vehemently disagreed with me made it clear that we would not be abandoning anything.

Accepting the fact that my surgical opinion meant very little to my supervising surgeon, I requested permission one more time to go to the bathroom, stating that if I could not leave, I would certainly pee in my scrubs. He told me to go. I broke scrub, removing my gown and gloves, and left the operating room to relieve my overdistended bladder. I managed to find two cups of grape juice in one of the hospital refrigerators, and I gulped them down, hoping to give me enough energy to keep working. Feeling much better after adding the handful of calories to my system, I walked back into the OR. When I returned, my heart sank. In my short absence, Mr. Breckenridge had been placed under general anesthesia and his abdomen was filleted wide open. The vascular surgeon was operating as fast as he could, hoping to get as much done as possible before I had returned. We promised each other that we would not do what was being done. But my boss was fed up, and he did what he knew our patient needed to heal his ankle. He was preparing for us to perform an aorto-bifemoral bypass.

We spent the next three hours doing so, sewing the large, bifurcating piece of artificial tubing to the lower portion of Mr. Breckenridge's aorta, and to portions of the previously placed artificial material in each side of his groin. After tying the last knot of my suture, I nearly jumped down to my patient's feet, hoping to God that I would be able to feel pulses. I did! *Hallelujah!* I was so happy that I could have nearly cried. After all that surgery, we finally restored pulsatile blood flow to our patient's poorly healing wound.

I spent the next three hours doing nothing more than closing all of the wounds I had created over the previous twenty-one hours. In total, I had been doing surgery for an entire day—twenty-four continuous hours of work on just one patient! That was a record for me. I nearly collapsed when I wheeled my intubated, bandage-covered patient into the intensive care unit.

The words I heard next were no more painful to me than if a wooden stake had been driven into my heart with a mallet.

"I don't feel a pulse," the nurse stated objectively. I saw her feeling my man's foot and looking inquisitively as if she thought about it hard enough, perhaps she might imagine a pulse. I had distinctly felt a brisk pulse in Mr. Breckenridge's foot before I closed, and I had to take a feel for myself. It had to be there. It *had* to be! But it wasn't.

I almost wanted to cry because I knew that when a patient lost his pulse immediately after vascular surgery, he needed to be taken back to the operating room. I dreaded telling my vascular attending, but I had to. It was my duty to inform him of the situation. Hoping that he might just as well tell me to forget about taking him back—hoping that he was as tired and frustrated as I was—I briefed my boss of the absence of our patient's foot pulse. Instead of any sort of condolence, he berated me for not having already taken our patient back in the OR. And so I prepared for yet another potentially long and grueling series of hours in surgery.

Back in the operating room, I reopened Mr. Breckenridge's right groin wound—the side where we had lost the pulse. I exposed the multiple sections of tubing all sewn together. Hoping to find a simple solution to our immediate postoperative failure, I removed the fine sutures in the most accessible portion of the synthetic tubing. Blood rushed out of the hole from above, which I controlled with the quick application of a vascular clamp. But blood only trickled back at me, suggesting that clot had formed somewhere downstream obstructing flow to the intended target.

Hoping for a little good luck, I passed a long catheter, about one millimeter in diameter, down the entire length of the artificial vessel. At the end of the tubing was a tiny balloon, which I carefully inflated with a small amount of air injected through an opening in the groin end. With air in the balloon, I slowly pulled back withdrawing the inflated catheter. With great joy, I removed a small piece of clot. I knew that where there was some clot, there would likely be more. I repeated the procedure several more times, each time removing additional bits of thrombus. With each successful removal of the obstructing material, the blood flowing backward and up toward me increased. I had hoped for a little luck, and I thought that I had received it. After feeling confident that I had removed all clot, I reclosed the area where I had removed the tiny sutures, and I reexamined my patient's foot. To my great joy, I again felt a strong pulse! I asked the anesthesiologist to begin infusing a blood thinner so that Stanley would not form additional clot. I knew that my decision was risky because it could cause Mr. Breckenridge to bleed from any one of the numerous wounds. But even the vascular surgeon agreed with me at that point.

I reclosed my patient's groin wound and once again took him back to the intensive care unit. The nurse who had given me the bad news before made me much happier when she had no difficulty finding her pulsating target after the second operation. Absolutely weary from my twenty-six-hour adventure, I wrote out a comprehensive set of postoperative orders and I proceeded to dictate the details of the endless operation.

Following my encounter with the badly burned man in the emergency room, I anxiously returned to Stanley's bedside. To my great happiness, Mr. Breckenridge's foot was warm and his pulse was brisk. I checked on him multiple times each day for the better part of the following week, and his foot thrived. He never needed to return to the operating room. I remember operating on Mr. Breckenridge as if it were yesterday. Our vascular marathon was a success, but strangely enough, I do not recall if his ankle wound eventually healed.

Although that endless operation was tiresome beyond words, I am not bitter or angry for having had to endure it. To the contrary, I am fortunate to have been allowed to take care of such a complex patient, and other patients like him. Without question, I was extremely fortunate to have trained at William Beaumont. My selection to the surgical residency in El Paso was a fluke, as I had never even applied to the program. And of course, William Beaumont was an *army* program. I was, by commission, a *navy* officer, and thus accordingly I should have trained in a navy program. Having been previously assigned to the eastern coast of Virginia, and to Southern California on the West Coast, I would never have favorably ranked what I considered to be the north Mexican desert of El Paso if I had been given a list of possible army programs prior to my applying for postgraduate training.

At the time, the navy only offered surgery training at three military hospitals in the United States: Portsmouth, Virginia; Bethesda, Maryland; and San Diego, California. Portsmouth was considered to be a workhorse hospital, where the surgical residents and staff were viewed and treated like blue-collar laborers. Portsmouth was a place with unlimited training opportunities, but the workload was infamously known as being exhausting. Bethesda—home of the National Naval Medical Center—was considered the flagship of the navy's medical commands. Presidents, senators, congressmen, and other dignitaries often sought care at Bethesda Naval Hospital, but opportunities for residents were somewhat limited. When most people of great influence requested that a resident not care for them, their wish was usually granted. San Diego Naval Hospital was a high-volume treatment facility in beautiful Southern California, far from the bureaucracy of the East Coast, and a frequent top choice among young doctors applying for residency training, but because it was so popular, few wishes were actually granted.

During the final year of my GMO tour with the marines, I submitted my application to the Navy's Bureau of Medicine and Surgery, hoping to get selected to complete my surgical training. Traditionally, representatives from each of the navy's postgraduate training programs assembled at a weeklong conference where they hashed over the applications, portfolios, medical school transcripts and board scores, and past performance evaluations to determine who among the group of applicants would be chosen for each of the navy's residency programs. However, during the year I applied, a joint, tri-service U.S. Army-Navy-Air Force conference assembled.

Apparently, during that application cycle, the navy had more qualified candidates capable of training as surgeons than it had residency training slots to offer. When I received my letter of congratulations from the Department of the Navy indicating that I had been selected to become a surgeon, it specified that my training program site would be at an "Other Federal Institution." Of course, I had no idea what that meant, but when I eventually learned that "Other Federal Institution" was a hospital in El Paso, Texas, my heart sank. My wife and I decided to fly out to El Paso to get a feel for the place. Leaving the lush, verdant, flower-covered lands of Southern California, and landing in the cracked-earthy, tumbleweed-strewn town in the desert southwest, I almost turned down the residency offer. But turning down a surgical residency at that time would have been a very bad decision and one almost unheard of. People wanting to become surgeons must be willing to sacrifice just about anything to achieve their lofty goal, and I realized this. So I accepted my training opportunity, and in July of 1994, our family moved to El Paso and settled in.

I do believe that God directs our lives, gives us certain challenges, and places us in situations for reasons that may not be clear to us at the time, but perhaps become evident years later. Years later, I am now quite certain that God sent me to William Beaumont for a distinct reason—to become a part of a truly stellar surgical training program under the leadership and direction of Colonel Stuart Goetz, M.D.

Doctor Goetz was a remarkable individual. The son of an Army Special Forces soldier, Dr. Goetz attended and graduated from the U.S. Military Academy at West Point. He then served as an infantry officer—a grunt leader, specializing in rifles, mortars, and human leadership. He then had a paradigm shift in his life's calling, and felt that he needed to become a physician. He changed gears and attended the Uniformed Services University of the Health Sciences, where he received his medical degree. After several additional tours of duty, including a surgical residency at Eisenhower Army Medical Center in Fort Gordon, Georgia, an overseas assignment in Landstuhl, Germany, and several additional years assigned to Fort Bragg, North Carolina, Dr. Goetz came to El Paso to head up the surgical residency training program—something he always told us was his professional dream come true.

Dr. Goetz was a gifted teacher, a skilled and talented surgeon, and a man of great integrity and honor. He was a trusted adviser, and a mentor both in and out of the hospital. Dr. Goetz taught us to be good surgeons, and he taught us to be good human beings. He stressed the importance of seeing patients not as "surgical cases," but as individuals with surgical disease processes, and to treat our patients at all times with compassion, dignity, and with all of the human kindness every individual who walks this earth deserves. And he taught us responsibility. From the moment we established a doctor-patient relationship with those who sought our services, we were responsible for their outcomes. We assumed responsibility for their preoperative workup, for the outcome of the operations we performed, and for any problems our patients developed after surgery.

He taught us that just because we *could* do various surgical procedures, it didn't necessarily mean that we *should* do the procedures. For some patients, especially the advanced in age whose lives were extremely frail, nonoperative therapy might better suit the particular patient rather than surgery. He reminded us over and over that surgeons are not superhumans, and that they are all prone to mistakes and human failures. But he also stressed that should we make a mistake, it must always become a learning opportunity so that our future patients' outcomes are as optimal as humanly possible. One of his many common sayings was, "Live and learn . . . live long, and learn a lot." I admired Dr. Goetz for all that he was, and I am grateful for that one fateful day at that tri-service conference, when one surgical residency slot at William Beaumont still needed to be filled, that he chose me sight unseen over all other candidates to be his next surgical trainee.

One day, very early on in my residency training, while Dr. Goetz and I were both washing our hands at the same scrub sink outside of the operating room, he asked me about my parachute experience with the Marine Corps. I didn't know much about my boss's past at the time and I answered his questions with all of the politeness and respect a program director deserved. I assumed that he was making small talk. He then asked me if I had ever had any problem jumps. I found that question particularly intriguing because indeed I did have one, very significant, problem jump, which I then explained to him.

On a moonless night at around midnight, I was slated to perform a mass tactical parachute jump over Camp Pendleton with the Marines of the First Air Naval Gunfire Liaison Company, or ANGLICO as the unit was commonly called. I was the second man in the front of a line of about sixty jumpers, all planning to exit the side door of a C-130 airplane in rapid succession. The goal in a mass tactical jump is to get as many men out of the aircraft in as short a time as possible. I was particularly excited that night and was eager for the jump to be a good one.

I stood with my chest pushed into the back of the man in front of me, himself being in the open doorway of the speeding aircraft. We waited for our signal—typically a boot in the rear end—and then exited one after another. As I had done so many times before, I jumped out into the sky and I quickly pulled my hands over my reserve parachute, awaiting my main chute to open. Unfortunately for me, however, having jumped out so quickly behind the man in front of me, my left arm became caught in his static line, and his line was still hooked up to the aircraft!

My arm was yanked from my body with the force of . . . well, the force of a speeding airplane. My arm went limp immediately, but I could feel my extremity somehow disengage the static line that tethered me to the C-130. As I was released, I felt myself twist and turn through space, as the force applied to just one of my arms caused me to spin while my main parachute was opening. I spun around countless times, causing the numerous lines connecting the harness strapped to my body and to the parachute canopy, to wind tightly. This decreased the surface area of my parachute, causing me to fall faster than I should have.

I was in a bad situation. I couldn't feel or use my left arm at all; it was essentially paralyzed. I knew I was falling fast, as I caught glimpses of parachutes near me rising quickly. I could see almost nothing in the pitch-black sky. I couldn't really tell just how close the ground was. I wanted to deploy my reserve parachute, but when the main chute is partially inflated, deploying the reserve parachute could cause both to fail, resulting in a screaming ride down to earth. What I needed to do in that situation—what I had been trained to do but couldn't do because of my bad arm—was to cover my reserve with my left hand while pulling the rip cord with my right, thus preventing the reserve parachute from flying out in a random, undirected manner that might foul the main chute. My training taught me to keep the reserve covered with my left hand and, reaching into the reserve pack with my right hand, scoop out a big handful of parachute material, and then throw it down and out to one side, resulting in a hopefully safe, twin-chute deployment, one alongside the other.

I couldn't do it. My arm was dead. I tried to twist, turn, and bicycle-kick my body, attempting to unfoul my lines, but my emergency actions were unsuccessful. I decided that I was going to have to ride that one in, and I hoped for the best. At that point, there was absolutely nothing I could do. And then, for no good reason at all, I began to spontaneously unwind. I turned about a dozen circles as my lines unraveled under their own power. After the lines unwound, I felt a sudden, braking feeling, as I was pulled upward. My parachute slowed down to a normal, falling velocity.

A few seconds later, I hit the ground with a hard, crumpling thud. I didn't quite expect it. I had been thinking of other things while falling. Once on the ground, I checked myself, specifically querying my dead arm, but it was too dark for me to see. I unclipped myself from my parachute harness, and with one hand I stuffed my used chute into my aviator's kit bag, which I hauled back to the rest of my unit. I could not see a thing, but I sensed where the rest of my group was gathered and I hiked on toward them. Once linked up with the rest of the unit, I ditched my parachute bag and walked away from the crowd with one of my corpsmen. I told him about my midair accident, and together we examined my arm. Under the luminescence of a Humvee headlight, I could see that my uniform shirt had been torn and the skin over my bicep was badly bruised and abraded. I had treated similar injuries in other jumpers before, most of whom had torn parts of their biceps muscles, and others who had stretched the brachial plexus of nerves between the shoulder and the arm. I figured that I was probably in the latter category. I knew that very little could be done for my injury at that point, and so I just hid my disability from the others for the rest of the training evolution, and I went home to my wife. Fortunately for me, by the next day, my arm function returned to normal. I was able to feel everything and I had completely normal motor function. I was lucky. And my arm never bothered me again.

Dr. Goetz listened to my story with seemingly great interest, and then he told me that he, too, had been a towed jumper. He extended his arm, causing his scrub shirt to draw up toward his shoulder, and revealing the scars of his own parachute mishap. His biceps had torn as a result of the same situation as mine, but his had occurred over the skies of Panama. In 1989, the United States military was ordered to capture de facto Panamanian president Manuel Noriega by parachuting into his country and overpowering the Panamanian Defense Force. Dr. Goetz jumped in, attached to the Third Ranger Battalion, serving as an airborne surgeon ready to render care to the combat wounded once on the ground. Unfortunately for him, however, he too had become a casualty. But somehow, despite his unfortunate circumstances, he still managed to operate with one hand and care for several injured soldiers.

From that day forward, I felt that Dr. Goetz and I had some sort of special bond. I knew that I would not only respect him for his position as my residency program director, but also for his past military, operational endeavors. Whereas most doctors, including military physicians, neither enjoy nor appreciate the uniqueness of military life and the hazards of operational duty, I knew that Dr. Goetz was the exception.

William Beaumont also afforded me the privilege of working for Dr. Sam Holbrook, who became a strong influence in my eventual commitment to trauma surgery. Dr. Holbrook came to El Paso as an army major in 1995, to provide additional influence and leadership to our trauma program. Two years prior, Major Holbrook was deployed to an expeditionary field hospital in Mogadishu, Somalia, supporting the military assault during the infamous "Blackhawk Down" incident. That was where at least one soldier slowly bled to death as he was taking cover from enemy fire in an abandoned building while being tended to by an enlisted army medic. The young soldier died in that building from an arterial gunshot wound to the groin—an especially difficult area to gain control of an actively bleeding vessel. Being barricaded in that building without surgical support, the poor medic was nearly helpless as he frantically watched his young casualty bleed to death, despite a truly heroic effort of handheld compression over the arterial pumper.

When Major Holbrook learned the details of that young soldier's demise, he became consumed with preventing future similar catastrophes by developing a product—a bandage, dressing, or clot-forming material of some sort—which could potentially prevent similar battlefield deaths. Dr. Holbrook became a man obsessively driven by the known science and future research of blood, clot formation, and hemorrhage control. He recruited me as his first research resident at William Beaumont, and together we studied the effects of his first major contribution to the field of trauma surgery—the dry fibrin sealant dressing.

I learned plenty from Dr. Holbrook, both from his teachings and his example. He was a meticulous stickler for details, and he was a feverish worker. One conclusion always seemed to lead to yet another question in need of answering from additional research and development. Dr. Holbrook's passion and seemingly endless energy exhausted me and the others who worked for him. He had a profound impact on my subsequent desires to treat trauma casualties in both well-equipped trauma centers as well as in the austere, expeditionary environment. I never knew at the time just how globally influential Dr. Holbrook would eventually become. Over the next decade, he was promoted to full-bird colonel. He was also selected to command the army's prestigious Institute of Surgical Research at Fort Sam Houston, Texas. He became the consultant to the surgeon general on all matters pertaining to trauma management, and he published over one hundred trauma research articles in well-read, civilian, peer-reviewed, medical journals. I was one of his earliest disciples, and I remain a humble admirer.

In that final year of my residency, the staff at William Beaumont polished my skills as a well-rounded surgeon. I treated patients with emergent, urgent, routine, and chronic surgical conditions within the full spectrum of surgical illness and injury. I also supervised and trained teams of residents junior to me, and I furthered my independence as a medical decision maker. In those last months of my training, I looked forward with great eagerness to the day when I would look back at my training facility only through the rearview mirror of my family's minivan as we departed to our next assigned duty station. Leaving William Beaumont would mean that I had finally completed my surgical residency.

Awaiting military orders directing me and my family to our next place of employment and opportunity was a source of both great excitement and anxiety to which most service members can personally relate. As the only navy man assigned to an all-army facility, I expected to be sent to either a naval hospital or to a ship, neither of which seemed particularly exciting. Despite the fact that by that time I had been commissioned as a Navy Medical Corps Officer for almost nine years—including my time spent as a reservist while in medical school—I actually knew very little about the navy. I had only spent one year assigned to a navy hospital, and I had never even set foot on a ship. My two years assigned to the Marine Corps paralleled an army experience so much more than were those typical of the traditional navy. Navy personnel who spent time with the marines called themselves "green-siders"—that is, they wore the green uniform of the ground forces stepchild of the navy, rather than the blue uniform of their proud parent. At that point in my military career, I was a true green-sider. I knew that receiving just about any set of "blue side" orders would make me feel like a proverbial fish out of water—no pun intended.

Strangely enough, one of my two residency peers—himself awaiting future orders—was an anomaly himself. A former Army Combat Engineering Officer, and an explosives and demolitions expert, he had an unusual penchant for the U.S. Navy of all things. Born and raised for much of his life in California, my residency-brother Matt wished that he could have the opportunity to serve aboard ship—an opportunity that I had absolutely no interest in. I wished that I was Matt, and Matt wished that he was me. Fortunately, my chances of remaining on the "green side" were unexpectedly elevated by an invitation extended to me in a closed-door meeting with my boss, Colonel Goetz.

Included in Dr. Goetz's list of professional accomplishments was the fairly well-known secret that he had been a former member of an elite group of military physicians who worked for a subordinate organization of the United States Special Operations Command, or USSOCOM. Only those in and formerly assigned to that particular organization really knew the details of what they actually did. I was not sure why Dr. Goetz had wanted to meet with me. As always, I expected to hear that I had done something wrong or that he had some new, time-consuming assignment for me to complete. But to my great happiness on that day, I was told that based on my past experiences with the marines as a military parachutist and diver, and my demonstrated skills as a physician and surgeon, that I was being formally offered the opportunity to join the elite and mysterious group within USSOCOM.

As I understood the deal, I could accept the offer if I could find an army surgeon willing to swap job assignments with me for the following two years— that is, I needed to find a surgeon in an army uniform who wanted to serve on a navy vessel. I knew that Matt might potentially be that individual, and when I approached Matt with the opportunity to trade spots, he couldn't have been more obliging. But the whole swap process wasn't exactly the smoothest, even by military standards. To make it all happen, we actually needed signed letters— Memoranda of Agreement—from the surgeons general of both the navy and the army to make it all happen. What ordinarily would have been an impossible, political obstacle to overcome, somehow all materialized in our favor. I always knew that Dr. Goetz was a man of great influence, but I never really knew if it was he or someone else who had persuaded the surgeons general to make things happen. But someone, somehow, had made that most unusual request a reality.

Our residency graduation ceremony was one of great joy and relief for all three of the graduating chief, surgery residents. We had each given the institution more than our share of sweat and human suffering, but in return we received our prized certificate of authenticity—each of us was officially anointed as *Surgeon*. We each shook a lot of hands and we posed for more than a reasonable number of pictures. And then, as if we had never even been there, we were done. We were officially discharged of our responsibilities at William Beaumont, and the other residents and staff went back to work—business as usual. The whole day was a bit anticlimactic for me, but it was made perfectly clear that we were to move on, and that life at William Beaumont Army Medical Center would not change a bit. With that final release from responsibility, my wife, Michele, kids, parents, and I went back to our home on Fort Bliss to relax, and to ponder my family's next career move.

10

The Independent Surgeon

Fort Polk Louisiana

Being the only navy surgeon assigned to the army had its disadvantages for sure. Whereas I had been given the great opportunity to work for USSOCOM—a job many surgeons considered to be an amazing privilege—my assignment to that special unit was really just a side job. You see, that particular group, which those of us on the team always referred to as The Unit, had a full-time cadre of operational members and staff. It received the bulk of its health-care support from medical and surgical specialists scattered throughout the United States, primarily east of the Mississippi River, stationed at various army hospitals.

Members of the group assumed our daily responsibilities as emergency medicine physicians, anesthesia providers, and surgeons at our assigned facilities, but we were tethered to our nation's needs by an electronic leash, which could summon us to our extracurricular duties at a moment's notice. Prior to graduation from my residency program, I didn't know where I would be assigned to work for the many months at a time between stints with The Unit. I had hoped to receive orders to a coveted base such as Fort Campbell, Kentucky—home of the famous 101st Airborne "Screaming Eagles"; or Fort Bragg, North Carolina, home of the illustrious 82nd Airborne. But I was the lowest man on the army totem pole, and I would get no such glorious assignment. My orders sent me to a place many still consider to be the armpit of the army: Fort Polk, Louisiana.

When most people think of Louisiana, they have visions of New Orleans: Bourbon Street, Mardi Gras, and great culture. But Fort Polk was located nowhere near New Orleans; it was in fact a good five hours west of the great city, located deep within the Kisatchie National Forest, in the absolute middle of nowhere. Fort Polk was developed during the Vietnam War era as a training post to accustom enlistees to the hot, humid, jungle environment where they would soon be sent off to fight. Now, I have never been to Vietnam, but people who have served in that Southeast Asia country tell me that Fort Polk *was* Vietnam—minus the Viet Cong and the booby traps. Every poisonous snake in North America slithered the grounds of our base, including the forested backyard of my living quarters. Bizarre insects the size of small birds darted at us on a daily basis. The climate was hot and humid, making a perfect home for the armadillos—bizarre creatures resembling miniature dinosaurs—which would bore holes into my front lawn at night, and scurry off at first sunlight.

Some military bases are huge, elaborate, industrial cities, surrounded by built-up towns whose businesses thrive on the patronage of the soldiers. But Fort Polk had no such good fortune. Our base consisted of a few small buildings and rows of houses scattered among the densely packed trees, creeks, and swampy marshland. Leesville was the town located just outside the front gate. It was an impoverished community of no more than seven thousand people, which never felt the need to expand or improve itself. Leesville had one main road, on which a few small-town restaurants, taverns, trinket shops, and strip joints were colocated. Shopping for basic essentials, such as groceries and clothing, all had to be done at the small, military exchange, at the Leesville Walmart, or at the pawnshop just outside the gate. If you couldn't find what you needed at any of those places, the only other option for nearly thirty miles was the Jack's All Ya' Need. Jack's was a well-furnished shack, complete with gas station, grill, and clothing aisle. I don't ever remember seeing more than a few people in that small shop. As the painted sign on the front door advertized, you really could find everything you might need at Jack's—assuming you didn't confuse the term *need* with *want*. If you needed a hunting jacket, a can of beans, a freshly grilled cheeseburger, or a stuffed alligator head, you could certainly find it all at Jack's.

But Fort Polk and Leesville each had unique charm for all of those who could recognize it. If you had ever wanted to get back to basics and live like a hermit or experience life like Tom Sawyer, Leesville would be the right place for you. People were very friendly and unpretentious. We were welcomed into the Fort Polk community with open arms. Despite my family's culture shock when we first arrived to the bayou state, I truly felt that the forest community of Fort Polk was one of the best-kept secrets in America. Despite its austerity, we were fortunate to have been assigned there for so many reasons.

My wife and my now four children immersed themselves in the Louisiana culture more than I did, as I spent more than my share of time away from the state. My co-assignment to The Unit within United States Special Operations Command kept me busy and gainfully employed. It would not be uncommon for me to be called away from my primary duty station to link up with USSO-COM on a few hours' notice. On one occasion, I was at Bayne-Jones Army Community Hospital—the small, military, health-care facility aboard Fort Polk—just completing the final wound closure after a two-hour operation to remove the cancerous thyroid gland in a middle-aged, active duty army officer, when I received a signal on my pager. It was a number to a phone far away, and a number I knew well. I wasted no time dialing the phone when the deep voice on the other end—the voice of a man known only by his two initials—told me the words I had grown accustomed to hearing, "Come to work."

That is all that was said, and that was all that was needed to be said. I knew that those words meant that I needed to get out to The Unit as soon as possible. On that particular day, I wrote some postoperative orders for my thyroid cancer patient, phoned one of my partners informing him of my leaving, and stopped home to kiss my wife good-bye. Michele knew the deal, and was supportive of what I did. She knew, however, that for an unspecified length of time she would be alone in that one-thousand-square-foot military home, with four small children, and with no husbandly support.

I grabbed nothing, as I needed nothing. I drove off to the airport, a forty-five-minute drive away from our military home. At all times I carried with me a set of special military orders. They were unique, open-ended orders, which authorized me to travel anywhere, by any means of transportation, in or out of uniform, with weapons, controlled substances, or classified documents. When I arrived at the airport, I would simply present the orders to the ticket agent, show my military ID and government-issued credit card, and then get on the next available flight to my destination. Once there, a van would be waiting for me, driven by a member of The Unit, who would then take me to our special compound where my gear was always waiting and ready. None of us ever knew what would be asked of us or when we would be called to special duty. We each kept a number of large bags in a locked cage, each bag packed with gear and uniforms for any conceivable climate and duty. Included in our cage was a "seventy-two hour bag," which contained just enough clothing, emergency food, and leisure material to sustain us for three days, regardless of what was asked of us.

Serving with the special members of The Unit was a privilege and an honor. I worked with special operations units both known and unknown. The basic, special operators included Army Rangers, Navy SEALs, and Green Berets. But I also served alongside others whose missions, team identities, and unit members remain truly covert—groups whose organizational names have been the subject of many fictional thriller novels, but whose true existence have never been officially acknowledged. I swore an oath and I signed a lifelong, binding contract to never divulge the crucial details of the secret organizations I served. Doing such could compromise the mission, the teams, and the individuals who risk their lives in selfless defense of our nation. However, it is no secret that such special operations groups exist, and thus my discussing them in a vague, generalized manner reveals nothing of importance.

I have worked closely with the members of unknown organizations, and I have trained with them on their ultrahigh security, secret compounds—places where over 99 percent of our nation's military have never seen but from the outside. I've parachuted and fast-roped—that is, slid down a three-inch-thick rope suspended more than fifty feet from a hovering helicopter—and I've fired truckloads of ammunition from automatic rifles and submachine guns, as well as from foreign-made AK-47s.

I've received both tactical training and intelligence training from the best of the best—an elite subgroup of quiet, mature professionals of the Special Operations community, who are America's truest patriots. They are men who don't seek recognition, and don't even talk about what they do. But they do their job with great passion, driven by a calling to protect the sovereignty of a nation they love selflessly. They are men who have been protecting our nation in battles that have been ongoing for decades, against enemies more than willing and eager to decimate the very existence of the United States of America and its interests. I developed a great affinity for these men, and I loved serving with them.

But, of course, I served as a military physician and surgeon. And as every member of the USSOCOM organization serves as a specialist in something, I, too, served as the specialist in my field. My role was to provide all levels of medical support to the members of that community wherever it was required of me or needed. I could do my job in any conceivable environment, with special gear and equipment that I and the other members of the medical team brought with us. Nothing limited what we could do and where we could do it. If we needed to carry in our gear strapped between our legs as we parachuted from the sky, then so be it. We never really knew exactly what would be needed of us, and where we would need to go. That was the thrill of the mission, and that was also the impetus for my subsequent unique passion—health-care delivery in the austere environment.

Military physicians are not considered as combatants. The Geneva Conventions of 1949 specifies the limitations of how doctors may use weapons and how they should be treated should they be taken as prisoners. Physicians are allowed to use weapons to defend themselves against their enemies and to protect wounded patients under their care. There is nothing that specifies the exact details of how that is to be accomplished or the exact limitations of how far doctors can go to provide the protection they perceive needing. Thus, while attached to USSOCOM, doctors like myself readied themselves for any possible situation, and maintained proficiency in the use of any and all weapons available to us. Knowing that firing a weapon in an offensive posture could potentially strip a doctor of any special rights or privileges typically granted to medical prisoners if captured, we had to choose wisely how we would use our firepower. However, not having much faith in our enemies' adherence to the rules of the Geneva Conventions, most of us followed our inner instincts and those we developed through working among the community. In the end, we trusted our conscience to guide the decisions we made.

If I had never been assigned to Fort Polk I might never have been able to do so many different types of surgery as the brand-new fully trained surgeon I was. I was fortunate to have been stationed at the only military hospital of any sort in the entire state. That brought a huge number of patients to our medical facility, and sent many referrals and surgical consults my way. Louisiana and the far-east portion of Texas had an abundance of loyal military retirees and veterans, who gladly traveled over a hundred miles to receive care at our military hospital. Fort Polk was also a large training post, hosting numerous military reserve and guard units who rotated through on a monthly basis, giving rise to various traumatic injuries and surgical diseases needing my partners' and my expertise and skills.

I was paired with two other surgeons, Steve and Chandler, and together we took care of nearly everything. Steve had completed his surgical residency in Georgia two years before me, and had been stationed at Fort Polk ever since. He was the senior surgeon on post. Chandler had finished his training in Hawaii at the same time I graduated from my program in Texas. Chandler and I were the two new guys on base, but we were both eager and aggressive surgeons. What we lacked in experience, we made up for in knowledge and confidence. Individually, neither Steve, myself, nor Chandler could do everything, but together, we seemed to be able to do anything. And that is exactly what we did. We operated on everything from head to toe. If the patients came to us and they were appropriate candidates for surgery, we operated on them. We did things many well-seasoned surgeons at greater institutions would refer away, such as pancreatic surgery, lung cancer resections, and even some plastic surgery. Having the pooled energy, knowledge base, and commitment of the three of us allowed us to achieve great outcomes and a pretty impressive surgical case log.

One of the reasons we did a lot was because no one else at Fort Polk could. Chandler, Steve, and I had very little physician support since there were very few other specialists at our hospital. We had no cardiovascular surgeons, cardiologists, gastroenterologists, or any other medical or surgical specialists, with the exception of one orthopedic surgeon, one oral surgeon-dentist, and one ear, nose, and throat specialist. For the most part, if someone came in through the Fort Polk Emergency Room with anything serious, it was highly likely that one of the three of us would get called for something. For the most part, we enjoyed doing all that we did, with the exception of a few things, including emergency colonoscopy. Ordinarily, when a patient comes into the hospital bleeding profusely from the rectum, a gastroenterologist gets called in to perform an emergency colonoscopy to identify the source of bleeding and to cauterize the source of hemorrhage. Without any gastroenterology support, however, we were called, usually several times per week, to do that unsavory chore.

But on occasion, we would get asked to do something extremely unusual. That was the case one early Sunday afternoon when I received a page from the hospital pathologist, asking if I could come in to help her do an autopsy. It just so happened that Chandler and his two boys were over at my house, and when I told Chandler of my most unusual request, he was too interested to let me go to the morgue by myself. We drove over together in our civilian clothes and went down to the basement hallway where we found the morgue door propped open. We knocked and walked in to find the only pathologist at Fort Polk sitting down, reviewing some notes she had prepared, wearing surgical scrubs and a heavy, black, plastic apron. She greeted us and asked us both if we could provide some insight as to what we thought killed the young soldier lying on the slab under a heavy opaque drape.

We put on gloves and pulled back the drape to reveal a young man, perhaps only twenty years old, with a classic high-and-tight haircut on his decapitated head! That was a particularly shocking and gruesome sight for us, as in my mind, the head should always be attached to the body. The pathologist apologized for not warning us ahead of time, and she explained to us that the soldier had been involved in a high-speed vehicular crash the morning before as he was driving with a friend down to Lake Charles to do some fishing. Their sports car apparently struck an early-morning bread truck, somehow causing a sharp edge of the truck's frame to cut through the boys' car, and slicing his head clean off at a level just below his jaw. His head was otherwise pristine and completely untraumatized, as if a giant, razor-sharp ax had been wielded with great force through a freshly sculpted figure made of clay. I was puzzled by her conundrum, as the cause of death seemed pretty darn obvious to me. And then she pointed out her second, important finding.

She peeled open the Y-shaped incision on his chest, revealing his perfectly dissected heart with all its arterial attachments. What she showed us was a massive tear—in fact, a compete separation—of a segment of the aorta on the left side of his body. That main tubular structure was a notorious source of immediate death in patients killed by very high-speed car crashes. Her dilemma was now a bit clearer. Was the completely torn aorta, or was the gruesome guillotining the primary cause of the young man's death? Personally, the answer to her question didn't seem all that important to me. Both choices were perfectly good causes of death. But she assured me that some bean counter somewhere mandated that a primary cause of death needed to be listed on the autopsy report. Secondary or contributory causes of death could be listed, but there could only be one, primary cause of death.

So Chandler and I pondered her question a bit as we examined the extensiveness of the corpse's injuries one more time. After talking it all through, we concluded that the decapitation *had* to be listed as the primary cause of death. We knew that even with complete transection of the aorta, the heart would need to beat at least five or six more times before it pumped all remaining blood out of the circulatory system. However, having seen numerous patients immediately lose consciousness when the heart stopped, we figured that by abruptly chopping off the head and severing the carotid arteries in the neck, the brain would receive no blood flow—as occurs in cardiac arrest—and the victim would immediately lose consciousness. We did, of course, realize that patients who lose consciousness from lack of blood flow to the brain rarely die if the head is still attached to the body. They usually regain consciousness and live to see another day. But we just couldn't stomach the thought of the possibility that the kid may have had even a glimmer of conscious awareness as his head rolled into the backseat. And so for our own sake, and for the sake of any family member who might ponder the same thoughts as Chandler and me, we agreed that decapitation *had* to be listed as the primary cause of death.

To the chagrin of my partners, I frequently departed Fort Polk with no notice for duty in places far away with my USSOCOM brothers, leaving Chandler and Steve to man the surgery service. Whereas those unexpected, temporary-additional-duty assignments were exciting breaks from the business as usual routine for me, they were temporary, additional burdens for my partners. Sometimes, the Special Operations community called me away for no more than a week, after which I slipped back into the hospital scene, going almost unnoticed by the nurses and other support staff. But at other times, I would be away for more than a month, making my absence very noticeable to everyone left covering for me back in the rear—most notably, my wife and small children.

One of my more lengthy duty assignments away from my Louisiana home did not involve any military activities at all, but in fact was to update and maintain my trauma skills while working as a trauma fellow at Ben Taub General Hospital, an affiliate of Baylor University in Houston, Texas. *Fellows* are physicians and surgeons who have already completed a residency program but who opt for additional training in a particular discipline. The trauma program at

Ben Taub afforded me a much needed bolus of intellectual stimulation, but also thrust me back into the world of never-ending work and every-other-night evolutions of sleeplessness. Ben Taub was one of two major trauma centers in Houston, both charged with caring for the worst injuries Houston's population could deliver. Trauma victims of every variety rolled into the trauma bays, often four or five at a time, and as a senior member of the trauma team, I laid my hands on every one of them and made the critical decisions of who went to the operating room, and in which order. Once in the OR, I supervised senior and chief surgery residents during routine trauma explorations. That was an enriching experience for me, as I always fancied myself a teacher, and being able to pass along my knowledge to junior surgeons satisfied me greatly.

I also played an active teaching roll on daily, intensive care unit rounds, where up to a dozen surgical residents, medical students, and several staff members strolled together as a group, stopping at each patient's bedside and critically analyzing lab and monitoring data, as well as the patient's progress. We then formulated individual patient care plans, which the junior residents faithfully executed.

While back at Fort Polk I was a fully trained, independently practicing, attending surgeon. However, while assigned as a Trauma Fellow at Ben Taub General, I was very much back down to the level of a trainee. Working at Ben Taub afforded me the great opportunity and pleasure to meet and work with legendary surgeons of the present and past. I operated side by side with Dr. Keith Major, a giant in the field of trauma surgery—the man who coedited and authored the Bible of injury texts. Dr. Major was a no-nonsense trauma surgeon, who operated fast and efficiently, envisioning every future, necessary step of the procedure well before we ever made an incision. He was also a man of great confidence and opinion. He would, often with uncanny accuracy, predict the time line and the ultimate outcome of his patients as he met them for the first time while they were under anesthesia, after the body cavity had already been opened. Dr. Major was one of those men wise people didn't argue with, and I had seen even the most intelligent individuals eventually cry "Uncle" when engaged in heated debate with the master, even when I thought those arguing with Dr. Major were correct.

I also briefly met the master of all master surgeons while at Ben Taub, Dr. Michael DeBakey. Dr. DeBakey had just turned ninety-one when I had the pleasure of sharing a short conversation with him. He was a man of incredible, historical importance—a pioneer of vascular surgery in the army during World War II and throughout the Korean War. Dr. DeBakey's contributions to vascular surgery during the wars allowed wounded soldiers with arterial injuries to keep their limbs rather than be treated with the surgical procedure of choice prior to that time: amputation. He was also the inventor of the roller pump, the device which led to the development of the first cardiopulmonary bypass machine making open-heart surgery possible. Dr. DeBakey also performed many firsts, such as coronary artery bypass surgery, and surgery to remove plaque in the carotid arteries. The mere fact that at age ninety-one, he was still working part-time and taking residents through meticulous operations, was an accomplishment in and of itself.

Being temporarily assigned to one of the busiest trauma centers in the United States afforded me great opportunity to see and treat a huge and complex variety of major trauma patients. One of my most memorable trauma cases at Ben Taub involved a middle-aged construction worker who fell at the job site. The majority of trauma patients get injured by blunt mechanism, most typically from car or motorcycle crashes. Falls are also among the most common in the blunt mechanism category. Included in the penetrating trauma category are gunshot wounds and stab wounds, but occasionally they get a little more bizarre. It is rare that someone falling from a height of twenty feet would suffer penetrating trauma, but that was the case on one particular occasion.

Only fifteen minutes prior, my patient had been walking along the steel framework of a building construction project. Steelworkers are accustomed to defying natural fears of height and falling, and often get somewhat cavalier when strolling on six-inch wide beams framed above the earth's surface. My patient had obviously taken that walk many times before. Although other men fell, it wasn't in my patient's plans or realm of possibilities. But, in fact, fall is exactly what this man did. Now, falling onto the hard ground would pose serious risk to life and limb in and of itself, but what lay below for my gentleman was a bit more treacherous. Rows of vertically oriented, half-inch thick, rebar steel poles, deeply and firmly embedded within a cement foundation, awaited like pointed stakes in the pit of a wild animal trap. The steelworker fell horizontally and could not avoid being speared in the abdomen like a whale on the open sea. He hung in midair with torso and legs folded over, screaming in agony as blood and bowel contents oozed down the steel bar. Rescue personnel were limited in their abilities to help until they could free the man from his spear. Eventually, a team with an industrial saw cut through the bar, leaving an entire segment of steel embedded deeply within his body, as a dozen men eased him down to the ground below.

When paramedics brought the man into Ben Taub, he was awake, breathing, and talking. He was not screaming, probably due to the multiple doses of morphine administered by the paramedics in the field to blunt the man's pain. His impalement looked gruesome even to me, bringing back memories of grotesque, killing scenes from the *Friday the 13th* movie series. The rebar was pummeled directly through his soft abdomen, just to the right side of his belly button. Several medics helped roll the patient onto his side allowing me to examine his back. I saw the tight tenting of his skin from the nonvisualized portion of the bar shoved almost completely through him. Although he had lost a fair amount of blood, he was not in shock. That was a good sign indicating that although his injuries were bad, the likelihood of an injury to a major blood vessel was low. I ordered some IV antibiotics, free-flow administration of intravenous fluids, a tetanus vaccine, and movement directly to the operating room.

The operating room nurses and technicians performed their routine duties of applying the topical antiseptic prep to both man and bar after the anesthesiologist had my patient deeply asleep. We draped my patient's body and I did what I had done so many times before—perform an exploratory laparotomy. That was my signature operation, where I opened what one of my former surgeon colleagues used to call the "temple of surprises." As expected, I found blood and liquid stool littering the usually pristine abdominal cavity. As I moved loops of bowel away from the metal, foreign object, I noticed that several segments of intestine had been speared like shish kebabs before the rebar implanted itself into the bulky muscle group lying parallel to the lumbar spine. I left the bar in place for the time being, and I surgically disconnected all intestine caught up in its grasp. The total length of injured bowel was only about two feet, and removing such a small amount would not cause any long-term consequences. I left the injured bowel attached to the bar, as there was no reason at that juncture to remove it. I carefully looked for a small, critical structure I knew was somewhere deep within the region and which was likely injured by the object of impalement. But I was quite happy to see that the ureter—the urine drainage tube connecting the kidney to the bladder—had somehow

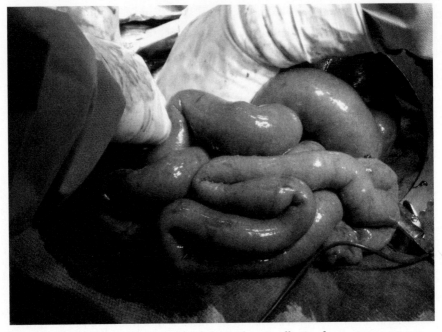

Loops of small intestine pulled out of the abdominal cavity, allowing for greater exposure as the author performs an exploratory laparotomy.

avoided harm by a margin of less than one millimeter. Once I freed up every-thing in need of such, I grabbed the bar with two hands and I pulled upward with all of my strength. It actually took two heaves to disengage the bar. When it was finally removed, I passed the complex of steel and pierced loops of intes-tine all as one heap to the back table for the circulating nurse to deal with.

After reconnecting the remaining bowel, a copious abdominal washing, and placement of a few rubber drains into the large gash within the deep muscles, I closed the belly. I then took my man to the intensive care unit. He did very well, and despite a minimal wound infection, he ended up being dis-charged in just over a week. I have no idea whether or not he eventually went back to work in the construction field, or whether or not he developed a fear of heights. I imagine that he never again looked at a piece of rebar in the same way as before his injury. And to this day, neither do I.

Back at Fort Polk, I was nearing the end of my two-year military orders and I had several options available to me. I could stay in the military and hope that my next set of orders sent me somewhere interesting and exciting, but kept me east of the Mississippi River in order to remain affiliated with USSOCOM.

Alternatively, I could get out of the service entirely, take a civilian surgery job somewhere, and settle my family once and for all. My wife and I discussed our options many times over and we prayed for guidance. It was a very difficult decision for both of us. But the navy pretty much made my decision for me. Whereas the surgeons general of the army and navy were all friendly and agreeable two years prior when they signed the Memorandum of Agreement, allowing my army colleague and me to switch job assignments, the navy was no longer being as cooperative. The army was happy with me, and they offered me the opportunity to remain in USSOCOM if I could secure a navy assignment at an East Coast navy hospital, such as Naval Medical Center Portsmouth in Virginia, Naval Hospital Camp Lejeune in North Carolina, or any other equally good choice. But the navy played hardball with me. They pulled the old "needs of the Navy" routine on me, and they told me that I could no longer affiliate with USSOCOM. They told me that I needed to accept one of two choices offered to me.

The first choice the navy offered me was the U.S. Naval Hospital Guam. Now, the navy couldn't have picked a more remote assignment for me and my family. Despite looking back at what likely could have been a tremendous opportunity to see a part of the world I may never choose to visit, I knew that if I accepted the assignment, I would likely never again practice trauma surgery. The second option offered to me was an LPD—a military ship, with a small operating room reserved only for the most dire of emergencies. I knew that the likelihood of me doing any real surgery on a ship was slim and far between at best. I didn't feel that either of the options was worth staying in the navy, and neither option supported my relationship with USSOCOM. I guess that I could have reaffiliated with USSOCOM two years after I completed whichever navy assignment I picked, but there was no guarantee that my follow-on assignment wouldn't be to Okinawa, Japan, or Keflavik, Iceland, or some other ship. Neither option seemed reasonable to me.

So I did what I thought was in the best interest of my family. Against my wife's better judgment, I decided to get out of the military and resign my commission from the navy. I did receive one last come-to-work call from The Unit at USSOCOM before I left, and I went on that one last mission with "the boys," knowing full well that serving with some of our nation's most elite warrior patriots would soon be just a memory. Two weeks later, the navy accepted my resignation without so much as a phone call to ask why I had chosen to leave—a poor public relations maneuver, which I believe was what caused the miniature, mass exodus of navy physicians, and the subsequent shortfall of surgeons over the following several years. Confirming my request, the navy sent me a letter stating that on September 31, 2000, I would no longer be a navy officer. And with that, I got out.

11

9/11—The Day That Changed Everything

Transition to Civilian Practice

On the first day of October 2000, I began the first day of my civilian career as a surgeon. No longer affiliated with the military, I was free to grow a beard or wear long hair if I had so chosen. But I had been a navy officer for a long time, and despite my newly acquired freedoms, I still chose to sport a short, well-groomed haircut.

I settled into my new job as a general surgeon in a rural community. The bulk of my patients were hardworking, blue-collar individuals or farmers. They presented me with a continuous stream of work of both routine and complex natures. I worked hard in my general surgery practice and I enjoyed living in the community. For the most part it was a very safe place to live. However, being situated ten minutes from a major state university, and about an hour from one of the larger cities in our state, brought occasional violence and violence-associated trauma to our rural hospital. Although I did on occasion treat some very complex and serious trauma patients, I maintained most of my trauma skills by moonlighting every other weekend at a Level I Trauma Center—the most comprehensive of the trauma referral hospitals—approximately one half hour east of our town.

I lived a short, three-mile drive from our community hospital, and I became known as the go-to guy by some of the emergency medicine doctors.

When they were told of a critically injured trauma patient being transported to their emergency department, I would often get a heads-up call requesting my presence, even when I was not necessarily on call.

On one such night, I was called about a SWAT team situation in evolution. As the story was relayed to me, a young woman from an urban community well north of our rural town had been staying with her sister in her home near the local university. Meanwhile, her estranged husband had apparently been seeking her for some time, and when he learned of her whereabouts, he planned to take revenge on her for some reason unknown.

He flagged down a cab in his own town and was driven the forty or so miles to where she was thought to be staying. When the man in the cab arrived at his destination, the estranged husband pulled a semiautomatic machine gun out from a gym bag and held it to the head of the cab driver, whom he then ordered to walk with him to the door of the home. At gunpoint, the cab driver rang the door bell as he was told to do and the woman's sister answered the door. When the woman answering the door recognized the man standing behind the cab driver, she attempted to slam the door shut, screaming for her sister to hide, but was instantly overpowered by the enraged assailant who forced his way into the home.

The hunted woman then ran up the stairs and barricaded herself into a small room, but the man with the gun pursued her, forced the door open, and emptied his entire rifle magazine into her body. Meanwhile, police were called and the SWAT team attempted to extricate the man—now a barricaded subject himself.

After a thirty-minute standoff with the police, the SWAT team entered the home and shots were fired, but fortunately, there were no additional injuries as a result of the police gunfire. In all of the confusion and pandemonium, how-ever, the shooter had somehow escaped through a back door and was free, on the lam. The police performed a room-by-room search and confirmed that the shooter was, in fact, no longer in the building. Once the home was declared to be safe, the paramedics were allowed entry where they found the woman, still alive but gravely wounded, riddled with bullet holes on nearly every part of her body. Her head and neck seemed to be the only areas not wounded in the melee.

She was nearly lifeless—dying—and had been lying in a pool of her own blood for the previous thirty minutes. It was an extremely serious situation as she had already lost a major portion of her Golden Hour of time, traditionally thought to be a critical factor in determining a trauma victim's potential for survival. Knowing this, the paramedics performed immediate, emergency life-saving measures, scooped her onto a gurney, and rushed her to our small community hospital without additional delay. I had already been awaiting their arrival among a nervous and anxious crowd of emergency room nurses, technicians, doctors, operating room staff members, an ICU nurse, a social worker, and a lone nursing supervisor. Victims of major trauma came to our place infrequently, but when they did, it was an all-hands endeavor, for both professional reasons as well as for purposes of human intrigue.

I assumed command of the situation immediately as the police-escorted paramedic crew rushed the gunshot victim in from the ambulance bay into our twelve-bed emergency room. They were directed over to an open cart where the majority of us had all been waiting since shortly after the entire barricaded-subject standoff began over half an hour prior. With the paramedic gurney pushed up tightly against the emergency room cart and all wheels locked down tightly, the bloody rag doll of a woman was lifted over by four sets of arms, eager to quickly involve themselves in the next day's front-page-news headline story.

As I had done so many times before, I rapidly assessed the airway, breathing, and the circulatory status of my patient. I directed our ER physician to secure our patient's airway with an endotracheal tube while I prepared to insert chest tubes into both sides of the women's thoracic cavity. I hadn't even yet performed a thorough survey, but I could see holes through both breasts—several on the left and one on the right—and without wasting precious time ordering and reviewing a chest X-ray, I knew that the patient needed bilateral chest tubes. Both lungs had to have been punctured by the bullet holes.

Once the chest tubes were in place and deep IV lines were infusing O-negative blood being squeezed by the strong and trustworthy hands of a young, wide-eyed nursing student from the university, I quickly but carefully assessed my patient's wounds. I counted two holes through the upper part of her left breast and one just above the nipple of her right breast. One hole pierced her right upper abdomen just below her rib margin, two entered her left, lower abdomen, and numerous holes peppered her thighs, hips, back, buttocks, calf areas, and arms. There were so many holes that there was absolutely no way for me to accurately determine the path of any of the bullets, to determine which might have passed completely through her body, or to even reliably predict which major organ structures might have been violated.

I envisioned the woman getting shot as she faced her attacker, then turning away and falling forward as the bullets kept pounding the back of her torso, buttocks, legs, and arms as she slumped to the ground in a tight ball. I imagined her pulling her legs tightly upward, folding her arms inward, and pressing her forearms together shielding her breast and face area. When I had finished my physical survey, I counted over thirty holes, but having counted so quickly, I wasn't sure if I had double-counted a hole or two, or maybe even missed one altogether.

Knowing that the woman had already been slowly dying on her bedroom floor for the previous half hour before ever getting to us, I had little time to waste. Recounting those holes was certainly not a priority of mine at the moment. My patient was cold, very much in shock, and her blood was starting to run thin, like dilute, cherry Kool-Aid from her numerous penetrating wounds.

Clotting factors—microscopic proteins circulating throughout the bloodstream which ordinarily promote clot formation and minimize ongoing blood loss—become dysfunctional after massive trauma. As a result of this fairly predictable phenomenon, massive bleeding and shock cause even more bleeding and shock, and eventually a situation develops where even the repairing of every wound and injury just isn't enough to prevent the continuous stream of blood from repaired wounds, needle sticks, and the damaged bodily tissues. At that particular juncture, our patient was already exhibiting some very bad signs— omens commonly seen in patients nose-diving into a clinical death spiral.

We could transfuse her with blood in the emergency room all night long, fire up the heated-air-warming blankets, and administer blood-thickening plasma, but the fact of the matter still remained that she would continue to actively lose blood from a source of hemorrhage deep to one or more of those numerous bullet holes. Based on my assessment of the scant volume of blood collected in the chest tube bottles, and the lack of massive or pulsatile swelling in either of her arms or legs, the major source of her ongoing blood loss just didn't appear to be from either her chest or extremity wounds. I knew that she had to be bleeding in her belly, and there was only one reasonable place for her to be at that point, and that was in the operating room. She needed to get there as soon as possible, and I planned on opening her abdomen to address whatever injuries I found inside.

I gave the order to make the move and two nurse anesthetists, two ER nurses, one OR nurse, and an ER technician all placed at least one hand on our patient's cart and wheeled it with great haste down the hallway into the operating room area. A large bloody trail followed our cart as it passed down the long hallway connecting the emergency room area to the operating room suites. Ordinarily, it would be unquestionably forbidden for inappropriately attired members to enter the operating room area in general, but during moments like that one, when a crazy killer with an automatic machine gun had come into our town, blasting a million holes through a young woman's body, no one— including the nursing supervisor—seemed to mind or even notice that some of the people escorting that victim into our OR were in their street clothes.

Once we got the woman transferred safely to the operating room table, however, mental clarity returned. Those unaccustomed to being in the operating room slowly backed away, thinking perhaps that if they remained quiet, they might not get noticed and not be told to leave. But they certainly were noticed as they were not part of the OR team, they weren't wearing scrubs, and despite their enthusiasm and interest, they just needed to leave.

I instructed the OR nurses to widely prep my patient with antiseptic paint, and I told the scrub technician to drape the patient so that I had access to every part of her body short of her head. I then went out of the room and washed for less than the six-minute scrub time usually recommended in those days. I rinsed the foamy soap off my hands and arms and backed myself through the doors of the operating room. In those few short minutes, our casualty had already been covered from neck to feet with brown solution, and all surgical drapes had been carefully laid. I grabbed a sterile towel and dried off. I then reached my arms forward as the gown was passed onto me, and I pushed my hands one by one into the surgical gloves stretched open for me. I handed the scrub technician the end of the waist belt attached to my surgical gown, and while she stood still, I turned a full circle, wrapping myself snuggly in my robelike, blue-green surgical garb.

The two anesthetists at the head of the table had already administered the anesthetic agents and were frantically hanging bags of red blood cells and plasma to help correct her low pressure and thicken whatever blood was still within her body. I sliced deeply and boldly through skin and fat, from just below her breastbone to just above her pubic region, in one rapid maneuver. I curved slightly around the belly-button area—a maneuver nearly always done by surgeons. I then divided all remaining layers of tissue in a matter of seconds, and I shoved countless surgical sponges, one after another, into her bloody abdomen.

I performed a rapid, exploratory examination procedure, which revealed a half-dozen holes in her small intestine, but they were small injuries and were not the source of the woman's instability. Deep within the right upper area of her abdomen was the smoking gun—so to speak—the major source of the woman's ill fate. One bullet had done extensive damage, as it had passed through multiple organs anatomically layered one atop the other. The bullet first blasted through the gallbladder and the portion of the liver connecting the two organs. It then blew a hole through the side of her duodenum—the small intestine emerging from the lowest portion of the stomach. The bullet continued its lethal path, blasting through and pulverizing the right kidney. But the most severe damage was done by the same bullet hole torn through the inferior vena cava—the largest of the body's veins—which lay immediately adjacent to the kidney, and was leaking blood at an alarming rate. One bullet had been so successful in causing so much destruction, as if directed by the Grim Reaper himself.

The repair I had to perform was not going to be easy—not by a long shot. Each of four necessary surgical procedures needed to remedy all of the destruction from that one bullet would ordinarily take at least twenty minutes or more—precious time that the woman's tenuous life just could not spare. I decided to work as quickly as I possibly could, and I dove right in to the traumatic area. That's about all that I could do other than pray that God would efficiently and expeditiously work through my hands.

I quickly incised whatever remained of the attachments that ordinarily plastered the duodenum down over the top of the underlying vena cave and kidney. The usual filmy, glistening tissues that connect all internal organs and create subdivided, little compartments deep below the surface of the skin were bloody, swollen, and grossly deformed in that young lady. The blast energy from the gunshot ripped more than just a narrow hole from the supersonic bullet. Instead, it tore a wide path of brute destruction. Fortunately, it seemed that the kidney had absorbed most of the blast energy, as I fully examined its shattered pulp after fully mobilizing away the duodenum. The cadaveric remnants of the dead organ lay sequestered within a gelatinous matrix of semiclotted and liquid-blue blood. I wasted no time in ridding the body of the useless detritus, and with a few applications of hemostatic clamps, surgical snips, and suture

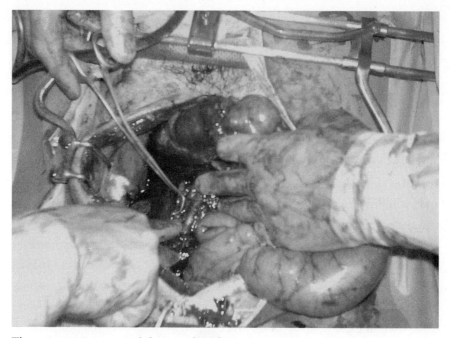

The arrow points to a curved clamp on the inferior vena cava.

ligations, the organ once previously called kidney, was now a mere specimen in the bucket on the surgical back table.

I scooped out handfuls of clot with my gloved hands, and I suctioned away about a liter of liquid blood, before I could clearly make out the limitations of the major venous injury. It was pumping like an old well, choking as it coughed another mouthful of dark-red liquid. I saw that the bullet had only passed through the side of the vena cava, creating an approximately one-inch tear from top to bottom. I maneuvered a curved vascular clamp into place over the out-side edge of the massive vein, isolating the injured portion yet maintaining an open channel within the majority of the uninjured segment of the vascular tube. I sewed carefully, but very quickly, with fine synthetic suture. I sewed until the wound was sealed water-tight and until I felt confident. When I anxiously released the vascular clamp I hoped that my sutures would hold. The restored blood flow bulged at the sutures and aggressively tested my repair, but thank-fully, my repair looked solid. I then took hold of the duodenum with two hands, and flipping it front to back, I examined the extent of the injury to that very unique segment of bowel. The duodenum is no ordinary loop of intestine. It is intimately attached to the pancreas, and is the recipient of the very important, common bile duct, through which drains the liver's digestive juices. One cannot simply remove the duodenum without doing major pancreas and bile duct surgery in conjunction. I just didn't have time for all that, and neither did my patient. Fortunately—as was the case with the vena cava injury—the duodenal injury was limited to just its outside edge, away from the pancreas and common bile duct. In order to do only what was necessary to save the woman's life, I applied a nine-centimeter linear surgical stapler oriented parallel to the duodenum, and I fired a row of microstaples, sealing the damaged bowel. I trimmed away the remaining damaged edges of the intestine outside of the staple line, and I withdrew the linear stapler apparatus. I had made great progress and I did so in record time.

Next, I had to deal with the damaged gallbladder and liver. Being a general surgeon, I had performed numerous laparoscopic cholecystectomies—that is, minimally invasive excision of the gallbladder—performed with long, miniature instruments inserted into the body through subcentimeter holes, all done while watching the progress of my work through a television monitor. Taking out a gallbladder through a two-foot hole was easy. Removing the gallbladder after clipping the bile drainage duct and its artery took me no more than five minutes, and electrically frying the bleeding liver injury with the electrocautery powered up high onto what I called "stun mode," concluded the right upper quadrant portion of the surgery.

Not forgetting the six holes I previously found in the small intestine, I quickly whip-stitched them closed one at a time, with suture that not only controlled bleeding but the seeping liquid stool as well. I finished the abdominal surgery by washing out the cavity with six liters of warm saline, suctioning out all remaining liquid, and removing all packs and sponges. A momentary touch of prideful arrogance overcame me, as I noticed on the anesthesia monitor that my patient's vital signs were looking quite acceptable. But a second glance revealed the dozens of used blood bags on the ground—red cell bags, platelet bags, and plasma bags—all infused by the anesthetists while I had been operating. The contents of those bags are truly what had kept that woman from dying on the table. I swallowed my shameful arrogance, closed her abdomen with lightning speed, and reassessed what I needed to do next.

She still had numerous holes in various places, and at best my patient could tolerate just one more operative procedure, but only if necessary. She badly needed to get off the OR table and into a warm, intensive care unit bed, where she could be further resuscitated with more blood and plasma, have her high levels of circulating lactic acid neutralized, and be aggressively warmed with hot-air blankets. Operating room staff members helped roll the young woman's still anesthetized body side to side as I tightly packed each bullet hole with several feet of iodine-impregnated, thin gauze. The gauze compressed the wound edges deep within each bullet tract, preventing further oozing and allowing clot to form. It also wicked away exuded blood and serum from the sites of injury, and it served as an antibacterial agent, minimizing the possibility of wound infections.

But after I packed all of her numerous holes and rolled her back down with her spine on the table, I noticed more bleeding. As if I had been watching a poorly made horror film, blood started to stream out from one of the wounds on her left breast, forming an expanding pool over her entire chest. Thinking that one of the bullets must have passed through her breast and into her chest, damaging an artery that hugged the lower edge of a rib, I cut down on the suspect wound to directly expose the bone. But before I even cut beyond my first slice, I could tell that the source of her bleeding was not coming from a rib artery. She was bleeding from the bullet tract that was directed not into her chest, but up toward her shoulder area. I expanded the bullet tract by creating a large cavity within her breast, until I could see that pulsatile blood was pouring from what I could only deduce was her subclavian artery—a large, arterial vessel that passes just under the collarbone and supplies all blood to the arm. It was another bad injury and, typically, a very difficult one to repair.

I cut horizontally, six inches long, just below her collarbone, through the upper portion of her breast, directly down to her chest wall muscle. I bluntly split the muscle fibers of her pectoralis major and I incised the dense layer of tissue below, exposing a few inches of the injured, subclavian artery pumping away at me. I hastily applied vascular clamps on either side of the injured blood vessel while my surgical assistant retracted the muscle fibers creating just enough room for me to see. My assistant was having difficulties because sheer, brute force was required to retract away the chest wall tissues. I sewed closed the hole as I had done to the injured vena cava. After completing my repair, I achieved satisfactory hemorrhage control. But a lot of blood was lost in the process. I didn't know just how much more that young women could take. I washed out the wound and I rapidly closed her latest incision. I then repacked the bullet tract in her breast, and declared the entire operation over. It was clearly time to move her to the ICU.

I backed away from the table and viewed the carnage of the room. Countless blood-soaked sponges littered the floor, and blood bags were laid out on the ground near the anesthesia cart in row after row like little corpses awaiting burial. Nurses and technicians taped gauze pads over my patient's wounds until she seemed almost completely covered in white. We then wheeled her over to the intensive care unit for additional resuscitative therapy.

She was anything but stable. Despite the heroic efforts of the entire team, she was still cold, profoundly anemic, and in shock. I stayed at my patient's bedside for six hours, giving orders for additional blood transfusions, drug infusions, and additional treatments. For that entire period of time she barely hung on, teetering on the edge of life. And then she coded.

She lost her pulse and blood pressure, and we started performing CPR. I knew in my heart that by that time, it was likely all over. She was going to die and we had done all that was possible. We pounded away at her chest, administered epinephrine, and transfused more blood. But despite all of our efforts in the operating room, my patient was in a state of irreversible shock and she had given up. She began oozing heavily from each of her bullet wounds and she was again bleeding to death before our very eyes. As the man in charge, I needed to make the difficult decision of deciding when enough was enough.

After nearly an hour of chest compressions, she never again regained a pulse. I knew that nothing else could be done for my patient and I finally called off the resuscitation effort. I then pronounced the young woman dead. I was physically and emotionally spent. I was down, but I knew that we had done well—in fact, quite well. We were a small facility, not ordinarily challenged with such significant, traumatic injuries the likes of which are usually seen only in the busiest of the urban-area hospitals and war zones. And because our casualty had been down for a good half hour before paramedics could even get to her, everyone trying to help her started out at a great disadvantage. Unfortunately, adversity is the very nature of trauma. Members of a trauma team get what's handed to them. In our situation, it was a young woman who tried her best to avoid trouble, but trouble sought her out. And now she was dead.

The following months' workdays were fairly routine for me. Clinic duties, patient rounds, and routine surgery—with an occasional trauma case—were my everyday activities. Some surgeons settle into a job right out of their residency training and stay there forever. But for others, events change their lives, which cause them to move on to greener pastures. I was in the latter category.

Just when I thought that I was going to settle into the life of a country surgeon, my world changed. That was when I woke up to the day that turned my life literally upside down.

That was the one particular day in my civilian life that I will never forget. Like most people, I can remember with great detail the events of my entire day on September 11, 2001. Less than a year after relinquishing my officer's commission, I was scheduled to perform several basic, bread-and-butter surgical procedures at the local community hospital. My first case was an open groin hernia repair. As I had done many times before, I made the incision, dissected out the surgical tissues, sewed in a custom-sized piece of synthetic mesh, and sutured the wound closed in several layers. The whole procedure took me less than one hour to complete.

As I exited the operating room and headed toward the patient recovery area to write postoperative orders, I saw a large group of people huddling in the anesthesia lounge peering intensely in the direction of where I knew the television was mounted. I figured that they were all watching some crazy talk show, like *Jerry Springer*, or something similar to that. It wouldn't have been unusual if that had been the case, because for some reason, the operating room staff at that hospital loved salacious television shows.

I walked into the room and asked in a lighthearted voice what crazy family was featured on *Springer* that day. But no one answered my question; nor did they take their eyes off the TV screen. I saw that what they were watching was a breaking news report of sorts, but I didn't know any of the details. Then one of the OR nurses whispered to me that an airplane had crashed into one of the World Trade Center towers in New York City. I was dumbfounded, and I found it to be almost unbelievable. My mind began to reel at the possible implications of what it could actually mean, and how the accident could have possibly happened in the first place. But I had more work to do, and I moved on to complete the paperwork from my last operation and to begin my second case that awaited me.

The second operation I performed was a minimally invasive, gallbladder removal. The laparoscopic cholecystectomy also went like clockwork and lasted approximately one hour. As I had done after completing my first operation, I again walked past the anesthesia lounge to see that the large crowd was still gathered in front of the television. When I again walked into the small room, I could feel the tension, and I asked what the latest news was regarding the crash. One of the older nurses then turned to me and told me that a second plane had struck the second Twin Tower. I was stunned to hear the news, and I glued my eyes to that television screen where I watched over and over as the first plane, and then the second plane sliced into those towers—either an impossible matter of chance, or bad luck on an unfathomable level. I already knew in my mind what I had just witnessed—an act of terrorism—but I didn't mention it openly.

After a few minutes, one of the people in the TV room stated that a commentator had suggested that it may have in fact been an act of terrorism. Without my even realizing that my thoughts were being expressed as words, I quietly stated, "Osama bin Laden ordered this."

"Who?" asked several people in the room. Realizing that I had in fact opened my mouth and had expressed my thoughts as words, I repeated my response: "Osama bin Laden ordered this, and it *is* an act of terrorism."

At that point most of the people in the anesthesia lounge turned toward me and wondered how I could be privy to such information, and just exactly who was this Osama bin Laden guy I had mentioned. They did, however, know that I had been in the military for over a decade, and that I might possibly have some insight into the matter. I revealed everything I knew about Osama bin Laden—nearly everything I had been taught about him when I was attached to United States Special Operations Command, and most of what I had learned of him from several members of my old unit. I then told them that I thought that there might possibly be additional acts of terrorism by the end of the day. And with that, I left the room to complete my work.

At that point, I was profoundly distracted. I could barely focus on the two surgeries I had yet to perform let alone the rest of my day's work, which included seeing an afternoon's worth of clinic patients. It took nearly all of my will to refocus my thoughts on my next two surgical patients, and away from the events of what I knew had just taken place. Fortunately, my next two cases were both breast biopsy procedures—minor excisions of suspicious breast lumps—each of which I completed in less than thirty minutes. I intentionally avoided the area near the anesthesia lounge prior to completing all of my remaining work at the hospital because I just couldn't afford any other mental distractions. What I had witnessed on that TV screen rattled me and gave me great anxiety. I wasn't yet sure why I was so bothered. I wasn't worried that my community would be the next one targeted by who I knew were terrorists on a religious jihad intended on indiscriminately killing as many Americans as possible. And I wasn't frightened personally. If anything, I was angry, and I felt a terrible sense of guilt over what had just happened—an illogical feeling considering I was just one person, and I wasn't even still in the military.

Once I was certain that all of my floor patients had been attended to, and that all of my postoperative patients' needs had all been addressed, I went back to the anesthesia lounge where I learned that both of the Twin Towers had fallen—a sight which I will never forget as I watched the video clips play over and over. I left the hospital and drove to the office where I knew that I would be tied up for the remainder of the afternoon seeing patients. Perhaps because of the tragic news reports of that day, many of my scheduled consults and follow-up patients were no-shows. They simply blew me off, all probably too wrapped up in their own emotions of what they had just seen on their own televisions to come in to see the surgeon on that day. Ordinarily, I might have been a little miffed by the great percentage of absentees, but on that day I was grateful because I just could not seem to keep my thoughts focused on anything other than my days back at USSOCOM and the job I once had protecting our nation's sovereignty.

During a lull in the schedule, I decided to call Matt, my former surgical residency brother who was still on active duty. Matt had been recruited into the Special Operations unit after I had left. I thought that he might be privy to some inside information that I could get out of him by asking the right questions, not overtly, but in a generalized clandestine manner. Yes, calling Matt was what I needed to do. I needed someone to talk to who could understand my concerns and interests and who was among the group of individuals that understood matters as I did. I grabbed my cell phone and called Matt's home. It was 1700—5 P.M.—on the East Coast where Matt was stationed, and I waited for Matt to answer as my heart pounded away. Mary answered.

Mary was Matt's wife, a woman I knew very well, like a sister-in-law. Mary's voice was stern and somber. I greeted her and asked if she had seen the news of what had happened. She stated nothing more than "Yes," which I knew was out of character for her to be so short on things to say. I then asked if I could speak to Matt, telling her that I needed to ask him if he knew anything that he could share with me. And then she broke the news to me.

"Jim, Matt's gone." I asked what she meant by the word *gone*. Was he away at a meeting? Was he stuck in the hospital, on call?

"No, Jim, Matt has already been deployed."

I asked a few more questions, but like all wives of members assigned to US-SOCOM, she was under strict orders to disclose nothing. I could tell by what she did say, and even more by what she *didn't* say, that Matt had been spun up by the Special Operations community to support what would soon become known as the Global War on Terrorism. I was soon feeling loads of guilt and immense pressure building inside of me that I was having terrible difficulty controlling.

"What had I done? Why did I resign my commission?" I asked myself over and over. I rationalized away some of my guilt by telling myself that I had done my time in the service, and that when I left the organization, the world was supposed to be at peace forever—at least that's what the pundits all said. And I knew that I was safer at home than over wherever Matt was going to be deployed, which was a plus for my family. But that was of little consolation for the heavy emotional burden I was bearing. I hung up the phone after wishing Mary well, and wrapped up my work that day. I was messed up, and I was having difficulty dealing with my feelings.

The next year were some of the worst months of my life. I was consumed by the memories of my past military service, and with thoughts and images of the people I had worked with and lived with, and of the military operations we had served on together. My comrades—people I would have died for—were now likely living in tents in some godforsaken country while I was living in a beautiful home far from harm's way. I felt like a traitor to my country, and a traitor to my friends. I was overwhelmed, and I was starting to mentally unravel. I was becoming profoundly depressed and began acting irrationally and fighting with the ones I loved most—especially my dear wife. I started hating the people I was working with, and I wanted nothing more than to quit my job and rejoin the military. But I had purchased a home and had settled my family. There was no easy solution to my problems, and I was spinning deeper and deeper into the abyss of hell on earth.

My wife was a saint, however. She knew me better than I knew myself. She was aware that my volatile ways and my irrational behavior were not that of the man she had married, and she went way out of her way to do everything possible to help me. She knew that leaving the military was a mistake for both of us, so when I proposed to her that I look into possibly joining the military reserves, she wasn't happy, but she knew that it was perhaps what was necessary to save me from my torment.

I talked to a military health-care recruiter—a navy recruiter. I often ask myself now why I talked to a navy recruiter. I, of course, had been previously commissioned as a naval officer, but I had always considered myself to be kind of an all-service military officer. I had served in navy, marines, and army commands, and I felt equally comfortable with each of the branches of service. I knew that I needed to be back with USSOCOM, and I knew that the organization I needed to serve was primarily run by the army. But being somewhat irrational at the time, I wasn't thinking things through completely. Having once been in the navy, I knew all of the right people to contact, which I assumed would make my rejoining the service a simple process.

Despite the navy's significant need for trauma surgeons at that time—*any* surgeon for that matter—reobtaining my officer's commission took many, many months. My application package was submitted to numerous review boards and committees making what would seem a very simple process a very lengthy and difficult one. But on July 1, 2003, after an exact thirty-three-month hiatus from the military, I raised my right hand and I repeated the Officer's Oath. When I was finished, I was again sworn into service as a lieutenant commander in the United States Navy Reserve.

12

Limb Lost, Life Saved

The Mutilated Limb

Several months prior to my recommissioning, this time into the military reserve forces, I left my community hospital group to begin the full-time practice of trauma surgery, critical care, and emergency general surgery at the Level I Trauma Center where I had previously worked only a few weekends each month. Changing to a full-time practice with increased complexity and urgency of the medical situations I encountered forced me to always be "on the edge," so to speak. I did not want to risk any possibility of losing my skills in the trauma or critical care arenas, and thus a major reason for my calculated move from the community hospital setting to the big trauma center. I had previously seen other surgeons' skills degrade over the years, as they became comfortable settling into what some call a bread-and-butter practice, where hernias and gallbladder surgeries became the most complex procedures on their surgical case logs. That was not going to be me, and being a surgeon in a nation engaged in war, I felt that it was my duty to remain as experienced as possible should I be called to serve in the combat zone.

As therapeutic as my career change to the trauma center was for me, so was my new navy reserve unit. Because of my previous experience with the USSO-COM group, I was assigned to Navy Reserve SEAL Team Eight. They were a great group of guys, nearly every one of them a bona fide wearer of the Navy

SEAL trident—a prestigious insignia and the largest of the navy warfare devices worn above the left breast pocket of the uniform, awarded only to the most elite navy warriors who complete the arduous, six-month Basic Underwater Demolition/SEAL training in Coronado, California, known as BUD/S. All of my new-unit team members welcomed and accepted me into their group with open arms upon my arrival. They were glad to have a doctor on the team, and even happier after learning of my background. Every war fighter feels a little more confident knowing that should he suffer a significant injury during combat, a competent healer will be there to patch him up. I was their talisman protecting them from harm, and they treated me well.

We would get together on a monthly basis for weekend drill, where we would spend most of our time telling genuine war stories, and the rest of the time hardening our bodies in the gym and on the roads. Running and weight lifting were SEAL Team requirements, and I relished those weekly drill periods with great anticipation. Many of the guys on the team had already been sent down range to Afghanistan, and to other adjacent lands in support of the Global War on Terrorism. I listened with great interest to their war stories and to their reports from the front lines. We would occasionally do something really "creative"—what others might call crazy—such as swim in the nearly frozen, 30-degree waters surrounding the navy base, clad only in wet suits, fins, and masks. I remember one frigid December day when after swimming one mile out and another back, I lost all feeling in my gloved hands, and felt the clinical effects of hypothermia. Safety crews standing on the beach gave us towels and blankets and walked us back to Building 52, where we assembled each month to drill. That was one of our many group-bonding adventures that hardened our minds, bodies, and our resolve to never become weak. I still keep a photo of our group taken on that day's ice swim and periodically admire it as a source of personal motivation as well as for the good memories it brings back.

Back at the trauma center, I was constantly challenged with complex trauma patients pushing my skills to the edge of my abilities. So exemplified was the burly, thirty-two-year-old house of a man, whose physical stature could easily be confused with any of today's National Football League linemen, who went by the name of Cedric White. Cedric lived his life dangerously, and was no stranger to trauma. His past included a prior hospital admission for a stab wound to the chest, which fortunately did not take his life. But in early October, Cedric was out riding his Ninja motorcycle—his crotch rocket—at a reckless

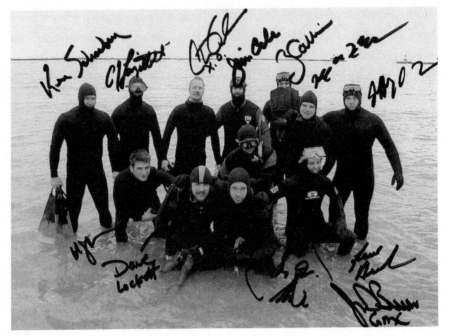

Members of Navy Reserve SEAL Team Eight. The author is fourth from the left in the top row. *(Courtesy Lieutenant Junior Grade Jon Burrow, LDO, USN)*

speed, when he caught a patch of loose pavement and skidded out of control into the back end of a multiton gravel truck.

He was, of course, not wearing a helmet, but despite that fact his head was unscathed, leaving his pelvis and his right leg to absorb all of the traumatic energy. As his motorcycle abruptly decelerated from a speed of about fifty miles per hour to zero upon striking the enormous vehicle, momentum threw his body forward, causing him to strike his pelvis against the rigid, motorcycle handlebar frame. To make matters worse, his right groin caught the right brake handle, causing the skin and underlying soft tissues of his thigh to tear away from the muscles, stripping everything away and leaving a massive, bloody limb. As if removing a pair of one-legged trousers, mounds of thigh skin lay accordioned down to the level of his deformed knee. His lower leg was bent sideways at the knee joint and dislocated backward, indicating a massive injury to the ligaments. His foot was ice cold and it had a mottled appearance suggesting a vascular injury.

He lay groaning loudly from the agony of the pain and from the sight of his leg he had viewed while lying on the street awaiting the paramedics' arrival.

His heart was racing from the pain and from surges of adrenaline, but his blood pressure and breathing abilities were normal. A full physical examination additionally revealed a crunchy, unstable pelvis, which gave way under the pressure of my examining hands as I pressed downward. The skin of his pubic region was badly mangled, and the shaft of his denuded penis was exposed. His left testicle was hanging freely outside of his torn scrotal sac suspended only by the cordlike structure containing an artery, several veins, and the sperm tube. His buttocks were torn on the right side just beyond the edge of his anal canal, through which a portion of his pelvic bone protruded.

A crunchy, unstable pelvis injury almost always translates to what is known as an "open book" pelvic fracture—as the right and left pubic bones, which are ordinarily held firmly together in the midline, separate widely, like a book opened for reading. The injury usually causes significant hemorrhage into the pelvis cavity and often results in hemorrhagic shock as the firmly adherent plexus of highly branched arteries and veins, physically resembling the root network of a mature tree, get shorn away from the bone in the traumatic process of opening the book.

I confirmed my suspicions with a quick, portable X-ray of the pelvis. Subsequently knowing my diagnosis with absolute certainly, I applied a simple treatment modality, which often prevents several liters of further blood loss. It was nothing more than a simple, rolled bedsheet laid under his buttocks, pulled tightly around his pelvis, and tied firmly across his pubic region to close down and temporarily narrow the large gap between the widely separated pelvic bones. Doing so decreased the volume of his pelvis and minimized the area in which bleeding could accumulate, in hopes it might eventually clot off on its own.

I performed numerous, additional diagnostic studies, including lab tests, CT scans, X-rays, and even a bedside abdominal ultrasound to look for additional injuries. Fortunately, his injuries were all limited to below the abdomen, but every one of them was quite bad.

The physical deformity of his knee joint and the X-rays I had performed confirmed a devastating joint dislocation. I was able to easily realign the disfiguring bony deformity by applying some brute force to his leg after amply administering both morphine and a heavy sedative. The maneuver, however, did not restore blood flow to his subsequently frigid and pulseless foot. Knowing full well that his dislocation had injured his popliteal artery—the name given to the femoral artery as it passes behind the knee—I rushed Mr. White off to the angiography suite where I would confirm with invasive dye testing exactly which segment of the artery had been damaged. Now faced with having to manage complex pelvic fractures, huge open wounds to the buttocks and scrotum areas, a major degloving of his entire right thigh, major ligamentous injuries, and a torn popliteal artery behind the knee joint with complete interruption of blood flow to the lower leg, I needed to triage the order of the operative procedures the other trauma subspecialty surgeons and I would be performing that afternoon.

Once in the operating room, six people including myself transferred our enormous patient from the trauma cart to the OR table. Once he was deeply anesthetized, we applied liberal amounts of liquid antiseptic from his chest to his toes, and prepared Mr. White and ourselves for a multipart, multihour operation.

I decided to work on his skin and groin injuries first, as they would take no more than thirty minutes to address. I thoroughly washed his thigh muscles and the massive, nearly detached skin flap, with a power irrigator—like a much larger version of a dental water pick—pulsing at least six liters of antibiotic instilled, saline solution onto the heavily contaminated body parts. Once done, I then hiked up the wrinkled mass of skin, pulling upward as if tugging on a massive, human stocking, covering the underlying anatomy that just shouldn't have ever been exposed under normal circumstances. I washed out the large wounds on the base of his penis and scrotum, and then popped the exposed testicle back into its sac. I spent the remaining time using a handheld surgical clip applier to close the several collective feet of wounds on his thigh, scrotum, and pubic areas, hoping that somehow we might all get lucky and that his skin problems could be managed expectantly.

The arterial injury needed to be repaired next, but to provide a stable joint over which to work, we needed our trauma orthopedic surgeon to insert a series of pins and rods and create a rigid, external framework around the knee joint. He obliged us without hesitation, allowing us to do what we all needed to do thereafter. After the orthopedic procedure had been completed, I turned my patient over to an awaiting vascular surgeon, who I spent the next four hours helping repair the injured artery behind the knee, hoping to restore blood flow to the tissues beyond. It was an unusually difficult operation, as the enormity of his body created physical difficulties even exposing the injured vessel. Despite numerous attempts to recreate a robust amount of blood flow to the tissues beyond the level of Mr. White's vascular injury, only limited blood flow could actually be restored.

Ordinarily, when surgeons perform meticulous vascular surgery—especially at or below the level of the knee—the entire bloodstream needs to be anticoagulated with the blood thinning agent heparin so as to maximize the likelihood that bits of clot will not form on the tiny sutures used to perform the fine repair. If a small amount of clot forms within an artery, it inevitably precipitates larger clots to form, which then often interrupt all blood flow through the limb entirely. But heparin could not be used on that day. Mr. White had a very bad pelvic injury, and the risk for torrential, pelvic bleeding if heparin was used was much greater than its benefit would be to the leg. I had to make a life-versus-limb decision. In order to save his life, I had to risk the very likely possibility that he could lose his leg. That was the kind of decision I was often faced with—a very difficult decision, and one I would have little time to sit and ponder beforehand.

Once the vascular portion of our surgery was complete, I turned the patient back over to our trauma orthopedist who spent the next hour stabilizing the pelvic fractures with an external fixation device similar to that which he placed across Cedric's knee. He placed six, heavy lag screws—each about an eighth of an inch in diameter and almost six inches long—deeply into the bony prominences of either side of the fronts of the pelvis. He placed three screws on the left and three screws on the right, each one left protruding several inches outside of the skin. To each cluster of the orthopedic "pins" he attached a screw-clamp apparatus, to which he attached a common, arched metal bar spanning from one side to the other firmly affixed to the embedded pins via the attached hardware. The orthopedic surgeon pushed inward on one hip as his assistant pushed inward on the other, reapproximating the damaged pelvic segments, then tightening all clamps to firmly affix the bones into a healthy anatomic alignment. When completed, it looked as if Mr. White had a towel bar permanently inserted onto his body, where washcloths could easy be hung in front of him if he so desired.

Finally, I had to deal with my patient's buttocks wound. The wound in and of itself was not a difficult problem to manage. Once the orthopedic surgeon realigned the pelvic anatomy, Cedric's protruding segment of bone had retracted itself back deeply under the skin of his butt cheek. The wound required a thorough washout with my handy irrigation device, after which I repaired the jagged tissues layer by layer.

Again, the wound itself was not the real problem. The real problem was inevitably yet to occur, sometime after Mr. White had his first, spontaneous bowel movement. Good critical care management always includes tube-feeding the gastrointestinal tract as soon as possible. Tube feedings always seem to cause diarrhea. Knowing that liquid stool would soon be flowing from Mr. White's rectum in an uncontrollable manner in just a matter of days, my patient's freshly closed buttocks wound with underlying pelvic bone would soon be placed in serious jeopardy after sitting in daily, albeit transient, pools of heavily contaminated, fecal material. Once even a tiny amount of stool—all of which is teeming with bacteria—found its way beyond my sutures, pus would form deep within the tissues and a life-threatening bone infection would be the inevitable result. I had to be proactive in order to prevent that disaster from occurring. An easy solution to my gentleman's problem was for me to create a colostomy.

A colostomy is a surgically relocated loop of large intestine—a new anus on the abdominal wall, if you will. And so I gave my poor patient one more thing to be miserable about. I opened the lower half of his abdomen and I divided his large intestine down toward where the colon transitions into the rectum. I sealed off both ends of the divided large bowel with finely placed rows of microstaples, thus preventing any contamination of the abdominal cavity. I created a two-inch-diameter hole in his left, lower abdomen, through which I pulled the large bowel and sewed its opening to the skin of Cedric's abdominal wall. From that moment on, any and all stool would be diverted away from his buttocks wound, allowing it to heal in a clean, uncontaminated environment.

I closed his surgical wound in the usual manner with sutures and skin clips, and I covered his colostomy with a bag. With every bowel movement—every soft, formed, or watery excretion—his stool would be collected neatly in the bag for the nurse to dispose of, rather than in the cracks and crevices of his obese, wrinkled buttocks.

When we all completed our nearly all day series of emergency operations, I walked out into the family waiting area, hoping to find some relative to whom I could brief of the events that had just taken place. I immediately saw Cedric's frazzled, young wife who had obviously spent considerable time crying. I introduced myself as she sat quietly with a deadpan expression, with black smudges of mascara below each of her puffy eyes. I slowly explained to her the injuries her husband had sustained, all that we had done, and my tenuous prognosis. I said everything in as gentle a manner as possible, but I made certain that I did not belittle the seriousness of any of her husband's injuries.

Mrs. White heard everything I said, then began sobbing as she explained to me that she was two months pregnant with Cedric's first and only child, and she wondered how she was going to support herself and her baby now that her husband had been so badly injured. She gave me a look of great despair, and wandered away from me slowly after I gave her every condolence I could think to say. I felt terrible for the woman, knowing that we had just had the first of many more devastating conversations we would share. I thought of my own wife and wondered how she would endure such horrible news, bringing on a genuine feeling of pain deep within my own chest.

Mr. White's ensuing critical care management and the numerous additional operative procedures necessary to keep him from dying became the mother lode of difficult cases. In a matter of twenty-four hours, it became apparent that our four-hour vascular repair had failed completely: Cedric's leg from the knee on down was becoming cadaverlike and dying, and it was questionable at best if

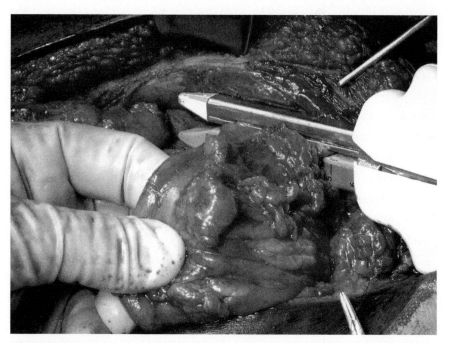

A linear-cutter-stapler applied across a segment of intestine. When fired, it applies several rows of microstaples, dividing the tissues between the rows.

the entire skin of his thigh would survive at all. The dying muscles in his calf were releasing copious amounts of toxic by-products into his circulation, plugging the microscopic, filter cells of his kidneys and sending him into what was to be certain, full-blown renal failure. It was clear that his leg would kill him if we didn't remove it, and so we did just that, removing it at the knee joint, not knowing if even further amputation subsequently would be needed. We decided to take things day by day, and to make any such decision when the situation declared itself.

Several days later, all of the wounds on Cedric's thigh, penile, and scrotal areas had broken down, miraculously leaving only his buttocks wound intact. A few days after that, all the skin that had stripped itself from his thigh muscles had become black and dead. Another trip to the OR was needed. I removed every bit of skin and fat from the far end of his femur bone to his crotch, leaving the badly jagged penile and scrotal skin intact as it had somehow found some blood flow from a stray source and had remained alive, albeit widely opened at all margins.

I wrapped his muscular thigh, now completely unprotected, in countless yards of saline-soaked gauze, and I packed the remaining genital wounds with additional dressing material. Day after day, my partners and I changed the dressings in the intensive care unit, while simultaneously managing his kidney and lung failure with mechanical ventilation, numerous medications, and dialysis prescribed by the kidney specialist. Every few days, one of us took Cedric back to the operating room for a more thorough exploration of his stump under general anesthesia, carefully trimming away bits of dead tissue as we identified it. But after several weeks of our unsuccessful treatments, it became clear that additional thigh tissues were now dying, and further amputation would again be necessary.

The orthopedic surgeons and I gave daily briefings to Mrs. White, who listened dutifully and sheepishly with great pain and anguish as we informed her of her husband's lack of progress. When we told her that more of her husband's thigh would have to be removed, she broke down and cried openly. She described the horror her husband would face once he became lucid, realizing that his once active and independent lifestyle had been irreversibly altered by our necessary butchery. Feeling her pain, we tried to be conservative over the course of three additional operations. At first, we removed all tissues and bone to the midthigh level, but then proceeded further amputating to the high-thigh level. Finally, we needed to remove everything up to a level just six inches be-low his hip joint. The resultant remnant of lower extremity was just a nubbin of bone and thigh muscle, still uncovered, as so much skin removal had been necessary.

Finally, we were able to declare some success, as the extent of our amputa-tions had started to make the rest of his body healthy in general. His kidney failure began to reverse, and his wounds stopped progressing in the wrong di-rection. He started to show signs of real healing. A healthy layer of healing tis-sue began forming over his thigh stump as well as in the depths of his penile and scrotal wounds. Healing tissue—which we call "granulation tissue"—is good, and seeing it gave us further evidence of Cedric's overall improvement. We placed a vacuum-assisted closure device (VAC) over all open areas and changed it every other day, marveling at the favorable progress each time we examined his wounds.

We eventually weaned Cedric from the breathing machine after we had exchanged his oral breathing tube for a tracheostomy, and it looked as if we might be nearing the point of maximal, inpatient benefit to our trauma victim. After two additional weeks of serendipitously good luck, his wounds had dimin-ished to a size we knew would close with the aid of a skin graft. Committing him to one more trip to the operating room, we harvested an ultrathin layer of skin from his good thigh and grafted it to his remaining open wound.

By this juncture, Mr. White's once hulking body had lost a tremendous amount of weight, and he had become terribly weakened. He wanted to help himself, but he could not even muster the strength to shift his body position. He was in terrible need of some aggressive physical rehabilitation. Under the direction of one of our physicians specializing in physical medicine and reha-bilitation, Mr. White was scheduled to spend the next three months recondi-tioning his limp, frail, body and mind at an inpatient, specialty rehab facility remote from our hospital.

On the day he departed our hospital by ambulance en route to the reha-bilitation center, his wife tearfully hugged each of us and thanked us for all we had done to save her husband and the father of her unborn child.

Nearly six months after first meeting Mr. White in the trauma room, while conducting morning wounds in the intensive care unit, I was approached by a gaggle of excited nurses eager to tell me of two visitors awaiting me at the op-posite end of our enormous ICU. I wondered who could be visiting. I was soon thrilled to be greeted by Mr. and Mrs. White, the latter pushing the former in a wheelchair. Cedric looked absolutely amazing, and I shook his hand firmly. He didn't remember me at all, but he smiled with gratitude as his proud wife—now with a large baby bump—introduced us with a joyous look on her face.

We reminisced over a few of the more difficult times we had all shared several months back, and Mrs. White praised her husband for all the progress he had made. She was a different person from the frightened, depressed woman I once remembered. She had become hopeful and confident that everything would eventually be all right.

Mr. White wanted to prove to me that he was still an independent man and began pushing himself up from his wheelchair. He struggled, and I almost offered to help him, but I recognized that he wanted to stand up on his own. Although a little shaky and obviously still quite weak, he managed to stand completely upright on his one good leg, showing pretty good balance considering what little we had left him with. He then plunked himself back in the chair and he told me good-bye.

I reminded the two of them that we would still be seeing each other again, as we still needed to do one more operation. We needed to reverse his colostomy once he had mastered being able to transfer himself on and off the toilet. After all, I told him jokingly, I didn't think that he wanted to have to keep buying new shoes to match that nice bag.

But the husband and mother-to-be had other plans. They told me that they were headed to Mississippi, where both had extended family who could help them and their soon-to-be new baby. I was happy that they had figured out how they were going to manage in what would inevitably be upcoming challenging times. I never heard from either of them again, but they will always be fondly remembered.

13

Cold-Blooded Killer

A Mother's Undying Love

I live in a small town within a county boasting a population of no more than 89,000 members. Many generations of people were born, raised, and died in our community, and most of the lifers in the area know each other in one way or another. I have only called the place home for the past decade, but I really enjoy the quaintness of my town, and appreciate the access to the heart of one of our nation's largest cities just over an hour's drive from my house.

I was driving home from the drugstore one evening and I noticed a sign taped to a light pole. It was a MISSING PERSON sign. I had seen others like it before, but I had not previously noticed that particular sign where it was hanging. It sported the photo of a smiling young man of about twenty-five years old. Included was the notice of a reward for any information as to the whereabouts of the individual who I know had mysteriously disappeared over three years previously. I didn't need to stop and read the sign as I had read identical ones posted in other places several times before. I knew from news articles I had previously read that the young man was last seen, prior to his disappearance, hanging out at a bar late into the night. He never returned home and no one has ever been able to give any good information as what might have happened to him after leaving the drinking establishment.

People in the town knew him, and they told me that he had been a trouble-maker for a very long time. He had apparently been no stranger to the police, having been arrested numerous times for fighting and for misdemeanor drug offenses, and he was even rumored to have possibly had alleged gang affilia-tions. The professional gossip crew wasn't surprised that no one had any useful information to volunteer. Everyone assumed that the man had been killed in a drug deal gone sour, and that his body was probably buried in a cornfield somewhere, likely never to be found.

I knew that the missing man's mother was almost certainly the one who hung the sign. Never having given up hope of finding her boy, his mom dedi-cated the rest of her life to finding him, or at least uncovering information that would give her closure. Every year or so, she stands out along busy intersections holding a large, hand-made poster similar to the small one hanging on the light pole. But when she makes her personal, roadside pleas for information, she in-cludes the words, "Have you seen my son?" I once read an article in our local newspaper that described how she makes her public appearances every year on special occasions, including on her son's birthday, and on the day he disap-peared.

I have come to the conclusion over the years that there must be no bond stronger than the one between a mother and a child. I have seen countless mothers grieve at the bedsides of their critically injured children, and I have seen the agony in women's faces when their young or even aged children die. I have seen little old, hunchbacked ladies, bent forward from advanced spinal arthritis, standing with the full assistance of walkers or canes cry openly and pound their fists with grief as they await the inevitable passing of the children they once carried in their wombs and raised as toddlers. I am certain that re-gardless of how old and independent a child becomes, and regardless of how successful or shameful their lives may be, mothers still worry about their chil-dren, and suffer terrible sympathy pains when faced with the severe injury or death of their grown-up babies. Hopefully, mothers faced with the loss or the grave wounding of a child have a husband or a close personal relative to help them cope, but I know from extensive professional experience that sadly it is not always the case.

On a cold, early winter's evening, while assuming my all-too-familiar in-house trauma surgeon duties, I was alerted to an inbound trauma patient. I sped to the emergency room where I was already gowned and gloved before the paramedics even arrived. The charge nurse informed me that a man had been stabbed in the chest and that paramedics were doing CPR en route. I pulled the chest surgery tray off the ER shelf myself, opened the carefully wrapped package, and awaited my trauma victim. Moments later, paramedics crashed through the emergency room doors. Two men were sweating as they pushed the gurney on which stood a third paramedic, feet balancing on a stabilizing bar between the front and back wheels, pumping vigorously on the chest of an approximately fifty-year-old man, who looked distinctly blue, and dead.

After expeditiously transferring the stab victim onto the emergency room trauma cart, I asked paramedics how long CPR had been ongoing, as an ER technician instinctively took over the responsibilities of chest compressions. They had been doing compressions for over fifteen minutes, which they began immediately on their arrival to the victim's house where they found him lying on his kitchen floor in a pool of blood. Doing some quick calculations, I surmised that our man had been without a pulse for at least twenty minutes, assuming someone made the 911 call the instant the wounding instrument entered his chest.

Taking a second, good look at the guy, I thought that he certainly looked dead, and with CPR ongoing I decided to check to see if his heart had any electrical activity—any sign of life whatsoever. His heart rhythm was an absolute flat line, and I highly suspected that he had bled out well before paramedics had even arrived. I knew that opening the chest in other patients under similar circumstances might save the patient's life. But I also knew from my experience that the man lying before me was well beyond any chances of saving. I decided to briefly check for signs of brain death before doing any cutting—what I knew would just be mutilation of an already dead body. His pupils were blown and entirely nonreactive to light. He had no brain-stem reflexes. He had no signs of life. The man was dead, and I knew that proceeding no further was the right thing to do. I ordered that chest compressions stop and his cardiac rhythm again showed nothing but a solid, flat line. I then officially pronounced him dead.

I looked down at his bloody chest and probed his wound with my gloved finger. While I examined his injury, I noted that he looked like an average guy: clean shaven, muscular but thin, with rugged skin. He was probably a hardworking man, I thought, based on the oil I could see ground into the ridges of his hands. Perhaps he was a machinist or a factory worker. And I wondered why someone could have wanted to kill him. I was impressed by how large his wound was, and with how much force his murderer must have used to kill the man, as the knife had obviously cut right through his breast bone and directly into his heart. I cringed as I envisioned a very violent death, similar to how I imagine Trojan or Spartan warriors must have succumbed.

After I finished my brief exam, but before I could even write a progress note or dictate the events that had just taken place, another trauma alert sounded. I hadn't even had time to grab an admission sticker to read my previous patient's name. I quickly removed my bloody gown and gloves, washed up, and grabbed a fresh set of protective overgarments to await my next trauma victim.

Rolling into the adjacent trauma bay was my next patient. He was much younger than the last, about twenty-five years of age or thereabouts. He was a thin, well-groomed, and generally healthy-looking guy. He was writhing about on the paramedic cart, being physically restrained by the crew so that the patient would not accidentally roll himself onto the ground. The paramedics gave us a brief history, shouting above the loud groans and nearly incomprehensible, foreign language utterances of our patient. They stated that our new trauma patient had just been involved in a domestic dispute where he had apparently stabbed his father and then fled the home in the family car, driving recklessly at high speeds throughout the city, striking three cars along the way, before finally coming to an abrupt stop as he impacted a large tree. Our new guy had apparently been incoherent and combative throughout the brief extrication process from the badly smashed vehicle, as well as during the hasty ride over to our hospital. I couldn't help but put two and two together, and I asked if the paramedics knew the guy's name. They handed me his driver's license, which bore a photo accurately reflecting the young man screaming on my table in front of me.

His name was Dmitri Zukov, and he was twenty-eight years old. As I began assessing my patient's injuries, I asked someone to check the name of the stab-wound patient I had just pronounced dead, and a chill went up my spine when they told me that my previous patient's name was Alexei Zukov. My mind was momentarily overwhelmed as I contemplated the fact that I was working on the alleged killer, and son, of the brutally murdered man I had just pronounced dead.

Dmitri's left foot and ankle were deformed and obviously broken, but his extremity injuries were the least of his problems. The guy was not doing well at all. My instincts as a trauma surgeon told me that Dmitri's life was in serious jeopardy. He was agitated, writhing about, and the color of a sheet. His skin was cold and I could not feel pulses in either his wrists or in his feet. I shouted out asking for a blood pressure but was told by the technician that she was having trouble getting a good reading. His level of consciousness was fading quickly, and in order to gain control of the situation, I ordered a nurse to administer a series of medications through his IV line. Within a minute, he was calm and his muscles were flaccid. I bag-ventilated him for another minute, then slid a plastic, endotracheal tube between his vocal cords and connected him up to the ventilator machine.

Still having not been given a blood pressure, I knew that it had to be very low. I ordered several units of O-negative blood to be infused immediately. Not seeing any blood on his body, I knew that the source of his shock had to be internal. So I checked a chest and pelvis X-ray while I performed a bedside ultrasound examination of his abdomen. The ultrasound revealed a belly full of blood. After both units of blood had been transfused I checked a blood pressure myself: eighty-five over fifty. The blood pressure was still way too low, and I needed to get the guy into the OR *stat!* I ordered two more units of O-negative blood and I instructed the ER crew to move the guy to the operating room pronto.

I wasted no time opening his belly once in the operating room. The anesthesiologist connected his anesthesia machine to the tube I had already placed through his mouth, the OR nurse poured antiseptic over his abdomen, we threw on the drapes, and I began cutting with abandon. Once through all layers of tissue, I packed his insides with a dozen packs to compress whatever it was that was bleeding deep within the swirling, red pool. I had never before sucked out as much blood from a belly as I did on that day. I removed five and a half liters—or almost a gallon and a half—of bright-red fresh blood, before the sucker had completed its job.

I gave the anesthesiologist a good ten minutes to rapidly infuse four more units of red cells into my patient's circulatory system with all abdominal packs in place before I would again pull the plug from the dike and look for the source of hemorrhage. One by one I removed the compressive packs, starting in the places where I figured to be the most likely sources for his exsanguination. I looked at the spleen, and then the liver, but found both areas to be pristine and uninjured. I removed more packs, finally exposing the center of the abdomen where the blood vessels formed a fanlike arrangement of numerous arteries and veins feeding the loops of bowel. In the main vascular fan, supplying blood to all of the small intestine, I found an arterial pumper spewing fresh blood, momentarily squirting me on my masked face before I clamped it with a hemostat. I also found a similar squirter in the fan of vessels supplying the sigmoid colon—the lowest portion of the large intestine just above the rectum. I was able to easily control the bleeding also with a similar application of a single hemostat applied carefully across the torn artery.

I tied sutures around the clamped vessels definitively controlling the bleeding and I removed the hemostats handing them back to the scrub technician. I then examined the entire small and large bowel where I found several segments of torn intestine in the vicinity of the damaged vessels. I looked up at the anesthesiologist and asked him how our patient was doing. I was given a lackluster "Okay" response, and was told that my patient had received a total of ten units of blood, several bags of plasma, and two packs of platelets. But he was cold—

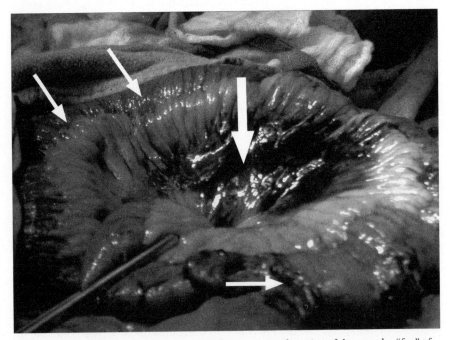

The large vertical arrow points to a large clot from an injured portion of the vascular "fan" of the small bowel mesentery. The small arrows point to the small intestine receiving its blood supply from vessels within the mesentery. The horizontal arrow points to a torn segment of bowel.

hypothermic—his temperature being only 90 degrees, and the combination of extensive blood loss, hypothermia, and bowel injury gave me only one good choice at that juncture. I needed to initiate Damage Control proceedings.

Damage Control is a navy term all sailors know well. When out at sea, if a ship is bombed or is burning and sinking seems inevitable unless unusually aggressive actions are performed, Damage Control goes into effect. In this scenario, all routine activities aboard ship cease and every sailor's actions are directed toward doing only that which is essential and necessary to save the ship.

From the trauma surgeon's perspective, Damage Control means doing only those procedures essential and necessary to save the patient's life. There is a saying among trauma surgeons: "Blood in the belly is like fire on a ship. You run toward it!" As opposed to typical situations when a surgeon performs all of the necessary steps of an operation at one setting, during Damage Control surgery, ongoing bleeding is controlled, ongoing abdominal soilage from leaking intestinal contents are interrupted with swift firings of surgical stapling devices across areas of damaged intestine, and the operation ceases. Patients are then expeditiously moved to the intensive care unit with the abdomen left open— bowel contents contained only by means of a few surgical towels and large, sticky dressings—and an aggressive night of active patient rewarming, transfusing of multiple blood products, and correcting of abnormal blood acidity ensues until the patient stabilizes. The ICU phase of Damage Control often lasts greater than twenty-four hours, after which the patient gets returned to the operating room for completion of all remaining surgery and definitive abdominal wall closure. The decision to convert a traditional operation to a damage-control procedure is a critical one. Failure to recognize the need to do so inevitably results in a perfectly performed operation and a dead patient.

Thus, having made my decision, I resected the two portions of damaged intestine leaving several segments of bowel unattached to one another. I then covered the abdominal contents with towels and dressings, and moved my patient to the intensive care unit with an extensive list of postoperative, resuscitation orders. Once he was safely transferred to the care of the entire team of critical care nurses awaiting my patient, I went off looking for a representative of the Zukov family, to whom I would have to relay some very bad news.

Speaking to patients' families may be the most challenging and difficult part of my job. When I get through working on a badly injured patient, some of whom die in the process, my next obligation is to brief the waiting family members. I often have to tell them the very worst news any person could ever want to hear. The most difficult part is deciding exactly how to phrase my tragic briefing. What always happens is, I walk into a room where one or perhaps up to twenty or more people are waiting. In a matter of seconds, I have to size up my audience in order to decide just how and what to say.

I have to control the look on my face, forcing a neutral expression before I even introduce myself. Walking in wearing a long, dejected face gives away bad news before I can ease the blow if needed. But smiling, although much more personable, can give inappropriate, false hope in addition to making me appear as a heartless doctor after revealing the sad truth. I have to decide based on momentary observations if the family members in the room are a closely knit group supportive of each other, or if their relationships are adversarial. I have to decide if I should use professional terms or simple terms, if I should ease the bad news out slowly in piecemeal fashion, or if I need to just inform them of the worst part of the news quickly up front. I have to decide if I should try to comfort those left behind with support from a religious perspective, or whether I should steer clear of mentioning God's name altogether. And I have to decide when relaying too much information might be more damaging to those left behind than just sticking to the basics. It is extremely difficult and often causes me my own pain as I sympathize with grieving families. It is my responsibility, yet one I do not at all relish.

I walked back to the emergency room where a hospital chaplain spotted me and told me that one family member was waiting for me in the counseling room. I was given a much appreciated heads-up that the person awaiting my briefing was Mrs. Zukov, the wife of my first patient, and the mother of my second. I was told that she was an immigrant from one of the eastern European countries, having been here in the United States for only seven years, leaving all of her other relatives behind in the old country. I knew this was going to be one of my most difficult briefings, considering the tragic circumstances.

The chaplain led me into the counseling room where I spotted an elderly lady, appearing much older than I had expected, dressed in heavy, loose, and simple clothing. A handkerchief covered her hair. Her head hung low and she looked blankly at the carpeted floor even as I approached her and as I extended my hand. She reminded me of my great-grandmother, looking as I remembered her as a young boy. My great-grandmother was a hardened Polish immigrant and a classic eastern European. She was widowed at the age of just twenty-four.

I decided to proceed slowly, and to break the bad news bit by bit. I started with the news of her husband, stating that the paramedics had been working heroically on him from the moment they arrived at their home right up to the moment they turned him over to me. I slowly told her in simple terms the details of what I did, but that despite my efforts he tragically just could not be saved. I concluded that short part of my conversation with a genuine "I'm so sorry for the loss of your husband." And that's when she looked up at me. She told me that she already knew. She said in broken English that she knew when the paramedics had left her home that her husband was already dead. She then asked about her son.

I told her in as optimistic of terms as possible all that had happened. I started by saying that he was alive, but that he was in very bad shape, on a breathing machine in the intensive care unit, and in critical condition. I told her when he arrived to our hospital that he was dying, but although very sick, he was still alive. He had lost a tremendous amount of blood, but I had stopped the bleeding, and still needed to do more surgery once he became more stable. I also told her that being a young man, he was more likely than most to make it through his terrible injuries and hopefully survive to lead a long life.

Thinking that I had presented the bad news in the best manner possible, I hoped to see some sign that she was at least comforted in some way, but I didn't see any such signs on her face. Instead, she started crying, telling me that she knew that if her son was going to live he would be spending the rest of his young-adult years in jail. My heart then began to ache, knowing that the words she spoke were the honest truth. Her son had killed her husband, and once he had recovered from his injuries, he would be put behind bars.

I sat silently, peering at her sullen face, offering her unlimited opportunity to ask questions or make comments. After several minutes of dead silence, she began to speak. She wept as she told me that her son was a good boy, but a troubled boy. Choking back tears, she told me that he had been going to college in the city for six years, but that he had to drop out several times because he could not handle the pressure of the classroom. She told me that her husband never understood her boy—he never understood why his son couldn't just make something of himself with all the opportunity he had been given. She said that her husband and son argued often, which made her boy go through periods of deep depression. She then began crying uncontrollably as she again reaffirmed that he was a good boy, but somehow must have just snapped.

It was clear that despite the horror of the events that had taken place that day, she still loved her son so very much. She would now have so much more than ever before to worry about. Moved by the woman's undying love for her son, the disturbed murderer, I asked her if she had any support at all. Being an immigrant with all related family members an ocean away, and having just learned the English language, she really hadn't developed any real friends in this country. I felt so bad for Mrs. Zukov, but I had little more to offer her. I told her that I would call her often, and I concluded my discussion with her by again offering my condolences for the loss of her husband. I then took her hand, established solid eye contact with her, and slowly said to her, "May you find peace." I didn't look away until I knew that she understood that I truly felt sympathy for her, and that I would be thinking of her often.

Over the course of the following week, the other trauma surgeons and I operated on Dmitri several more times. Once he stabilized in the intensive care unit, I reconnected his unattached segments of intestine and I closed his abdomen tightly with heavy sutures and staples. Orthopedic specialists performed operations on his complicated foot and ankle fractures. Their surgeries included applying plates and screws across the broken, lower leg bones, and thin, wire pins through the numerous broken pieces in his foot and toes. Small pieces of metal protruded from each of his digits, each capped by a small plastic covering. His entire foot and ankle were collectively wrapped in a bulky, gauze dressing requiring twice daily nursing care to remove and reapply the bandages. The foot-and-ankle orthopedic specialist managing his limb injuries directed that the wires would stay in Dmitri's foot for six weeks, after which time they would be removed and he would hopefully be able to begin applying some weight on his leg. In the meanwhile however, Dmitri would have to learn to get around using a walker, and be careful not to bear any weight on his badly broken foot, lest he risk causing permanent injury to himself and lifelong disability.

I spoke to Dmitri often about what he remembered about the day he became injured. Throughout, he acted distant and aloof, supposedly not remembering anything. He often mentioned his mother in conversation, but he never once discussed his father. Occasionally, I asked if he knew anything of his father's status, and he simply answered me by saying that he had heard that his father became injured. Dmitri never mentioned an argument, an altercation, or the violent assault he had already perpetrated against his dad. He also never acted as if he knew that his father was dead. I never really knew if Dmitri had in fact blocked the events of that fateful day from his consciousness, or if his apparent lack of awareness was an intentional ruse, perhaps part of some defense strategy he would eventually use in court. While conducting daily patient rounds, I would occasionally notice business cards from attorneys sitting on his bedside nightstand, and legal pages of handwritten notes, the contents of which I never read.

I made good on my promise to contact Mrs. Zukov often, but she rarely answered her phone and she never visited the hospital during regular work hours. When we would talk, she remained distant and said very few words. She was always very gracious and she thanked me for caring for her son, but she rarely contributed anything to our conversations. I would occasionally hear that she had slipped into the hospital late at night to visit her boy, but would usually leave after only very brief stays. I know that she dropped items off for Dmitri—a Bible, prayer cards, and perhaps those attorney business cards—but she never made a habit of remaining in the hospital long enough to talk with any of the nurses, doctors, or social workers.

After about a month, it became time to release Dmitri from the hospital. Ordinarily, that would mean discharging him to a rehabilitation institution, and eventual release to home after several weeks or months of inpatient therapy. But Dmitri was on police hold, and jail was the next place he would be going. For days prior to his release, I spent hours talking with jail health-care workers and prison administrative officials, making sure that they would be able to provide the necessary pin-site care to his foot, while the legal authorities wrangled over where the most appropriate place would be to confine my still injured, yet historically quite violent individual. Mrs. Zukov, who had been conspicuously absent and nearly impossible to reach by phone for the previous several weeks, had finally resurfaced after hearing of her son's imminent transfer. I was given a message that she had asked to speak to me personally, and she asked that I call her at a number left for me.

When she answered the phone, she was still the broken, despondent woman she was on that first night. We discussed the reasons why it had become time for her son to be transferred. She pleaded with me through heavy tears and open sobs, using every argument—logical, illogical, and purely emotional— why her son should stay in our hospital until he was completely recovered from all his injuries. She was so terribly worried about Dmitri's well-being, and she dreaded the thought of her boy being locked behind bars. Mrs. Zukov was clearly unraveling emotionally, and I asked her if she had found anyone to share her suffering with. She told me that there was no one she could talk to. She said that she was too humiliated and mortified to even share her thoughts with her one good acquaintance with whom she worked part-time as a nurse's aide at a local retirement facility. I suggested that she fly back home to be with her own family for a while, but she said that she didn't have the money, and that she didn't want to leave her son who needed her more than ever.

On his last day at our hospital, two police officers handcuffed Dmitri's arm to the frame of the wheelchair as emergency medical technicians working for a contract ambulance transport company escorted him outside to the awaiting rig destined for the medical ward of the county jail. Dmitri seemed strangely upbeat without any noticeable apprehension or look of fear. He waved good-bye to the floor nurses as he was wheeled away by the medical crew and the armed policemen. Mrs. Zukov did not show up to the hospital that day and she did not see her son off to his new confining quarters.

I never again saw or heard from her, nor did I ever receive contact from the police or attorneys regarding Dmitri's medical condition. Although I never learned how the legal proceedings against him were resolved, I still imagine Dmitri behind bars, and his mother still holding a silent vigil for her son's well-being. She will forever remind me through her dutiful example during that cold, winter month just how a mother's love and concern for her child persists even in the most extreme of trying times. Because of how Mrs. Zukov's example enlightened me, every time I notice one of those MISSING PERSON signs asking the whereabouts of our missing, hometown young man, I think about his mother, and I say a quiet prayer hoping that she one day finds her much needed source of peace.

14

Broken Minds and Damaged Bodies

Mental Illness

I am, for the most part, proud of the profession as a whole which I chose. I know that I was called to be doctor at a very young age. I cemented my plans to attend medical school before I had even graduated high school, motivated by the exceptional experiences I had working as an emergency room technician at a large, suburban, community hospital. Once in medical school I decided that unlike some of my student peers, I would learn everything taught to me, in every subject. Some students knew that they would never pursue a particular career specialty path, and got by learning only the bare minimums to pass certain clinical rotations. I knew that I would never go into pediatrics, or obstetrics, or a number of other specialties for that matter. But regardless of the rotation I was assigned to, I learned everything I could, figuring that whatever specialist I would eventually become, I would be a better one by understanding the nuances of all medical specialties.

Now that I am an attending trauma surgeon, I appreciate and respect those who chose to master the obscure specialties I would never want to practice—like the kidney specialists who practice the minutia of nephrology, the anesthesiology subspecialists who practice chronic pain management, and the bug chasers who practice infectious disease. I know people in each of these areas, whom I admire and respect, and as a whole are more than happy to become involved in the care of my trauma patients when I need their expertise, regardless of an injured patient's insurance status, social status, or ability to pay. I have always felt that whatever a man or woman chooses to pursue as a specialty, he or she should pursue it with all available energy and dedication. I have complete and total respect for good physicians in every realm of medicine. God knows that this world needs good family physicians just as much as it needs good surgeons, and it is nothing more than disingenuous arrogance to look down on another physician's chosen specialty.

But I have begun to lose a great deal of respect for an entire specialty of medicine, having been let down over and over by their lack of helpful input and commitment. I am sorry to admit that I am losing respect for many psychiatrists. Having just stated that this world needs all good physicians, it might sound hypocritical for me to say that I don't have a lot of respect for the mental health providers, and I recognize this. But I have met so few psychiatrists who are willing to reliably take on the responsibilities of caring for my mentally disturbed trauma patients, even when my patients really need them—even when I can spoon-feed my mental health colleagues my patients' psychiatric diagnoses.

One patient clearly failed by the psychiatric profession was Elizabeth Barlow. Elizabeth was an emotionally labile manic depressive who often had terrible periods of great dysfunction. She struggled throughout her young adult life with self-imposed isolation and loneliness, exacerbated by a tremendously low self-esteem due in part to her morbid obesity, and reinforced by the constant remorse she felt for the ramifications of her repeatedly poor life decisions. Elizabeth was also of limited intelligence, having never gone beyond high school, and thus her employment options were sparse. She worked on and off over the years in grocery stores, strip-mall shops, and fast-food restaurants, but was usually fired during her employment probationary periods as her mental illness often prevented her from reliably showing up for work. During her manic phases, she would spend her money with abandon on clothing inappropriately provocative for her rotund figure, and on alcohol and drugs, which she would share with strangers she would meet at places like the video store or in the laundry area of her subsidized housing complex. During her depressive periods she would sequester herself in her apartment for days at a time, ignore her obligations to go to work, fail to pay important bills, and contemplate suicide repeatedly.

In fact, she had attempted suicide several times before. Twice previously, she had seriously cut her wrists—once while still in high school and living with her parents, and once since moving out on her own. Both times she ended up in the hospital, requiring treatment for her wounds, and several weeks of inpatient psychiatric stabilization. Her previous suicide attempts were apparently not gestures but bona fide attempts at taking her own life. She bore deep, disfiguring scars on her wrists, constantly reminding her of her past. She was at times seriously disabled by her demons and she often struggled throughout her young life. She saw several different psychiatrists over the years, and had been diagnosed with various disorders including major depression, bipolar illness, and paranoid schizophrenia. She had been prescribed multiple different medications and she had attended numerous counseling sessions. But she had little continuity of care from her mental health care providers.

Each time she would develop a comfortable relationship with one of the psychiatrists or psychologists to whom she had been assigned, she would soon be told not to come back, either because her health insurance had lapsed due to her numerous job changes, or because she had apparently achieved "maximal psychiatric benefit," and allegedly no longer needed routine mental health care and counseling. But Elizabeth never really became stable. She merely achieved periods of normal thinking and behavior in between abnormal highs and lows. Her parents described her as seemingly "normal" as her mood elevated from a state of depression en route to her predictably inevitable manic episodes. For every period of mania she experienced, a painful, potentially suicidal, disabling crash of emotions always followed.

On one particularly bad day, Elizabeth sank into a deep depression, filled with irrational thoughts and overwhelmed by voices telling her how to end her life. Ordinarily, Elizabeth would be powerless to help herself, as she would suffer silently, painfully toying with thoughts of ending it all. But on that one particular day, for the first time ever, she mustered just enough courage and strength to seek the help she knew that she needed. She drove herself to the emergency room of the hospital where she had been admitted a few years before. After detailing her thoughts of suicide to the emergency room doctor, she was admitted to the hospital's psychiatric unit where she spent five days on suicide watch, and where the mental health doctors started her on a different regimen of medications. Apparently, after five days of therapy and observation, the psychiatrists felt that Elizabeth was again well and they informed their patient that she would be discharged from the psychiatric facility.

Elizabeth apparently did not agree that she was well, and she supposedly informed several people that she was still feeling suicidal. As she would later recount, the thought of being abruptly discharged from the hospital had caused her to panic and she began having overwhelming thoughts and visions of her own death. Elizabeth was crying and feeling desperate. She told a staff nurse that if they discharged her, she would surely kill herself before she got home. Whether this was or was not passed along to the psychiatrists is unclear, but regardless—the psychiatrists had made their final decision, and Elizabeth was released from the mental health facility later that afternoon.

Elizabeth was escorted out of the hospital and she walked herself to her car, which she had left parked in the visitor's lot five days before. She was anxious, frightened, and at that point obsessed with putting an end to her mental anguish once and for all. Consumed with dying, and driven by psychotic voices directing her self-destructive actions, she drove herself to an overpass and parked the car on the shoulder. She looked down at the interstate expressway below, where cars zipped under her one after another. She saw visions of herself jumping down into the traffic below, being struck by a speeding car, and paramedics covering her with a shroud, as she lay dead on the road. Feeling unable to control her destiny any further, she made good on her earlier promise to the psychiatric nurse, and Elizabeth jumped down nearly thirty feet into the path of the speeding cars on the busy thoroughfare below.

But as fate would have it, Elizabeth was not struck by any cars. Certainly shocked at the sight of a falling body, automobiles and trucks braked, swerved, and dodged as she impacted the pavement and lay limp on the otherwise busy roadway. She was not dead, as she had hoped. But she was in terrible pain— pain in her back that made taking a breath feel like a knife was sticking her between her ribs. She couldn't move, as her legs felt numb and heavy. She didn't even realize that both bones of each of her lower legs had snapped like dried tree limbs and had pierced through the overlying flesh, leaving both extremities twisted into bloody, serpentine configurations. She couldn't feel the pain in her legs because she had broken her spine in the fall and as a result, her spinal cord had been severed.

Meanwhile, I had just finished operating on a young girl with a very puzzling condition. Monica DeSilvia was my twenty-four-year-old patient who just a few hours earlier had called paramedics to a home where she had been visiting friends. She had not been injured in an accident, nor had she been involved in any other trauma for that matter. Monica called paramedics with a chief complaint of severe abdominal pain. She was taken to the ER and was evaluated urgently by the hospital's emergency room physician who had become quite alarmed by her presentation and felt that an emergency surgery consult was warranted. Because a trauma surgeon is always in-house at our hospital, there are times when we are called to emergently address patients having potentially life-threatening, nontrauma conditions that required a surgeon's intervention immediately. That was felt to be one of those situations.

I walked into Ms. DeSilvia's ER room after being briefed by the emergency room physician who was genuinely concerned. Taking one look at the girl concerned me as well. She looked sickly and malnourished, like a cancer patient in her last few months of life. She had a look on her face that reflected some source of torture deep within her, and she groaned miserably between rapid, shallow breaths. She was able to tell me that for no apparent reason she abruptly began having excruciating abdominal pain. I pulled up her hospital gown to examine her abdomen and was quite stunned to see evidence of numerous previous operations, with scars running vertically, obliquely, and horizontally. I had never seen anything quite like it in such a young girl. The scars made me both curious as well as nervous, as multiple previous operations increase the likelihood of a very serious problem brewing in her belly. Multiple scars also make surgical operations much more difficult. I asked her what all the scars were from, and she gave me a meticulously detailed explanation of having been diagnosed with a rare disorder while vacationing with her mother in Italy two years previously. She knew her medical history well, and she described with precise detail her multiple operations and reoperations for various complications, which developed during her nearly one year long admission to the Italian hospital.

To complicate matters, she said that she had also been involved in a car crash the day before while she and her husband were visiting a friend about one hundred miles away. She told me the details of the accident: a head-on collision on a two-lane road versus a car that had swerved into her lane of traffic. She described the damage to her vehicle and the ambulance and the crew that drove her to a small hospital, where she was examined by a doctor and had X-rays and lab studies performed prior to being discharged. That piece of history certainly threw a wrench in the works, because all of the abdominal scar tissue from her previous operations could easily have tugged at a soft loop of intestine during the crash impact, causing a potential minor tear. If such a small tear did exist, it would slowly leak intestinal juices, causing her to eventually develop severe pain from a slowly brewing peritonitis. But her lab tests were all normal arguing against anything very bad at all.

She repeatedly told me how frustrated and angry she was, as she had thought that her abdominal problems were all behind her. She expressed how upset she was that the setback would interfere with her job, which she stated she had successfully held for the past seven months, working as a firefighter in some downstate, small-town community. I was surprised to hear that she was a firefighter. Frankly, I didn't think that she looked strong enough to pull a garden hose let alone a fire hose. Regardless of my suspicions, she did appear to be in terrible distress, both physically and emotionally. She was crying. It seemed that she knew that she was again headed down a road she had traveled so many times previously—a road she stated she had hoped to never again see.

But her emotional state wasn't my primary concern at the moment. What bothered me most was the girl's excruciating pain—her relentless, writhing agony—despite without what I would consider to be any solid, objective findings or convincing data pointing to a specific cause of her misery. A particular, very serious entity does exist, which presents itself in a very similar manner as the girl who had been perplexing me in that emergency room. The entity being considered can be catastrophic, and often fatal, if missed and not operated on early. Pain out of proportion to physical findings by the examining surgeon is the hallmark description of the potentially devastating situation called ischemic bowel. When present, intestine gets twisted in such a manner that the adjacent blood vessels flowing toward the bowel get strangulated cutting off all blood supply to the digestive organ. If not recognized and surgically untwisted urgently, the entire length of small intestine can turn black and literally die, leading to a situation which is usually fatal if untreated, and can still be fatal even if treated appropriately by surgically removing huge segments of the dead bowel.

I knew that the girl had the potential of having ischemic bowel, or perhaps less likely a segment of torn intestine from the previous day's crash. I knew that despite having no clear-cut evidence of what it was that was causing Monica's pain, I had no alternative but to operate on her. I spent an additional ten minutes with Monica, explaining in great detail my diagnostic dilemma, what I needed to do, and why I felt that I needed to operate on her urgently. I also explained to her that there were several potential risks associated with the operation which both she and I would have to assume. She didn't seem to care in the slightest about any possible risks. She was sick, in tremendous pain, and she told me that she felt as if she was dying. She wanted me to operate on her as soon as possible, and quickly signed the surgical consent form giving me the authorization to do so.

I had Monica on the OR table in about half an hour, and exhaled a large sigh as I incised atop one of the many scars on her belly wall, badly mutilated from all of her previous surgical procedures. I encountered dense webs of internal scar tissue, matting together loops of small bowel, large bowel, and stomach. Carefully snipping a few millimeters of scar tissue at a time, I freed up every inch of her gastrointestinal tract from beginning to end. It was a technically difficult, painstaking process. Hasty cutting would have been a mistake, as inadvertently injuring a segment of intestine could have complicated matters greatly. After dividing all areas of scar tissue, I examined the insides of her entire abdomen, stymied and frustrated to find absolutely nothing which could have caused her pain. I wasn't sure if perhaps the scar tissue itself was the culprit, but I found not even the slightest hint of intestinal obstruction—one of the primary sources of abdominal pain caused by intestinal scar tissue. Perhaps her intestine had been twisted prior to my operating and perhaps it spontaneously righted itself before I had actually opened her up. However, I knew that was highly unlikely, and I suddenly felt that I had somehow been duped by my young patient into operating on her for no good reason—but why?

After she had fully awakened and recovered from surgery, I talked to her about my negative, intraoperative findings. Immediately postop, most people are in a fair amount of pain and require several doses of intravenous narcotics before they are usually comfortable enough to talk. However, numerous doses of even our most potent narcotics did not relieve Monica's pain. In fact, I saw no difference in the wincing, crying, and writhing exhibited by her before or after surgery. Her behavior was most peculiar and my suspicions that the girl was mentally disturbed were rising.

After telling her of my absence of findings, I asked if she would like me to call anyone, perhaps her husband. She declined, however, stating that her husband was the sole owner of a small business who worked long hours and would not have time to talk with me at that hour of the day. She assured me that she would call him later that evening. I then asked if I could call her mom or her dad. She told me that her parents had separated several years prior and that they had lived apart ever since. She stated that her mom could no longer handle hearing about her medical problems as a result of their yearlong nightmare in Italy. Her father, she stated, was a telephone lineman. She said that she had been told to never call him during the day, as answering his cell phone might cause him to fall while working, potentially causing him injury. Most of what she said made perfect sense, but I wasn't satisfied that Monica was being entirely truthful with me.

Less than an hour after leaving Monica in the recovery room, my trauma alert sounded and summoned me back to the emergency department. That is where I first came into contact with Elizabeth Barlow—the poor girl who tried so hard to kill herself, now unable to move or feel below her waist with broken bones protruding through the skin of both her legs. Despite suffering a broken spine with spinal cord damage, as well as two mangled legs, she was really quite stable and I couldn't find any physical evidence of additional injury. But spinal cord injuries are notorious for masking other injuries, especially those deep within the abdomen, as patients rarely feel pain below the level of their damaged cord, which made diagnoses based entirely on physical examination unreliable. In addition, she was fat—morbidly obese fat. Patients that large who *don't* have spinal cord injuries are often difficult to examine reliably.

In the case of this obese woman with a spinal cord injury, performing a hands-on abdominal exam is almost an exercise in futility. So, to rule out any potentially hidden injuries, and to get a good look at her broken back, I ordered CT scans of everything—brain, neck, chest, abdomen, and pelvis—so as not to miss anything. To get Elizabeth into the scanner, and to keep her calm and quiet, she needed a sedative. I ordered a dose of Vitamin V—Versed, otherwise known as midazolam—which put her into a restful slumber. Taking advantage of the sedative's effects, I quickly washed out, bandaged, and applied custom-formed, fiberglass splints to her badly torn and broken legs. Once the splints had hardened, the crew took Elizabeth for her plethora of scans and X-rays.

All scans and X-rays were negative, with the exception of the spinal injuries and the leg fractures already diagnosed based on clinical examination. The twelfth thoracic vertebra—the lowest of the spinal bones in the chest—had completely burst from the impact of the fall. Numerous bone fragments were in places they should not be, including one large chunk of bone pushed directly back into the canal ordinarily occupied by the spinal cord. Clearly, that large, stray bone fragment had either crushed or cut her spinal cord, and neither gave her very much hope of walking again. When her leg X-rays revealed broken leg bones on both sides, I sighed quietly at the twisted irony of having to surgically treat broken legs in a person who unfortunately may never walk again. At that point, she was breathing well on her own, her blood pressure was stable, her leg wounds and fractures were dressed and splinted, and all diagnostic studies had been completed.

Even though the girl needed three surgical procedures, I would be performing none of them. Her injuries required a spine surgeon and an orthopedic surgeon. My trauma surgery partners and I would still remain in charge, however, of all critical care management and the overall coordination of her required care. Having nothing more to do, I wrote a full page of admitting orders and told the emergency room staff to get Elizabeth into an intensive care unit bed.

Not long after Elizabeth had arrived into the ICU, I began receiving pages from the nursing staff telling me that my patient was emerging from the sedative we had administered in the ER and that she was becoming quite uncontrollable. I ordered additional sedation, and I contacted the spine and orthopedic surgeons who were taking subspecialty trauma call that day. By the end of the night, Elizabeth had received all of her necessary surgery—both legs fixed, and spine fracture stabilized through an incision along the midline of her back—and she was back in the intensive care unit.

But Elizabeth was inconsolable and overly needy. The same mental illness that had destabilized her life for all her years had again reared its ugly head and was making the nurses' job of caring for her in her postoperative period nearly impossible. After receiving more pages requesting additional sedatives than I cared to answer, I decided to walk down to the ICU and see just how bad things had become. By that time, the ICU nurses had learned of the tragic details of all that had happened to the girl, including her recent stay in the other hospital's psychiatric ward, her past psychiatric history, and her suicidal past. I tried to console my patient and to determine her current mental state by asking her some basic questions included in any cursory psychiatric examination.

Elizabeth's answers gave me ample insight into the depths of her psychiatric disability. She described hearing voices, and she tried to convince me that cameras were spying on us, monitoring our conversation. She cried inconsolably and she wouldn't let either me or the nurse leave the room, convinced that someone was waiting outside the door, intending to do her harm. Elizabeth was psychotic and she needed a lot of help. I became angry at the other hospital's psychiatrists who discharged her less than one full day prior from where it had become clear to me that she had needed to stay. But none of that mattered much subsequent to her injuries. My patient's condition warranted another professional psychiatric evaluation, and the sooner the better.

I consulted the psychiatrist taking call at our hospital that day and I relayed to her all the information I knew. The particular psychiatrist happened to be on staff at the facility where Elizabeth had just been discharged from, and she decided to access Elizabeth's records from the other hospital before evaluating her at the bedside. That would take longer than I wanted at the time, and having no choice but to initiate psychiatric treatment on my own, I prescribed one of the latest generation, antipsychotic medications, wrote for additional sedatives, and I waited for the psychiatrist to arrive. Unfortunately, the psychiatrist did not arrive until late the next day, which did nothing to bolster my respect or confidence in the psychiatric profession.

When the psychiatrist finally did evaluate Elizabeth, the mental health diagnosis assigned to her that day seemed to be based more on politics than on good medicine. Elizabeth was clearly psychotic, and the psychiatrist's prescription of Geodon—an effective antipsychotic medication—seemed to support my assessment. But the psychiatrist diagnosed Elizabeth with "Suicide Attempt Due to Acute Grief Reaction." That, in effect, stated that something abruptly had caused Elizabeth to grieve, which caused her to lose her will to live. As far as I was concerned, that diagnosis was nothing more than a load of garbage, and a very diplomatic attempt at deflecting blame for Elizabeth's attempted suicide, and now paraplegia, which I felt was certainly due to her being prematurely discharged from the other psychiatric hospital on the day she promised that she would kill herself—assuming that what she told me was true.

In a bed on the opposite end of the intensive care unit lay my other, now recently postoperative patient, Monica. Her vital signs, laboratory studies, and physical exam findings all indicated that she was recovering nicely without any complications from the surgery I had performed. She continued to complain of pain. According to Monica, her pain required doses of intravenous narcotics every two hours. If the nurse missed asking Monica by as few as five minutes whether she needed another dose of medication—at the time ordered to be administered on an as-needed basis only—Monica jumped on her nurse call light and whined until she got the drugs she demanded.

Four days postop, I was more than suspicious of Monica's integrity. I suspected that she had a drug-dependency problem. Although Monica admitted to having taken painkillers for over a year, which included her extended stay in the Italian hospital, she denied vehemently that she had had any narcotics in the previous twelve months. Since having operated on her, I never once saw her husband, her parents, or anybody else for that matter. I desperately wanted a family member's input to corroborate my patient's stories. I asked on several occasions if Monica wanted me to call someone, but she kept giving me the same story of how her husband was extremely busy at the shop, and how her father was probably working up on a pole fixing the telephone cables. Each time, she told me that she had spoken to both of them the night prior on her cell phone, and that I shouldn't worry about them. By now, I was having difficulty believing anything Monica told me, but I just didn't have any proof to support my suspicions that she was being deceitful, as her stories were so detailed.

Later that afternoon, Monica asked for her dose of morphine and complained to me angrily that her nurse had skipped her last dose of painkillers entirely. I knew that Monica hadn't really slept in over four days, always watching the clock day and night, awaiting her scheduled dose of narcotics. I knew that the nurses were trying to space Monica's narcotics farther apart to wean her from what was almost certainly a narcotics addiction. I happened to be in the area, hearing the arguing between Monica and her nurse and I tried to intervene.

After talking with Monica, we agreed that we would give her another injection, but that she needed to give me her husband's cell-phone number so that I could call him. She agreed, and immediately after she received her drug, I asked her to give me her husband's phone number. Her eyelids were heavy and she seemed to be drifting off to sleep. We had a deal and I was persistent about getting that number. Finally, after slapping her hand enough to keep her attention, she mumbled a ten-digit phone number, and she told me that it was the phone number of a man named Frank. But Frank was not her husband's name according to the nurses. Wanting to know exactly who it was I would soon be calling, she told me that Frank was her father.

I dialed the phone number given to me by Monica, and a man answered. I introduced myself and told him that I was the surgeon who operated on his daughter. The man on the other end of the phone asked me to stand by for a minute as he walked to an area where he could speak to me privately, as it sounded as if he was out working at a job site. A minute later, he asked me to repeat my name again and he asked me which of his daughters was in the hospital. "Monica DeSilvia," I replied.

"Who did you just say? Monica DeSilvia?" he responded, obviously somewhat shocked and surprised by my news. I affirmed that it was, in fact, Monica who I had operated on four days prior. And that's when the whole, twisted charade started to unravel.

"Doc," the man said. "Her name isn't Monica DeSilvia, it's Samantha Acardo." I was stunned, but not completely surprised to hear that I had been lied to by Monica . . . Samantha. The man on the other end of the phone then gave me the sordid details of the bizarre life of his daughter—and my patient—Samantha Acardo.

"First of all, Doc, Monica DeSilvia is the name of my daughter's exboyfriend's fiancée, and I have no idea why she is using Monica's name," he stated. He then spent the next twenty minutes or so explaining that his daughter had serious psychiatric problems and that she had spent the previous two years going from hospital to hospital, telling stories of a trip to Italy where she contracted some disease or illness, and that she tells every doctor she meets that she is in severe pain. He told me that she has literally convinced a halfdozen surgeons to operate on her for some bizarre reason, and when she gets released from one hospital, she hitches rides, takes cabs, or asks people she meets to drive her to a different town where she goes to a different hospital looking for more treatment for a disease she is convinced she has, but which is nothing more than a figment of her mentally disturbed imagination.

He said that Samantha had never been married, she doesn't have a car, and the motor vehicle crash story is one she had been using for over a year. With his voice cracking ever so slightly, he also told me that he had spent several hours every evening over the previous two years calling hospital emergency rooms in a three-state area asking if they had seen or heard of his daughter, Samantha. He said that when he had occasionally located her, she always seemed to get away before he could get to the hospital. He was relieved to hear that she was still alive, but he also told me that he had absolutely no idea how to help his daughter. Apparently, every time she became confronted with her web of lies, she abruptly signed out of the hospital against medical advice, leaving the area. Floored by the incredible story I had just been told, it became clear to me that my patient had what is known as Munchausen syndrome.

Munchausen syndrome is a psychiatric disorder in which patients fake a particular disease or illness for purposes of secondary gain, such as attention or pain medication. Munchausen patients are often extremely knowledgeable of the disease entities they feign, and in extreme cases, convince consulting surgeons to perform exploratory operations. I had never before met a true Munchausen patient, but I was convinced that if there ever was a classic case of it, Samantha Acardo was that case. I thanked Samantha's father for all the information, gave him our hospital's phone number, and hung up the phone.

Still very much shocked after my conversation with the father, my trauma nurse making rounds with me that day saw the bewildered look on my face and asked me what the girl's father had told me. I gave her a fragmented, thumb-nail version of our conversation, and together we walked directly into Samantha's room. With a pleasant smile on my face, and in a soft, compassionate tone, I put my hand onto my patient's and I asked, "So how are you feeling this morning Samantha?" Unscathed by my use of her real name, she answered in small whimpers that she was finally starting to feel a little better. I then told her that I had just spoken to her father, and that he was heartbroken that he had not seen her in two years. I also told her that I knew she had never been to Italy, that she made a habit out of bouncing from hospital to hospital, and that I knew that her real name was Samantha Acardo. Now wide awake and very defensive, she quickly sat upright and blurted out with an angry look on her face, "What the hell are you even talking about?"

For a brief moment I wondered if what I was about to do next was the right thing. Knowing that she had swindled at least five other surgeons before me, I told her in no uncertain terms that I was angry—*very* angry—that she had lied to such an extent that she put not only her own life at risk, but the careers of the surgeons she had deceitfully convinced to cut on her. I told her that her dad had been crying nightly for years, and that she was a selfish, insensitive person for doing what she did. She then told me with great indignation that she wanted the Against Medical Advice paperwork, and that she wanted to sign herself out of the hospital as soon as possible. But I told her that knowing her story, I was going to force her to stay. I told her that I would be filling out a Certificate of Commitment, which was a legal document forcing people who have psychiatric illness causing them to be a risk to themselves or others to be involuntarily confined to the hospital, and that the only person who could reverse my order would be a psychiatrist.

Samantha looked nervous and puzzled by my aggressive actions, and she no longer resisted me. She lay back down in her hospital bed and she pulled the sheet over her face. I grabbed the hospital chart and wrote a lengthy note detailing the revelations of the past hour. On the Certificate of Commitment, I described that Samantha Acardo met criteria for involuntary admission as her psychiatric condition caused her potential risk and harm to herself as she had convinced several surgeons to perform unnecessary, invasive surgery on her for secondary-gain purposes. I also stated that she had no home, she was terribly malnourished from always being in the hospital, and that she was not capable of caring for herself. I signed the papers making her commitment official, and I then called the department of psychiatry.

At our hospital, it is difficult to speak directly to a psychiatrist, as they are apparently always engaged in some sort of therapy session. A very competent psychiatric nurse liaison, however, is always available for initial consultation. As is the custom, the liaison then briefs the on-call psychiatrist of the details. After relaying the crazy story, the psychiatric nurse liaison was nearly as shocked as I was, and she told me that she looked forward to meeting the girl, as she, too, had never actually met a true Munchausen's patient. She agreed with me that the Certificate of Commitment was entirely appropriate, and that the psychiatrist would see her just as soon as possible at Samantha's intensive care unit bedside. Feeling that I had dotted all of the I's and crossed all of the T's, I felt comfortable leaving the hospital later that evening and turning over my in-house trauma and critical care responsibilities to my partner who was taking over.

The next morning, I arrived at 6:45 A.M. to again assume my in-house duties. I met up with my partner who had been in-house all night and I asked him specifically what the psychiatrist had said about Samantha. He took a deep breath, and then told me that the psychiatrist had reversed my Certificate of Commitment. Shocked and furious over the matter, I pulled up the electronic chart on one of the hospital computers and I read over the psychiatrist's commentary. Her dictated note stated that she agreed with my diagnosis of Munchausen syndrome, but that contrary to my opinion, the psychiatrist felt that Samantha posed no harm to herself, and that she was perfectly capable of caring for herself. Having reversed my Certificate of Commitment, there was nothing officially preventing Samantha from leaving the facility. Astutely picking up on that fact, Samantha signed herself out of the hospital, and she hastily departed the area.

Meanwhile, taking care of Elizabeth—a morbidly obese, mentally unstable, paraplegic—was a nightmarish burden for the ICU nurses, and a painful, daily chore for me and the other surgeons. Elizabeth's paralysis only further exacerbated her anxiety, depression, and paranoia. Realizing the unpleasantness of Elizabeth's condition, the psychiatrists were the first ones to sign off her case, documenting in the chart that Elizabeth's physical injuries and her resultant paraplegia would be too great a challenge for the psychiatric staff to handle. Clearly, they were not willing to accept Elizabeth to the psychiatric ward once we were ready to release her from our trauma service. She desperately needed psychiatric help, but once again it didn't seem that she would be getting what she needed. Her physical wounds had sufficiently healed after two weeks time to get her into a physical rehabilitation program. She was accepted into a local facility where she left, never to be seen by me or my partners again. I was frustrated and angry at the psychiatrists who discharged Elizabeth from the other psychiatric hospital on the day she then later tried to kill herself. But I was equally disappointed in our own psychiatrist.

Still reeling as well over how the psychiatrists had refused to treat my Munchausen patient, I requested that the chief of psychiatry review Samantha Acardo's case, hoping to gain some clarity as to why they reversed my Certificate of Commitment. I heard nothing for almost six months, and then one day I received a confidential letter in my professional mail box. It was a letter from the Chairman of Quality Improvement in the department of psychiatry.

His letter stated that a board of psychiatrists reviewed Samantha's case and that they all concluded that the psychiatrist who interviewed Samantha met the standard of care regarding her psychiatric recommendations. The board also concluded that Munchausen syndrome is a disorder that requires extensive psychiatric therapy, and could not be adequately managed over a short period of time. There were no additional comments pertaining to the case, and no specific answer as to why they reversed my Certificate of Commitment. The letter was short and cold. I was completely dissatisfied by the Psychiatry Department's response but I also didn't want to create a war between our professional services. I simply laughed with disgust as I tore the letter in two and tossed it into the shredder. If the author thought that this letter might have somehow regained my confidence and trust in the professional opinions of mental health providers, the author was certainly mistaken.

15

The Illegal Alien Problem

Everyone Has an Angle

My family and I enjoy watching old movies and one of our annual favorites is the 1954 Bing Crosby classic *White Christmas*. There is a scene in the movie where Bob Wallace, played by Bing Crosby, chuckles at Rosemary Clooney, telling her that he has figured out her "angle." Clooney, playing one of the two Haynes sisters in a singing-dancing duo seeking their big break into the show-business world, invited Crosby and his show partner played by Danny Kaye to watch the girls' performance under the false pretense of an alleged favor to the Haynes sisters' brother, who had served with Crosby's character in Europe during World War II. In the movie, Crosby's character figures out the girls' ruse, and when gently confronted by Crosby, the mildly disturbed Clooney retorts that she and her sister certainly did not have an angle. But Crosby, neither upset nor disappointed by his being lured to the performance hall by two girls just wanting to become noticed, simply cozied up in his chair, lit his pipe, and told Clooney not to worry because "everybody's got an angle."

One person who I remember having a very mischievous angle was Mr. Jumoke Okuwa, the estranged husband of Kapinga Okuwa, both immigrants from Nigeria, and in America on an unauthorized, self-extended traveler's visa. Both visas had been expired for more than six years.

I barely knew Mr. Okuwa, as he rarely made visits to the hospital and he never answered his phone when we attempted to call him. One morning an extremely well-dressed, black man with a heavy African accent came to our Trauma Services office and asked to see one of the trauma surgeons. I was in-house and on call that day. When notified of the visitor, I came down to meet him. He introduced himself to me as an attorney representing Mr. Okuwa, and he requested that I sign a document stating that his wife, Kapinga, was mentally incompetent as a result of her brain injuries. The attorney also asked that I might render the medical opinion that the husband should have full power-of-attorney rights over all matters pertaining to Mrs. Okuwa.

Immediately smelling a rat, I asked the attorney why his client had suddenly taken an interest in his estranged wife's well-being. He answered me by stating that his client eagerly wanted to get his wife all of the government benefits entitled to her—financial benefits the attorney would see got paid to Mrs. Okuwa.

Flash backward about six months when Mrs. Okuwa, the forty-four-year-old driver and sole occupant of a car, crashed into a tree at a moderately high rate of speed. Paramedics found her unconscious at the scene, but she partially regained consciousness in the field, and began to vomit multiple times. She would not open her eyes, she could not speak, and her arms and legs extended and rotated inward when the paramedics poked her skin when starting her intravenous line. She was comatose when she arrived at our trauma center. In order to prevent her from further inhaling her saliva and stomach contents, I quickly placed a breathing tube through her mouth and into her trachea, securely connecting it to the ventilator. Her blood pressure was normal and the only place from where she was actively bleeding was a large scalp wound. I easily controlled the non-life-threatening bleeding by quickly stapling together the cut, bloody edges after a several minute scrub and washout.

I ordered the usual complement of X-rays and CT scans, which revealed several injuries, none of which seemed likely to be life-threatening. Her most serious injury was a traumatic, subarachnoid hemorrhage of the brain, seen on the CT scan images as wisps of white material serpentining through the shallow crevices on the surface of the brain's cortex. As opposed to several other types of traumatic brain hemorrhages, subarachnoid bleeding is rarely a surgical condition. Whereas localized collections of blood between the brain and skull can cause life-threatening brain compression, increased pressure within the skull, and downward herniation of the brain through the two-inch-diameter opening at the bottom of the skull—an inevitably lethal event—subarachnoid bleeding almost never behaves in such a manner.

Traumatic subarachnoid hemorrhage rarely causes death, but it does cause serious and often protracted disability. Injured patients often do not wake up for weeks. Once out of their comatose state, they often have serious impairments in their abilities to think, concentrate, and perform even the simplest of tasks, such as feeding themselves, and going to the bathroom. They often have profound behavioral disturbances, crying out when hungry or agitated, and frequently require soft restraints placed on their wrists to prevent them from pulling out their intravenous lines and their indwelling bladder catheters.

In addition to her brain injury, Kapinga also had a fractured bone in her neck. Some cervical spine fractures—as we call them—can be fairly trivial re-quiring essentially no treatment at all. However, some can be profoundly dev-astating, with associated injuries to the spinal cord causing quadriplegia of both arms and legs. Fortunately for Kapinga, her neck injury was not very seri-ous, and her spinal cord was not injured. Unfortunately, however, the fracture did extend through several parts of her fourth of the seven neck bones, making it critically important that we keep her neck immobilized in a rigid collar for perhaps up to two months.

Her chest CT scan demonstrated numerous broken ribs on her left side and an accumulation of blood between her lung and her chest wall. The amount of blood in her chest was concerning, but not alarming. I was quite confident that I could manage the problem by inserting a chest tube into her thorax and drain the bloody fluid into a set of collection bottles connected to the chest drainage tube. Inevitably, the bleeding would stop on its own, after which we would dis-continue the chest tube, and Kapinga's ribs would be allowed to heal.

Once back in the emergency room, I inserted a half-inch-diameter tube through a small incision cut into her chest and I evacuated the four hundred or so milliliters of blood, which had collected in her chest since the crash. I stitched the tube to her skin, securely taped the tubing into position, and I re-viewed the rest of my diagnostic data.

I found no other hidden injuries so I concluded that Mrs. Okuwa would not need any glamorous or sophisticated trauma surgery. Performing surgery is usu-ally the highlight of my day, but there would be no surgery for Kapinga, since all of her injuries would be amenable to nonsurgical, critical care management in the intensive care unit and eventually on the general hospital floor once she was definitively stabilized and off the ventilator.

Contrary to what most people likely imagine, but all too familiar to trauma surgeons, a large percentage of even critically injured trauma patients require no surgery at all other than minor bedside procedures, such as suture repair of skin lacerations or the placement of chest tubes, which I had done for Mrs. Okuwa. The very nature of trauma care, however, necessitates that those caring for trauma patients be well versed in all aspects of surgical as well as non-surgical treatment. Without a doubt, the nonsurgical, critical care aspect of trauma management can often be just as arduous as the complicated surgeries trauma surgeons and the subspecialty surgical consultants perform.

Mrs. Okuwa's brain injury would likely keep her in the hospital for a while. Having treated thousands of brain-injured patients with injuries similar to Kapinga's, I knew that her disability would not be short-lived, and would require extreme patience and understanding by the family members who would be caring for her long after discharge. Wanting to brief Kapinga's family and prepare them for the future, I looked for anyone in the waiting room who might know Mrs. Okuwa.

But no one had come to the hospital inquiring about my patient's injuries. The chaplain on duty that day spent several hours poring over the contact list found on her cell phone, making call after call and trying to identify a relative to whom I could brief. Finally, the name of a man sharing the same last name as Kapinga was reached. He identified himself as Kapinga's husband.

Despite the fact that most spouses come to the hospital immediately upon notification of an injury of that magnitude, Mr. Okuwa did not show up until the following day. When he did arrive, he spent only a few minutes at his wife's bedside before abruptly leaving. According to the intensive care unit nurse caring for Kapinga, Mr. Okuwa stated that he and Kapinga had not lived together for over four years, but they still were in fact legally married. He showed very little interest in his estranged wife's injured condition. After that first visit, he never again came back to the hospital to visit and he never once called to inquire about her condition or about any progress she might be making.

Mrs. Okuwa became a serious challenge for our social workers. They quickly established that she was an illegal alien. Like so many other illegal aliens brought into our trauma center, there were no relatives to be found who would come forward and provide us with any information as to her past medical history or potential family support system. Such information is critically important when figuring out how and where we would eventually be able to discharge her once her stay at our hospital was no longer necessary.

Kapinga was just one of many illegal aliens I have treated over the years who strain our health-care system. She was uninsured, and being an illegal alien, she was not even eligible for long-term, state-funded Medicaid support. Her status guaranteed that neither I nor any of my trauma associates would ever receive so much as a dollar in financial compensation for the numerous hours of care we would provide to her. Fortunately, Medicaid would cover some of the hospital administration's expenses, as the tax-paying citizenry would be charged for her care and for the care of others like her by way of tax deductions from the citizens' semiweekly paychecks.

But the state doesn't pay for any necessary aftercare, and I knew that there would likely be no rehabilitation center or nursing home that would be willing to care of Mrs. Okuwa after she no longer needed to be at our facility. I knew from countless past experiences that Kapinga would be unable to care for herself long after she didn't require inpatient hospitalization. With no source of funding, she could not go to a rehabilitation center or a nursing home. With no family willing to help her, she would have no place to go. Unable to help herself, I knew that we would be the only ones left interested in her overall well-being. As a result, I knew that she would be staying with us for a very, very long time.

Mrs. Okuwa did not wake up even after a full week in our intensive care unit. She remained intubated, breathed for by the ventilator, with her neck rigidly immobilized in a custom-made, cervical spine collar. The collar was provided by a local orthotics company at no charge to our patient. The costs would undoubtedly be passed along to the many other patients they served who did have the means to pay.

Because her progress was so slow, I ordered an MRI scan of Kapinga's brain to look for evidence of additional injuries too subtle to be picked up by the faster, yet less sensitive CT scanner. In fact, she did have additional injuries—diffuse axonal shearing injuries, which we often just call *shear injury*—which were still nonoperative in nature, but portended an even poorer prognosis for recovery. Shear injury occurs when traumatic twisting occurs deep within the white matter tracts of the brain. The white matter contains billions of microscopic linear

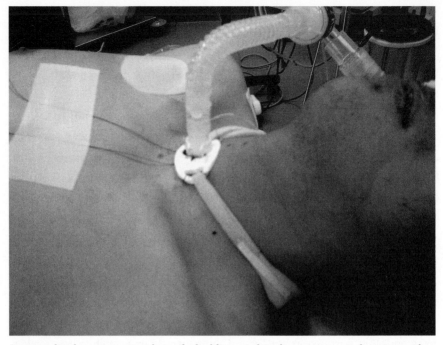

An immediately postoperative photo of a freshly created tracheostomy in a male patient with a traumatic brain injury.

fibers connecting the brain cortex—which initiates and processes brain activities—to the muscles and organ systems below. The neuronal, white matter fibers are densely compacted and pass through an area within the upper brain stem called the Ascending Reticular Activating System, or ARAS. The ARAS is one of the areas of the brain that controls whether a body is awake or asleep, and thus comatose or alert. When the densely compacted white matter tracts get twisted, microscopic interruptions—tiny little tears—occur in random areas, which dampen the higher brain's input to the rest of the body, including the ARAS. Patients with sheer injury often remain comatose or obtunded for prolonged periods of time, and remain in a semisleep state until spontaneous healing starts to take place. There is very little anyone can do to speed the healing process, and there is no guaranteed time line predicting if and when healing will actually take place.

Knowing that Kapinga's sheer injury would be keeping her comatose for an even longer period of time than originally anticipated, I began to consider her long-term, breathing status. She had been on the ventilator for over a week and she had shown no signs of waking up. She was in no condition to have her breathing tube removed, as it was the only thing guaranteeing that she would get appropriate amounts of oxygen to her already injured brain. But like all things in medicine, every drug, surgery, and treatment modality has its potentially harmful side effects in addition to its benefits. Leaving the breathing tube in for more than about two weeks time increases the chances that the patient's trachea—the natural structure through which air passes between the mouth and lungs, and in which the artificial breathing tube sits—could develop potentially irreversible injury. The injury is almost akin to the pressure sores, which develop on the backsides of bedridden people too weak to reposition themselves. Well aware of the potential problem, I scheduled Mrs. Okuwa for a tracheostomy as well as for the placement of a semipermanent feeding tube, which I would perform if she continued to show no signs of improvement over the course of the ensuing few days. The time passed without any change, and as planned, I performed the two minor operations on Mrs. Okuwa.

Over the next few weeks, we were able to wean Kapinga from the ventilator, and eventually allow her to breathe through her tracheostomy tube, unassisted

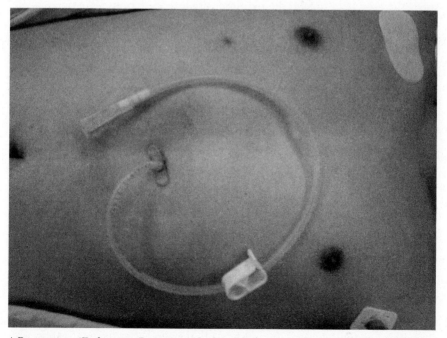

A Percutaneous Endoscopic Gastrostomy feeding tube—commonly referred to as a PEG tube—placed in a male patient with a traumatic brain injury.

by the machine. I subsequently was also able to remove her chest tube. My partners and I continued to round on Kapinga every morning. We reviewed her vital signs and we ensured that her neck brace was appropriately adjusted. We examined her heart, lungs, abdomen, and limbs for any evidence of potential complications not uncommon to the chronically ill, bedridden patient. For a good week she had nightly fevers. We searched diligently for the source of her hidden infection, performing blood cultures, sputum cultures, and urine cultures. We performed several ultrasound examinations of her arms and legs, looking for inflammatory blood clots, but for several days none of our tests revealed anything useful. Finally, one of Kapinga's many blood and sputum cultures grew out an infectious organism, allowing us to treat her pneumonia with the appropriate antibiotics, which eventually made her well. We fed her continuously throughout her stay with liquid nutrients through the feeding tube I had placed through her abdominal wall directly into her stomach. I tried to stimulate her mind daily by attempting to engage her in conversation, but never received any real indication that she was able to mentally process anything of that which I had been saying to her.

Kapinga was still semicomatose. She was no longer critically ill, nor was she really even sick. In fact, she required very little care from a physician at all. My partners and I still rounded on her every day, as is required of us, but we rarely found anything requiring a physician's order. She didn't even require much skilled nursing care. Most of the care she needed could have been provided by anyone with compassion and a kind heart. Kapinga could not care for herself at all. She was completely dependent on the nurses and nurse's aides attending to her and feeding her, bathing her, and maintaining her basic hygiene standards. She exhibited no control of her bowels or bladder and she required frequent diaper changes. Being a woman still within her reproductive years, the nurses even needed to attend to Kapinga's feminine hygiene needs.

About six weeks into her stay with us on the trauma service, Kapinga finally starting showing some basic signs of improvement. She demonstrated minimal interaction with those who cared for her during brief periods throughout the day. She became less agitated and impulsive, allowing her periods of time free from the protective bondage of her soft restraints. Having been bedridden for so long, she was very weak, and getting her out of bed required the brute strength of several physical therapists. At that stage of her hospitalization, she had still not walked even one step.

And then one day, nearly two months after her initial admission, Kapinga started to show some real improvement. I was making my usual, morning floor rounds and I was about to go into Mrs. Okuwa's room, expecting to find the same, moderately vegetative woman I had seen on so many previous mornings. Just prior to my entering her room, a nurse stopped me and, with a big smile on her face, informed me that Kapinga was doing a lot better. I smiled at the nurse politely, thinking that she was obviously more optimistic that me, and doubting that things could have improved much, if at all, over the past day or two.

But to my surprise, Kapinga had, in fact, improved markedly. As if blinders had been removed from her eyes, my once blank-staring patient looked directly at me. She smiled at me and tracked my movements as I moved from one side of her bed to the other. I began talking to her, telling her that she had been involved in an accident, and that she had been with us for over two long months. Looking a bit dismayed, she gave me a wide-eyed, surprised look. She was obviously confused, but she was clearly more awake than ever before.

Seizing the opportunity, I engaged the physical therapists to begin an aggressive rehabilitation program. The entire therapy team was more than happy to oblige, as they too became fascinated with the fortuitous and favorable turn of events. For the next several weeks, the entire team of therapists—physical therapists, occupational therapists, and speech therapists—went above and beyond helping Kapinga regain her independence, with a clear understanding that there was little to no possibility that an outside rehabilitation center would be willing to accept her considering her illegal alien status.

Other than Mr. Okuwa's five-minute appearance at the hospital the day after his wife's accident, no one else had come to visit Kapinga throughout her stay with us. We knew by her list of cell-phone contacts that she had plenty of acquaintances, and we had hoped that her husband would have told somebody of his wife's accident. Yet, no one came. It was as if no one outside of the hospital cared at all about Kapinga. The nurses, doctors, therapists, and technicians seemed to be all that Kapinga had, and all who cared about her.

Our social workers did make several attempts to get rehabilitation institutions to accept Kapinga on a charity basis. Although several facilities were willing to consider taking her despite her lack of a funding source, they would only accept her if we could assure them that there was a family willing to take back Kapinga once the goals of the rehabilitation facilities were met. They, too, didn't want to be stuck with a long-term resident with no ultimate place to send her once all therapies had been completed.

I began trying to reengage Kapinga's alleged husband. He continued to remain elusive, never returning my calls. One day, a minister from Kapinga's church presented himself to us and offered to help however he might be able. The minister seemed to be an honorable man truly interested in Kapinga. He genuinely wanted to help, and he listened intently to our plight. He told me that both Mr. and Mrs. Okuwa were members of his congregation, but although Kapinga routinely attended Sunday services, Mr. Okuwa was rarely seen. The husband apparently paid little attention to his legally married spouse, and they had lived apart for years. Trying to seek help for our patient, the pastor went back to his congregation, asking parishioners to volunteer their services after Kapinga's discharge. Unfortunately, despite the minister's genuine willingness to help, he could not get any of his parish members to reliably commit to what we and the rehabilitation personnel needed. Kapinga still had no place to go, and she remained with us on the trauma service.

For weeks, the therapists gave extra special attention to our patient, truly taking her under their wing. They would often take Kapinga on walks down to the cafeteria and eat lunch together. After a while, the occupational therapists— trying to prepare Kapinga for independent living after discharge—would give her handfuls of change and watch as Kapinga counted her money as she paid for the daily meals. It was becoming quite clear that Kapinga would soon be ready to leave us.

Seeing the progress his parishioner had made with his own eyes, the pastor went back to his church again seeking help for Mrs. Okuwa. Finally, someone did step up to the plate and offered to take her into their home. And finally, after spending three months in our hospital, Kapinga was discharged to the home of a kind, good Samaritan.

The hospital graciously paid for a nurse and a physical therapist to visit their home three times per week, and we saw Mrs. Okuwa in our trauma clinic several times before she just stopped returning altogether. Although Kapinga had made great improvements since her admission, she still demonstrated evidence of significant disability. She acted in a slow and juvenile manner, and she was emotionally very labile. Her behavior, however, was not unexpected and was a usual consequence of severe, traumatic brain injury.

Flash forward back again to my meeting with Mr. Okuwa's slick attorney in our trauma office. I found it rather intriguing that Kapinga's husband would have suddenly developed a conscience, wanting to protect his wife's interests by securing disability funds on her behalf. Remembering how her husband had refused to visit, how he never answered his phone over a period of several months, and how he wouldn't return a single one of the numerous voice mails left by me or the other staff members made me even more suspicious of his intentions. I thought about signing the attorney's document just to get him to leave me alone. But I decided not to enable his client's almost certainly nefarious—if not fraudulent or illegal—activities. I owed Mr. Okuwa and his attorney no favors, but I did feel a need to look out for Kapinga. For all I knew, Kapinga had fled the area, or perhaps she was in hiding from the man who had abandoned her. I decided to not cooperate with the lawyer.

I smiled at Mr. Okuwa's attorney and told him that I had no knowledge of his client's wife's current degree of disability at that time. I told him that Mrs. Okuwa hadn't returned to our clinic in a long while. I did offer to accommodate the attorney if his client might be willing to help us. I stated that if Mr. Okuwa would be so kind as to bring his wife back to our clinic for a follow-up evaluation, I would be happy to give my professional assessment of his wife's disability status.

Frustrated by my position and by my unwillingness to blindly cooperate, the attorney had nothing to say. He gave me a half-cocked smile, nodded his head slightly, and then politely departed the trauma office. I never again heard from either of the Okuwas, or from the attorney. I suspect that Mrs. Okuwa had been whisked away by one of her parishioners, or perhaps had even gone back to Nigeria. As for Mr. Okuwa, I believe that he was disappointed that I hadn't secured his opportunity to profit from his estranged wife's injuries. And I believe that to his chagrin, I had in fact figured out his angle.

16

Off to War

Deployment to Afghanistan

In 2004, my regular life was put on hold after I received a set of military orders sending me overseas to support the war in Afghanistan. Several months prior, my reserve SEAL team sent me to the East Coast for a short period of service to provide medical support to one of the active duty, special operations teams. For the most part, I managed minor orthopedic injuries incurred by the elite military members pushing themselves beyond their reasonable, physical limitations. I also gave several lectures to the enlisted medical crew on various trauma topics. While teaching, I did my best to enlighten the corpsmen on my favorite, military medical topic, "Delivery of Trauma Care in the Austere Environment."

My audience was a group of seasoned, Special Operations war veterans. They were also enlisted corpsmen with medical training commensurate with that of civilian paramedics. They received my teachings well and they expressed gratitude for having an experienced trauma surgeon willing to share civilian experiences and advice with them. I, in turn, was happy to have had the opportunity to teach to an audience so eager to learn. They listened to everything I had to say, and they eagerly soaked up my impromptu lectures like human sponges. The corpsmen and medics were fascinated by my stories of real-world trauma care. They appreciated my sharing several of my pearls of wisdom, which might help in their management of future casualties during their inevitable return to the battle zone. And they enjoyed regaling me with their own stories.

I worked out at the SEAL team gym every day, and I socialized with the commandos regularly. My brief stint on the East Coast was quite enjoyable, and was a much-needed restful break from my usual mental grind. It provided me great relief from the endless responsibilities of the trauma service, and it allowed me to reconnect with the active-duty, special operations side of the military I had enjoyed so much in my past years.

On the last day of my short period of time assigned to the unit, the senior medical officer of the group told me that things were getting complicated in Afghanistan, and that I was again needed by my old group at United States Special Operations Command (USSOCOM). I was even asked to consider going back onto active duty full-time, but my family and I were settled and I respectfully declined his offer to uproot my wife and kids again and make yet another geographic move. After listening to the senior medical officer, however, I knew that it would only be a matter of time until I received a set of deployment orders activating me from reserve status to active duty status. And I knew that I would soon be going to Afghanistan. As I anticipated, about one month after returning back to my home and to my civilian job, I received my orders.

My orders to deploy did not trouble me. The acts of terrorism committed against my homeland on September 11th, made me deeply regret leaving the service in the first place, and I saw the orders as an opportunity to contribute to the war effort I believed in wholly. I felt fortunate to be able to again serve with my old unit at USSOCOM, and in a strange sort way, I looked forward to joining my former brothers in arms in the war zone. Several weeks before I was to be forward deployed, I was mobilized to my old military unit where I received numerous briefings on multiple military matters of importance to the mission overseas. They included intelligence updates, security briefings, and the most recent rules of engagement.

I drew my weapons from the armory and I spent several days sighting in my M-4, semiautomatic rifle as well as sharpening my pistol skills. I drew my deployment gear from the supply chief and I custom configured my rucksack and my body armor. I updated my ISOPREP data card, which gives the list of questions I should be asked—along with the appropriate answers I should give in return—should I be captured by the enemy and my nation require proof-of-life verification. I received an extensive list of contacts with whom I would link up with in Afghanistan, and I waited for the day when the military airlift command would take me to where I needed to be.

On the morning of my deployment, at 0400, I stood on the tarmac waiting to board the massive, C-5 Galaxy—one of the largest military aircraft in the world. The monstrous gray jet, with its twenty-eight wheels and its four mammoth engines was an eerie sight as I walked up the ridged planks and boarded the plane's open rear clamshell. I thought that my five-foot, seventy-pound rucksack, my two duffel bags, and I would have had plenty of room in that spacious airbus, but to my dismay, I shared my nineteen-hour flight not only with several hundred other men and their gear, but also with a fifty-two-foot long MH-47 Chinook helicopter, chained to the floor of the transport plane by large, heavy links of steel. I found an empty section of web seating toward the rear of the aircraft along the wall of the fuselage, set my gear down by my feet, and settled into my cramped, little space. Barely able to hear above the deafening whine of the turbines, I closed my eyes trying to sleep away the next day of my life while in transit to the war zone.

Several hours into the flight, my muscles were in spasms and I could not find a comfortable position. I noticed that during my interval of slumber, several service members—obviously having made the painful trip before—had sprawled about lying recumbent on whatever piece of flat ground they could find. They found creative sleeping areas such as their neatly arranged gear bags, and even the large, flat engines of the helicopter. Wanting to get in on the action, I saw my desired area—an unoccupied space of floor underneath the huge, tethered bird, next to one of its wheels. I quickly grabbed my camouflage poncho liner from my rucksack and pulled it and myself under the helicopter. I arranged my thin layer of padding exactly how I wanted it, and I snuggled next to the rear tire. After taking a look upward at the underbelly of the rotary aircraft, I closed my eyes and managed to get several more hours of needed sleep.

To my dissatisfaction, I found that sleeping under a helicopter was neither comfortable nor restful. I awoke after about seven hours into the flight and needed to use the bathroom. Knowing that the latrine was located near the front of the aircraft, I crawled out from under my hiding area, and I walked along the outcroppings of the helicopter so as to not step on anyone, making my way to where I needed to be. After I relieved myself, I made my way back to my piece of hard ground where I lay for two more hours until we made a refueling stop in Germany, where we all disembarked the aircraft to stretch our legs.

After about an hour and a half delay, we again boarded the winged behemoth and we headed off to war. The next ten hours were torture, as I negotiated short bursts of sleep, pangs in my bladder and stomach, and fears of both what lay ahead of me as well as what I left back home. The C-5 crew chief informed us when we had entered the unfriendly airspace of the combat area, and I knew that we would soon be landing in a place completely unfamiliar to me. But *soon* turned out to be more like two hours. When we finally made our nighttime approach to the expeditionary runway, I wanted nothing more than to get the hell off that aircraft. We landed with an enormous thud, as the 850,000–pound flying machine set down onto the crudely constructed runway on the Bagram Air Base.

We landed on a moonless night and I was more than happy to disembark my flying prison cell. I exited the aircraft, adorned in military body armor with my M-4 rifle slung across my chest and my nine-millimeter pistol holstered to my right thigh. I looked among the many silhouettes for my initial contact. I could barely see, and I wouldn't have recognized him even if I had full use of my sight, but thankfully I heard someone call out my name.

"Lieutenant Commander Cole—over here," shouted one of the USSO-COM corpsmen. I walked over in the direction of the voice calling my name and met my escort. He was a pleasant young man who informed me that he had been waiting for me for several hours, as my flight had apparently landed later than scheduled. I was unaware of the in-flight delay, and I never heard why we had been apparently been diverted from our original flight path. I was happy that he had waited for me, for without him, I wouldn't have had the slightest idea where to go. The corpsman introduced himself to me as "Tom," and he told me that everyone was pretty much on a first-name basis aboard the USSO-COM compound. Tom helped me load my rucksack and my two bags into an awaiting military vehicle and together we drove to my quarters.

While en route, Tom told me that the operational tempo was high, with missions being conducted every few nights. He told me that after I got some sleep, he would introduce me to the group I would soon be working with, and to the man I would be working directly for. We arrived at the heavily fortified and well-guarded USSOCOM compound—a base within a base. After showing the guard my credentials, I was escorted to my living quarters. My new home was a wooden hut I shared at times with as few as two other members, and at other times with as many as five. I dragged my gear into the wooden structure and was introduced to my hut-mates, all of whom were wide awake, some reading and others playing cards. It was well after midnight.

I was tired and I desperately needed some sleep. The guys who shared my hut told me that they would keep quiet and let me get some rest, but they advised me to sleep only briefly, as the USSOCOM group was on what they called a reverse day-night operations cycle. They explained to me that they slept when the sun was up, and they lived and worked when the sun was down. I recognized that if I slept too long I might never acclimate to the time-cycle change. But I was so exhausted. I was experiencing an extreme case of jet lag and I needed to get at least some rest. I opened my rucksack and laid out my sleeping bag on the hand-constructed plywood bed I was directed to. I closed my eyes and quickly drifted off, getting some much needed shut-eye.

Feeling refreshed after only a few hours rest, I awoke. By my watch, it was only a few hours until sunrise, but the guys were still up and they offered to give me a tour of the Special Operations compound. The USSOCOM area consisted of a large network of interconnected tents, wooden huts, and box toilets. Portable showers were also scattered about, and the whole array of structures sat on a thick pile of medium-size rocks, which kept the underlying dust and sand from kicking up more than our lungs could bear. Our special compound on Bagram Air Base was completely surrounded by ten-foot-high walls of HESCO barriers topped with two layers of razor studded, concertina wire. The HESCO barriers were the ingenious invention of a now undoubtedly rich person. They were simply constructed boxes of heavy cardboard—each large enough to hold a standard-size refrigerator, and each surrounded by a chain-link-fence-type outer covering. Each HESCO was filled to the brim with earth, and when stacked one atop the next, it served as a protective barrier against potential rockets, mortars, and small-arms gunfire.

The encampment was dark and I couldn't appreciate any of the area details, but I was eager to see more of my new surroundings after the sun rose. But aware of the reverse, day-night operations cycle, I decided to follow the lead of my hut-mates and again lay down just as the sun was breaking the horizon. I was still suffering from the effects of transoceanic jet lag.

I slept soundly despite my several-hour postflight nap and I was awakened by the sounds of the others in the room. They were getting ready to migrate to the daily command briefings in a tented area of the compound, which I wondered if I, too, was supposed attend. My question was answered after a knock on the hut door revealed Tom, my arrival escort, who told me to quickly get dressed as we would be on our way to the command briefing. I threw on my uniform and together we walked out into the blinding sunlight. I had no idea how powerful the sun's rays could be. I was thankful that I had been issued a pair of black Oakley sunglasses, which I quickly affixed to my face. We trudged through the rocks over to the tented area in which sat the large, Tactical Operations Center—known as the TOC.

In the TOC (pronounced *tock*), several dozen individuals were seated in metal folding chairs behind long cafeteria-style tables. The tables were littered with a complicated array of monitors, screens, and computers. Several key people maintained a twenty-four-hour presence in the TOC, including the operations officer, the intelligence officer, and representatives from each of the various elements of the Special Operations community. In the back of the tented area were several dozen loose chairs and plenty of standing room, where non-key individuals congregated and listened passively to the daily command briefings. I grabbed one of the backroom chairs and sat down, but I was soon directed to the main area of the TOC, where I apparently had an assigned seat awaiting me. I was led to my place of honor in front of a table marked with a sign reading TASK FORCE SURGEON. Hoping that no one would ask me to make a statement, I sat down and I introduced myself to the people around me.

Moments later, a firm hand smacked the back of my shoulder. I looked around and I saw a very familiar and welcome face. It was Will, and I was so very glad to see him. Lieutenant Colonel William Flanner was a trauma and critical care surgeon, enthralled by the minutia of research and scientific publications, but with enough of an adventurous side to enjoy the Special Operations lifestyle. He was one of my past USSOCOM brothers and a former close friend with whom I had served on missions past. Greeting each other with a traditional man-hug, we did our best to catch up on the four years since I left The Unit, knowing that the meeting was soon to start. Will was the current task force surgeon, and I would be replacing him. He and I would spend the next week together as I would transition into his job, and he would transition out of it.

All conversation in the room was abruptly silenced as someone loudly shouted, "Attention!" Instinctively, we all stood rigidly with arms locked down at our sides, as our commanding general swiftly entered the room.

"As you were, gentlemen," the general ordered calmly. We each took our seats and remained quiet. What followed next was a fascinating, two-hour meeting—a detailed and well-orchestrated series of presentations from representatives of each of the key elements of The Unit. The briefings covered everything from the local weather forecast, the number of personnel from each of the subunits onboard, recently gathered intelligence information, planned operations, and logistics issues. At the appropriate time, Will gave a two-minute speech reporting on the medical status of the unit personnel as well as the health of the enemy prisoners held in the Bagram prison. When all of the key presentations were completed, the general spoke. I was immediately impressed by his command presence, his insightful thought process, and his demonstration of in-depth knowledge in every one of the areas briefed. I felt very comfortable with the man in charge, and I looked forward to working for him.

At the end of our meeting, we were again called to attention when the general departed. He exited into a small side tent, which was obviously where his command office had been established. After the general had cleared the confines of the main area, chatter again started up among the group, and Will and I talked some more, each very happy to see the other. He briefed me on my responsibilities as task force surgeon, which basically boiled down to the fact that I was soon to be in charge of all health-care matters of the entire Special Operations Task Force, including hundreds of men, and dozens of enemy prisoners. Writing down numerous details and feeling a little overwhelmed with my newly assigned responsibilities, Will decided to stop with the briefing and introduce me to the man I was directly responsible to: the commanding general.

Major General Steve McCormick was a thin but muscular man with chiseled facial features. I guessed by his appearance that he was about fifty years old, but well aware of his rank and position of leadership, I'm sure that he was at least several years older than he appeared. He sat behind his simple desk, wearing reading glasses and looking down at a document he had already begun poring over. Will rapped on the general's tent flap and requested permission for us to enter. The general quickly welcomed us in, and Will introduced us, informing the general that I would soon be talking over the task force surgeon's position.

General McCormick extended his hand and introduced himself to me simply as "Steve." I shook his hand firmly and responded by saying, "It's a pleasure to meet you, sir." Regardless of how the general had introduced himself to me, there was no way that I would ever consider calling a general officer anything other than "sir." We engaged in cursory conversation before it became clear that the general had things more important to do than chitchat. Recognizing the appropriate time to excuse ourselves, we again shook hands, and Will and I left the command tent and ambled back into the Tactical Operations Center.

By that time, I had been awake for only about three hours but had not eaten anything of significance for almost a full day. I confided to Will that I really needed to get some food, and he told me that we had just enough time to get to the chow tent before it closed. We exited the main tent complex and went outside, heading over for some sustenance. When we exited the synthetic gathering place, I was a bit confused by the fact that the sun had fallen. It was dusk and the sun would soon be fully below the horizon. Remembering that we were on a reverse, day-night operations cycle, the lack of daylight quickly made sense to me, but I knew that it would take me a few days to fully get used to.

The Bagram chow tent was a welcome sight, for I was absolutely starving. Will and I pulled back the tent flap of the entrance area and each of us grabbed one of the cardboard trays, compartmentalized so as to separate each of the servings of food issued to us by the food personnel. After they filled my tray with several scoops of military rations, Will and I found a spot to sit, and we inhaled our meals. Between mouthfuls, we talked more about each of our past four years, and Will and I caught up on old times.

When we had finished eating, we walked back to the hut area and we headed toward his living quarters. Inside were a number of men who I would soon be working with very closely. I didn't know any of the guys, unfortunately, but each of them was a member of the elite USSOCOM medical team to which I had once belonged, and to which I again belonged for the duration of my Afghanistan assignment. I introduced myself to each of the guys and we engaged in cordial conversation.

I knew that they were a tight group—as we had all been when I was a full-time regular—and that we would have plenty of time to get to know each other. I looked forward to what I knew would be some very interesting times spent with those guys. Not wanting to wear out my welcome too soon, I told them that I had some unpacking to do, and Will and I left. Fortunately, my hut was just a stone's throw away from theirs, and I told Will that I wanted to get to know the guys in my own hut a bit more. I also needed to unpack some of my bags. He told me that he still had a lot to show me, but that we could meet up again in a few hours. We planned to again link up at midnight, which was when the chow tent served the final meal, where we would eat some more and continue my briefing.

After socializing with my roommates, Will and I went back to the chow tent to get some more to eat. He then took me to a place he stressed that I keep very close tabs on. He took me to an out-of-the-way area surrounded by yet one more wall of HESCO barriers and concertina wire. The building was clearly not built by the U.S, military, but was obviously some sort of storage facility constructed by the Afghanis or perhaps by the Russians during the occupation years several decades before. We walked inside the hardened area, where we were greeted by an armorer to whom Will handed over his weapons and ammunition magazines. Following his lead, I did the same. He then removed his uniform top thus wearing only his brown undershirt and camouflage pants and he told me to do the same. I asked him why we were undressing and handing over our weapons. He told me that we had entered the enemy-prisoner-holding area. No one wanted a prisoner to accidentally get ahold of one of our weapons, and we didn't want any of them to know our identities. Because our names were embroidered onto our uniforms, every person doing business in the holding area removed his shirt.

A prison guard then opened a heavy six-inch thick door, and we walked down a short flight of stairs into a narrow hallway lined on either side with small, individual cells. Each cell held a high-value prisoner captured on military raids. The facility was only a temporary prisoner-holding area, where high-value targets were kept for several days after capture, hoping they would divulge important intelligence information to the specialized officers who interrogated them on a daily basis. As the task force surgeon, it was Will's job to ensure that each of the prisoners was kept healthy, and that any of their previous medical problems were being adequately treated.

Since the overthrow of the Afghan government by the Taliban, nearly all of the nation's hospitals had been completely destroyed. Most of the Afghan doctors had been either killed or forced to leave the country, fearing torture and death. As a result, disease was common among the Afghan people, and many captured jihadist prisoners had various chronic medical afflictions, including tuberculosis and other communicable diseases. All prisoners were screened for illness and injuries and appropriately treated with standard of care medications to keep them healthy, and to hopefully gain their trust so that the prisoners would begin to feel comfortable enough to provide good intelligence to our interrogators.

As we walked the prison hallway, I peered through the small openings in each of the prison doors, noting how thin and sickly all the prisoners looked. I asked Will if they were being given enough to eat and he laughed, informing me that the prisoners were fed better than we were. Four times daily, each prisoner was given a complete, Halal meal—food considered lawful to eat by Islamic standards and approved by the local, religious leaders. He told me that the country of Afghanistan that I would soon come to know was a desolate wasteland with little food and water. I would apparently soon learn that most Afghanis were seriously malnourished and underweight. He also told me that most Taliban prisoners gained between five and ten pounds between the time they were captured, and when they were released to a more definitive prison. Will strongly recommended that I briefly check on every prisoner daily to ensure their well-being, as activist groups and protestors back home were becoming very critical in their perceptions of how the United States treated its enemy prisoners. Will assured me that the prisoners were all treated quite well at our facility, but that I needed to keep it that way.

He told me that immediately after any prisoner was captured and brought into the holding area, I was required to perform a full medical examination on him. I was required to note any injuries, wounds, or existing disease, and document a care plan for each abnormality identified. He told me that during each examination, several prison guards and intelligence officers would be present should any useful information be voluntarily leaked by any of the captives.

Will then took me to the rear of the holding area where the makeshift shower had been erected. He told me that every prisoner was offered a warm ten-minute shower every day—a luxury which none of the servicemen on the compound were entitled to. It wasn't that we couldn't shower, but we were strictly limited to no more than five-minute "navy showers," where we were to quickly wet down, turn off the water, soap up, and then quickly rinse off. We were allowed to shower no more than every other day, as water was a precious commodity in the desert. If we were lucky on any given day, the rubber bladders holding our nonprisoner shower water might be sufficiently warmed by the beating of the sun's rays, but often our showers were cold. Intrigued by what I had just learned, I realized that modern war was a politically complicated endeavor, and I knew that I would soon learn so much of what never gets publicized by the media.

Will and I left the cell area and we reclaimed our weapons, ammunition, and our uniform shirts. He next took me to the medical compound where I would spend a part of my day seeing various service members afflicted with the maladies common to any encampment or any other closely quartered group of individuals for that matter. The enlisted medics and corpsmen provided most of the sick-call care, treating diseases such as diarrhea, upper respiratory tract infections, and skin abscesses. The medical area was heavily stocked with antibiotics, ibuprofen, bandages, and many other necessary items, which would get readily dispensed to service members on a daily basis. Interestingly, I would soon learn that many healthy warriors develop asthma while in Afghanistan, as heavy clouds of fine dust are inescapable in that country—a problem that afflicted me personally while on deployment. Boxes of inhalers sat in the medication dispensing area and became a popular treatment item issued.

Noticing that there was nothing resembling a real hospital within the US-SOCOM compound, I asked Will where people with serious illness or disease, or perhaps those casualties needing surgery, were treated. He then walked me outside our compound to a military encampment on the Bagram Air Base a few hundred meters adjacent to ours where the regular army had set up a Combat Support Hospital, abbreviated by the letters CSH, and pronounced *cash*. Recognizing Will's and my USSOCOM identification badges, the gate guard at the CSH compound let us enter without being questioned. We walked into the large tent hospital unescorted. We were permitted to roam the place with carte blanche privileges.

The medical facility was actually a complicated arrangement of large tents, connected to one another, each having a unique and special purpose. There were intensive care unit tents, general medical holding tents, several operating room tents, and a large, emergency treatment tent. Pharmacy tents, equipment sterilization and processing tents, storage tents, laboratory and radiology tents, and administrative office tents complemented the treatment areas. I was impressed by how comprehensive the expeditionary medical facility was, despite its austerity. Will was recognized by several of the CSH hospital staff, including surgeons, anesthesiologists, nurses, and even the commanding officer of the medical unit. I was introduced to many of the key players in the group, and I felt certain that I would be seeing more of them in the future.

But I knew that my mission did not specifically include working at the Combat Support Hospital per se. I was assigned to USSOCOM, and my role in supporting the war was rather unique, for in addition to providing care and medical oversight to the enemy prisoners, providing oversight to the medics and corpsmen treating the everyday ailments of the unit members, and providing guidance and consultation to the commanding general on all medical matters pertaining to the Special Operations personnel, I was tasked with providing far forward medical support to the Special Operations commandos.

When combatants go to war, every one of their mothers, fathers, spouses, and children old enough to understand the risks of battle hope that there is a competent group of medical providers readily available to treat serious wounds should they be fallen by the enemy's weaponry. I was one of those medical providers. When actionable intelligence guided the elite USSOCOM assaulters to a battle site, I and a handful of other co-professionals accompanied them on their mission, always ready to provide life-saving medical care as close to the battle as possible. My team and I were usually staged in an area just adjacent

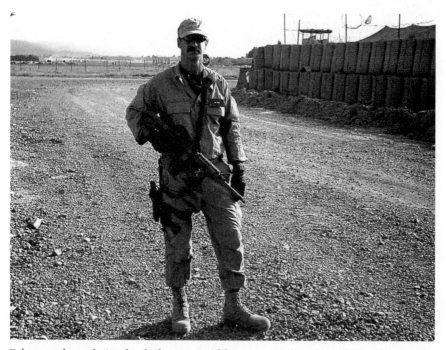

Cole, several months into his deployment to Afghanistan, standing aboard Camp Salerno near the Pakistani border. Hesco barriers in the background protect the tent area.

to the assault zone, flown in by heavily armed helicopters, where we remained vigilant, awaiting the delivery of any gravely injured casualties.

We carried specialized equipment allowing us to temporize our casualties' wounds, and to perform emergency surgery if necessary—on captured prisoners as well as U.S. service members—in one of several prepositioned mobile medical facilities located a relatively safe distance from the battle area. I would soon learn that one of my favorite areas to do emergency surgery would be in a three-tent medical unit, operated by the regular army aboard Camp Salerno—a remote encampment along the Afghanistan-Pakistan border.

I acclimated to the responsibilities of my new job and to my living conditions quite quickly. By the time Will left, I felt quite confident that I would be able to handle whatever lay ahead of me. Will departed Bagram Air Base as scheduled, leaving me in charge. I was certain that the months ahead of me would be interesting and challenging, and I eagerly awaited my new experiences.

17

A Desolate Wasteland

Afghanistan

Afghanistan is for certain the most godforsaken place I have ever been. My military career has taken me to many Third World countries over the years, but if ever there was to be a land known as a Fourth World country, Afghanistan would be that place. I flew numerous missions while on deployment, and most of those were at night. I spent my entire deployment in the southern region of the country, never having made it north of the Hindu Kush mountain range. With the exception of a few flights over Afghanistan's capital city of Kabul, I never once saw any evidence of electrical lighting—the country looked like a black abyss, as if I was flying over the ocean at night. On several occasions, however, I flew on daytime missions, usually to provide medical escort to enemy prisoners from one holding area to another, or occasionally to visit one of our injured unit members being temporarily held at one of the army's three-tent medical facilities.

Southern Afghanistan is a desolate wasteland, with miles upon miles of blowing sand dunes bordered by some of the most rugged mountains I have ever seen. Roads are sparse and are rarely paved. I saw many winding, narrow pathways hugging the rocky edges of cliffs passing through narrow channels between mountains and earthy hills. Dried riverbeds cut deeply into the scorched earth, and small packs of malnourished camels and long-haired goats wandered about looking for food and water. Wild dogs were as abundant as cockroaches, and at night their incessant howling haunted the darkness. Nomads, sometimes traveling individually and at other times in groups, could be seen from above, wandering the vast dunes and usually walking alongside one or several of their animals. They gave no hint as to where they could have possibly come from or to where in the world they were going. Reminders of the previous war with the Soviets could be seen everywhere. Carcasses of blown-up old tanks and Soviet aircraft shot down from the skies lie like beached-whale skeletons throughout the Afghan desert.

Whereas many of the buildings in the larger, named cities resembled fairly modern structures, every domicile in the hinterlands was as primitive as the clay and mud huts topped with hay roofs, which were built during biblical times. Every one of them was riddled with bullet holes and many had entire walls blown away from rockets and tank fire from wars past and present. Sadly enough, most of the structures considered uninhabitable by most people's standards, served as homes to countless Afghan families. Perhaps one of the main reasons why many local citizens rarely ventured away from their villages, tens of thousands of active land mines still lied buried in open areas, often detonated by unsuspecting, wandering children or nomads.

The Afghan people themselves were as rough and weather-beaten as the land in which they lived. Nearly everyone was thin—very close to what I might call severely malnourished—by American standards. Their skin was dry and leathery from many years of exposure to the hot, dry desert climate. Many Afghans seemed to be prematurely gray. Their collective, aged features made the people appear old in general, as their actual age was often a decade junior to how their features presented themselves. I'm not sure if any of the Afghan people really knew their exact age. The Afghans I met didn't seem to have much concern for time like we do. They awoke when the sun rose and they retired when it became too dark to see. I once asked a well-educated Pashto translator—Pashto being the native language in southern Afghanistan—how old he was. He gave me a puzzled look and he didn't even seem to understand why I would ask him such a strange question. It was as if he had never been asked this before. When the translator finally seemed to understand what it was I was asking, he answered by telling me that his mother had told him that he had been born in the great winter before the war began. I was quite sure that his mother had been referring to the war when the Soviets invaded in 1979, but I had no idea when

Afghanistan experienced what I guess they called the great winter. The guy clearly appeared to be older than twenty-five, but the truth is I had absolutely no idea how old our translator was.

Health care in Afghanistan was essentially nonexistent. In my travels down near the Pakistani border, I met a man named Dr. Ali. He was the only portly Afghani I ever saw. Dr. Ali received his medical training in Kabul, before the Taliban killed or drove out the intellectuals. He then went to Finland where he received some additional training, which sounded much like a medical internship to me. Sometime later, he returned to southern Afghanistan where he set up a clinic in a small but named village. The clinic was truly quite pathetic, but it was all that Dr. Ali could offer the people of his homeland. The clinic was actually just a large, four-walled building, with a roof overhead but with only dirt covering the ground. Wounded or sick Afghans too ill to be anywhere else, lay on Dr. Ali's clinic floor, receiving the most basic of nursing and medical care from the few untrained workers employed by the good doctor.

Dozens of metal boxes lay stacked in the primitive clinic, stuffed with bandages, vitamins, and various medications donated by the United Nations for Dr. Ali and practitioners like him to use. I saw Dr. Ali hand out packs of medications to patients who often traveled great distances to visit. However, the pill packs Dr. Ali handed out were usually either the wrong antibiotic for the particular infection being treated, or simply not enough of the drug to affect cure. The United Nation's supply boxes contained large numbers of old-generation antidepressants and ulcer medications. As a result, almost every visitor to Dr. Ali's clinic received a handful of each of the drugs, whether or not the prescriptions were indicated.

Many of the Afghan people were afflicted with chronic disease, including respiratory tract infections and diarrheal illness. Many suffered disabling, disfiguring injuries from land-mine explosions or flame burns from kerosene heaters, which tipped while they slept. I saw men with crudely amputated limbs dragged in and left by family members, ostracized by the community for their inability to work as men should. Of course, there was nothing Dr. Ali could do in these cases other than build the men simple crutches from tree limbs, as there were no prosthetics manufacturers in all of Afghanistan. I saw grotesquely burned children dropped off in front of Dr. Ali's clinic with festering, infected burn wounds over their faces, torsos, and limbs. Dr. Ali's hired help dressed and rebandaged the wounds to no avail. On a few occasions, I used some of the

Afghan doctor's crude, surgical instruments to trim away infected, nonhealing tissues from patients' wounds, which I knew could never otherwise heal.

Cultivating food was an ongoing priority for the Afghan people. Most homes had pitiful little gardens growing either in the dirt floors of the unroofed portions of their housing areas or in the outside, adjacent land spaces. There was never enough to eat. Humans and animals alike—with rare exception as in Dr. Ali's case—showed ribs tenting through the skin of their fatless bodies.

Men who had been recruited into the Al Qaeda or Taliban organizations were often just as pathetic as the peasants they terrorized. On several occasions, I escorted groups of enemy combatants captured on raids or assaults to prisoner-holding areas. I easily manhandled the skinny men, blindfolded and flex-cuffed by the American service members. I carefully guided them onto heavily guarded helicopters or fixed wing aircraft, which would take them far from the places in which they conducted their nefarious deeds. The men often had so little muscle mass that I could wrap my hand entirely around their biceps areas as I escorted them, sometimes two at a time, onto our airships.

I remember one prisoner falling as I walked him up the rear ramp of an idling helicopter. I had no difficulty keeping him suspended in midair as he regained his footing. I carefully sat the prisoners down on the floor of the aircraft and observed them throughout the flight to their prison destination, while U.S. military guards hovered over them with automatic weapons. Whereas I assumed what I would consider to be a typical seated position on the cold, aircraft floor, the Afghan prisoners never sat. Instead, they balanced on their feet in a deep crouch with their knees pushed up into their chest. Flying was obviously something very foreign to the Afghans, as they often fell from their bizarrely perched positions and periodically vomited from motion sickness as the helicopters rolled and twisted through the sky.

Despite the fact that I was assigned to a Special Operations organization engaged in a war with the Al Qaeda and Taliban terrorists, I never forgot that I was a doctor first. I treated each of the prisoners with the same compassion and dignity with which I treated my American patients and casualties. In fact, I did more life-saving, emergency surgery on the captured prisoners than I did on American servicemen, owing to the fact that we had superior body armor, weaponry, and shooting skills.

When captured enemy combatants were initially brought to the fixed, prisoner-holding areas, they were brought in one at a time into an interrogation room. There they were unmasked in front of a group of American intelligence officers, guards, and myself. That was the time when the greatest amount of useful intelligence could be obtained, as the shell shock of their capture often caused the weak and scared prisoners to blurt out loads of information useful to our intelligence officials. I never witnessed a single act of physical violence against a captured prisoner, although my comrades' screaming and shouting was often quite intimidating and effective.

My presence during those interrogations was a necessary requirement, as I carefully examined each prisoner before any actual questioning took place. Prisoners were ordered to disrobe completely and I examined every part of them looking not only for evidence of illness and wounds, but also for hidden weapons or explosives, which I occasionally found in some of the strangest places.

Despite my associates' requirements to speak harshly and with great commanding authority to the prisoners, I never spoke with anything other than a calm and civil voice. I moved slowly so as not to frighten the captives, believing that if they trusted that I would be a compassionate doctor, they would be more compliant with my treatment over the days spent in the prison cells. Many of the captured prisoners were frightened and meek, but others seethed at me with devilish looks of anger and hatred. These were the hardened terrorists who had been well trained by their leaders to resist the American tactics at intelligence gathering. We did not use any form of torture. I never saw anything done to them that hadn't ever been done to me. As a result, we often gathered no information of significance from those who firmly resisted.

I became fascinated by the commanding general's daily meetings, which I attended each morning in the Tactical Operations Center. I was most intrigued by the daily intelligence briefings given by some of the most fascinating people who presented information deciphered during prisoner interrogations. Human flow charts were displayed showing photos of enemy leaders of the various sub organizations—who the leaders were, who served as their lieutenants, and who carried out the low-level thuggery. When word was passed that a major player had been killed in battle, intelligence would be offered as to who would likely fill the void and assume command of the particular terror cell, and who would then become the priority targets.

I learned more about Al Qaeda and the Taliban than I could have ever hoped to, and it was all so very interesting to me. I learned that Osama bin Laden had a vision and a well-thought-out plan to reclaim the historical Caliphate—the

Islamic kingdom of the prophet, Mohammed, which began in the seventh century AD. The Caliphate once extended throughout all of Arabia proper and extended into the lands of northern Africa and Spain, as well as east into what is now Afghanistan and Pakistan. Bin Laden's plan, promulgated throughout his discipleship, was to again reestablish strict, Islamic control of the historical kingdom, and then expand the borders of his controlled land as far as possible. Bin Laden's executive officer, the Egyptian physician Ayman Al-Zawahiri, was likely the one giving most of the orders during my tenure in Afghanistan. He, in addition to his boss, remained elusive throughout.

When a large-scale military raid was scheduled, I and other medical professionals went out with the assaulters. Often with as little as a few hours' notice, we hastily loaded our medical gear into the back of a waiting assault helicopter. We donned our body armor and weapons, and we flew off into the darkness of battle. I usually sat idle in the back of a hovering aircraft for hours. Occasionally, I sat on the ground of an open clearing a reasonable distance from the actual fighting, awaiting receipt of wounded friendly or enemy combatants. Through the green illumination of my night-vision goggles, I saw many places so very strange to me—places like Jalalabad, Asadabad, Kandahar, and additional unnamed land areas. At times, I didn't even know where I really was, only able to identify my location by the military grid coordinates indicated on my handheld Global Positioning System device.

I distinctly remember one such place, somewhere near the southeast, Pakistani border, where it seemed that no locals had been for a very long time. I thought that it must have been an abandoned, village airport as our airlift of opportunity was a combat-modified C-130 transport plane, which touched down on a cracked landing strip with thick weeds growing between the crevices. Exiting our aircraft, a handful of medical folks and I, accompanied by four USSOCOM assault personnel, hunkered down in total darkness among a pile of rubble just off the landing strip near the idle turboprop, awaiting word of potential incoming casualties. It was a moonless night, and despite billions of stars scattered throughout the heavens, I could not see the hand in front of my face without looking through my night-vision devices. The small team and I scoured the area, each peering in separate directions. Each of us had our long guns at the ready should we be unexpectedly ambushed by an angry group of jihadists who sometimes came from nowhere seeking trouble and revenge. I recognized the rapidity of my breathing, acknowledging that I was indeed nervous being well within the enemy's territory.

I felt perhaps inappropriately confident in my marksman skills, as I patted the ammunition pouches affixed to my body armor. They contained six additional thirty-round magazines, which would, should I need it, supplement the ammunition already locked and loaded into my M-4 assault rifle. I counted on that confidence to keep me alive should we get ambushed. I was damned sure that I would take out as many of the terrorists as possible before they got me.

The stillness of the night was eerie, but was suddenly interrupted by the deafening screams and thunderous cracks in the atmosphere as the A-6 Intruder jets whipped overhead to unload some explosives, perhaps at the assault site. I hoped all was going well for our guys, and my heartbeat was becoming noticeable. I could hear the fast pounding of my pulsating blood within my ears.

Radio silence then broke. We were told that several rotary aircraft were to be landing at our location. After a few minutes I heard the distinct sound of helicopter blades chopping through the night air but I could not see any of the incoming birds. The sound of the rotors became louder and louder but I still could not see the helos. I then turned my night-vision goggles from starlight mode to infrared mode. Suddenly, beams of light led me to the otherwise invisible, approaching two aircraft, which I clearly watched as they touched down not fifty feet from me. Obviously, the aircraft were equipped with illumination gear, which emitted electromagnetic beams outside of the visible light spectrum. I was previously aware of this, but I had forgotten about it altogether. Once safely on the ground, precious cargo was quickly transferred from the rear helicopter onto our fixed wing, now with props turning at high speed. Minutes later, our medical crew and the assault team members boarded the plane we flew in on, and we made our hasty exit to our final destination.

I felt truly honored to be able to work with and care for the commandos of USSOCOM. My true value to them was in the operating room where I performed emergency surgery in austere, surgical sites. One such site was in southeast Afghanistan, located aboard Camp Salerno—an expeditionary, but well-supported encampment just a few clicks north of the mountain range bordering Afghanistan and Pakistan. Prepositioned on the small camp was a small army medical team—a group of folks from the regular army tasked with running a three-tent, forward medical facility. The team included two general surgeons, one orthopedic surgeon, two nurse anesthetists, two operating room nurses, and several additional army nurses and medics. They worked out of three general-purpose tents, each sixteen by thirty-two feet in size. One tent served as an emergency room of sorts, where casualties were received and resuscitated by the doctors, nurses, and medics. A second tent served as a holding area, where patients awaiting movement to a more robust military medical facility remained sometimes for as long as three days. And the third tent was reserved solely for use as an operating room.

In the operating room tent, two modular operating tables, each able to be broken down into about twenty pieces and easily moved in no more than about ten minutes, served as the platform for all of the surgical procedures I performed in Afghanistan. The two tables were arranged in a V configuration, with the heads of the tables canted toward each other, allowing one anesthesia provider to administer anesthetic agents to two surgical casualties simultaneously. Surgical technicians and circulating room nurses provided the necessary assistance to me and the other surgeons as we performed the whole gamut of trauma operations in the combat theater tents.

All of our needed equipment was stored in long, hanging bags, which when zipped closed could be stored or moved without worry that the equipment within would become contaminated. When unzipped, each hanging bag hung from cord strung around the inside perimeter of the OR tent, allowing the team easy access to their contents. The hanging bags contained all of the basic equipment needed to perform most trauma operations, including exploratory abdominal procedures, surgical operations within the chest cavity, neck explorations, and emergency vascular repairs. There was also a complement of basic, orthopedic fixation hardware, and even a kit allowing us to do basic neurosurgical procedures, should a wounded combatant need emergency evacuation of bleeding from inside the skull.

I loved operating in those small tent facilities scattered throughout Afghanistan. The true owners of the tents and equipment were always very gracious, allowing me and the others in my group to barge in on them and use their equipment and space.

The medical team at Camp Salerno was especially gracious, and I maintained friendly relationships with several of the doctors, a few of whom I still contact periodically. Whereas some surgeons might rebel at having to perform surgery in crude, dimly lit, dank tents, I relished the opportunity. There were no surgical scrub uniforms, and so I operated in my military T-shirt and uniform pants, with disposable shoe covers slipped over my desert boots. I covered up with a sterile, surgical gown after scrubbing my hands at the portable handwashing station situated in the corner of the OR tent. I rinsed the soap off my hands with bottled water squirted via a rubber-bulb foot pump located on the floor of the tent. We had masks and surgical head covers, and for the most part the place was very similar to a real operating room. The obvious exception was the fact that a real war was ongoing just outside the camp, and rocket and mortar explosions occasionally rocked the ground we stood on.

I operated on Americans and foreigners alike, some of whom were innocent civilians or United Nations workers, and some of whom were enemies sworn to kill us. Regardless of the language they spoke or the organization to whom they swore allegiance, we took care of all comers. That was understood and supported by all levels of the U.S. military. I did chest surgery, abdominal surgery, and extremity surgery. And I cut off a lot of legs—often missing feet and portions of leg below the knee, with strips of burned muscles draped like limp ribbons attached to broken bones stripped clean of any healthy flesh. Land mines were an especially precarious enemy of the casualties I treated, and were the primary reason why I performed so many amputations.

I never lost a single patient brought to me with a pulse. My most proud save was a serviceman gravely wounded by a single shard of shrapnel, which caught him just below the lowest limit of his body armor, piercing his abdomen and cutting through his vena cava. He lost enough blood to become just a few red cells away from dying. With bold cuts of my scalpel, I opened his abdomen as fast as I could. I freed up and rotated from right to left the intestine, which was covering his deep, vascular structures and was preventing me access to his source of bleeding. Once the bowel was rotated out of my way, I immediately saw the hole in the massive vein and I stopped the bleeding with direct pressure while awaiting the anesthetist to transfuse enough blood to get my patient's pressure from nearly undetectable to acceptable. After a good ten minutes of pressing down on the huge, venous tube, I slipped a curved, vascular clamp around the damaged portion of the vena cava and sutured the vascular wound closed. My casualty quickly stabilized once the hole was repaired. I then washed him out, closed him up, and shipped him out via medical evacuation helicopter as soon as I could.

I know for certain that he ended up doing fine and that he suffered no complications, all of which was really quite amazing. Perhaps the reason he did so well was because of his body's superior physical condition prior to his wounding, allowing him to tolerate the extremely low blood pressure without suffering the typical consequences. Or perhaps he was just meant to live—with God intervening, preventing one more mother from having to grieve on that particular day.

Mentally decompressing after going out on dicey combat missions or after performing harrowing, meatball surgery in a war zone was difficult. Sometimes after making it back from an all-night escapade, with the sights and sounds of gunfire and blood still on my mind, and with adrenalin still flowing through my veins, all I wanted to do was relax and gulp down an alcoholic beverage. But there was no beer in Afghanistan—at least none that I had ever found. There were no military clubs where one could sit back and crack open a cold one, there were no televisions to mindlessly sit in front of, and most important, I had very limited access to phone calls home to my wife, and essentially no personal e-mail access. At best, I was able to access a phone bank a couple of times per week where I often waited for up to an hour to place a fifteen-minute call back home. When out on a mission or when away from the confines of the Bagram Air Base, I had no phone access at all. I did read a lot of books, did some basic exercising, and smoked a lot of cigars.

I know that I smoked well over a hundred cigars out there, some of which were Cubans, which I had procured from nonuniformed, government agents who had paid occasional visits to the capital city of Kabul. There were many occasions when I wanted nothing more than to just set one of the prized Cubans ablaze after our mission bird set us all down on tierra firma once safely back at Bagram—my body reeking from the smell of enemy prisoners and JP-8 aircraft fuel.

I became close to a few of the guys on the USSOCOM team. One of my closest buddies was a former commando turned physician assigned to more of an administrative position rather than a health-care provider job. Lieutenant Roy Leutren—an Undersea Medical Officer and SEAL by all rights and privileges—was a rather religious man and he always had something spiritually uplifting to say. He often put my thoughts into perspective after a wild mission. He rarely got out into the fray with us but he always wished that he could. Instead, he was relegated to watching our engagements real time from his seat in the Tactical Operations Center as unmanned drone aircraft took live, photo imagery of the missions below. Roy wasn't the only religious guy I met out there. In fact, there were several others who were openly devout Christians. It seemed ironic to me at the time that some our nation's most elite war fighters were also some of the most religious men I had ever met. I guess I shouldn't have been too surprised as every man I knew on the team was extremely dedicated to the defense of our nation and I hadn't met a one who wouldn't have given up his own life if necessary to save the life of his brother in arms. I guess they each needed something to give them the inner strength necessary to carry on their calling. To many, that source apparently was God.

Just before the Christmas of 2004, my period of duty in Afghanistan was over. Another man came to replace me and I extended him the same courtesies Will had extended me when I arrived. I showed my replacement the ropes as best I could. I was more than happy to leave Afghanistan behind me and oh so eager to again see my wife and kids. My wife drove out to the East Coast to pick me up when I got back to the States and our reunion was sweet. After spending an obligated length of time at the command, where I received a series of debriefings, I was allowed to depart back to my hometown. I was released from active duty to return back to my family, to my reserve unit, and to my civilian job. I was proud to have served with my teammates, but I was also very happy to leave them and the war behind.

18

Suicide by Crossbow

Treating the Full Spectrum of the Ages

After returning from Afghanistan, I saw many common, everyday things in a very different light. Many things I once considered essential to maintaining a comfortable lifestyle suddenly seemed trivial and insignificant. Subsequent to my return, a spacious home, easy access to restaurants, and the Internet all seemed like luxuries to me. I began to feel that if I needed to, I could be happy living in the pop-up camper I stored in my garage in which I periodically spent nights with my family, relaxing at local state parks. I lost my former appreciation for high-end restaurants. I realized that as long as I had access to any basic source of palatable food, I would be just fine. Although I still enjoyed the Internet's easy access to any and all information, I became increasingly frustrated by the dozens of daily, unsolicited e-mails sent to my online account.

After being in a place where there was very little food or water, essentially no means of reasonable health care, and decades of armed conflict and violence, I realized that Americans are, in general and by comparison to many other nations, so very well off. But I was frustrated at how many of my fellow countrymen seemed to be so disengaged from the events taking place overseas. Many people seemed to be oblivious to the fact that our nation was at war. I did my best to not be bothered by the little things that annoyed me. I did my best to focus on my renewed appreciation and gratefulness for the things and for the people to whom I was able to safely return.

Whereas some veterans have disturbing dreams or nightmares after returning home from a war zone, I had none. I feel that I came back pretty much unscathed by my experience, only one time having had a mildly disturbing flashback, which took me back to where I had been. Strangely enough, it was at a Notre Dame football game, of all places. Less than a year after getting back from Afghanistan, my wife and I met up with one of my former college roommates and his wife at our university's alma mater. Being back on the Notre Dame campus was a wonderful and refreshing experience, which brought back many good memories of the four years I spent living in Grace Hall and majoring in preprofessional science.

On that day, Notre Dame was playing the Naval Academy—one of the great football rivalries on campus. We sat midlevel in the southern end-zone section, giving me a great view through the north goalposts of the enormous library. The building served as the canvas for an artist's huge mosaic depiction of Jesus Christ, spreading his arms up toward the heavens. The artwork has been affectionately known for years by all on the Notre Dame campus as Touchdown Jesus, raising his arms skyward signaling another score. Although the religious depiction may seem somewhat blasphemous to some, most of the Notre Dame students and graduates have felt great respect for all that it represents, and don't seem to have any problem with it.

Before the game even started the announcer asked that everyone stand for the singing of our national anthem. I took to my feet, and like any good military man in or out of uniform, I instinctively stood at a position of attention as the music played. I felt great admiration for the country whose sovereignty I was proud to have helped protect. And then, as if I had been instantly teleported back in time, I was suddenly back in Afghanistan as four navy fighter jets performed an overhead flyby. I felt mildly anxious as if I was back on a mission with the old unit, and I wondered in a transient state of confusion if any of the people I knew were perhaps engaged in a firefight with the enemy, possibly in trouble, requesting that the fast-movers flying overhead drop munitions to scatter their attackers. I quickly came to my senses as the images in front of me were again that of a football stadium, and not of the Taliban-infested desert. My racing pulse gradually slowed, and I became pensive as I had never before thought that such an occurrence could ever happen to me. The kickoff, which commenced just a few minutes later, redirected my attention and I soon became fully engaged in the gridiron battle. Notre Dame won the game, and I made our long drive back home with my wife thereafter, never again to be momentarily bothered by a single flashback. I know that I am one of the lucky ones not bothered by my deployment, having met and read about so many others who have not been so fortunate.

Returning back to my civilian trauma job was an easy transition. For the most part, I felt as if I had never left. My experience treating war casualties and impoverished Afghani nationals—all people with extremely limited resources—gave me a whole new perspective on how we in America care for our patients. I began to realize that a disconnect separates people's expectations of our health-care system and the medical outcomes that can actually be achieved. For the most part, I have become convinced that regardless of how many chronic medical diagnoses a person accumulates, there will always be at least one family member who feels that his relative's medical problems are all completely manageable. Regardless of how old or sick a person's family member gets, the fact that their relative was once young and healthy convinces them that there must be a medicine, a procedure, or a fairly benign treatment plan out there somewhere that can restore the body's function for many more years. I began to feel troubled at how chronically ill people in their seventies, eighties, and even nineties would get transferred great distances to my trauma center. The transfers often seemed to provide nothing more than additional expense to an already costly medical adventure for treatment of what would ordinarily be considered to be trivial injuries. However, due to the patients' advanced ages and their numerous, preinjury medical conditions, their otherwise little problems became potentially lethal situations.

There comes a time when all people must die, and hopefully for most, that will only be after living a long and otherwise healthy life. But when our advanced seniors do get hooked by the claws of aging body failure, reasonable people—family members and health-care providers alike—need to recognize when enough is enough, and when the care we provide does far more harm than good. Tens of thousands of people living in nursing homes get sent to emergency rooms annually, for evaluation and treatment of serious conditions such as stroke, pneumonia, congestive heart failure, fall injuries, and numerous other maladies well represented in the geriatric population. Often, these conditions come on suddenly, and often occur in the numerous patients who suffer from mild to advanced states of dementia. These situations results in patients not being able to express to their caregivers just how much longer they really want to continue their suffering. I often wonder whether perhaps they would have preferred a compassionate, gentle hand to hold, rather than what inevitably occurs. Quite typically, patients get transported to a strange, frightening place where people insert tubes and catheters into their bodies, perform painfully invasive surgical procedures, and extend their otherwise unproductive lives for yet another few months or years. All of this is done despite what often appears to be a complete loss of any reasonable quality of life.

At times, I have been frustrated by seeing how people who have previously lived long and memorable years, now stricken with irreversible, chronically life-threatening diseases, get sent back and forth to hospitals to receive treatment for end-of-life conditions, with no hope of restoring any decent quality to their frail existence. I'm talking about people who should die—people tortured within their own bodies, and those whose minds left them long ago. I wonder how many of them would ask us to let them die in a compassionate manner if they only had the mental and physical abilities to speak for themselves. Yet, all too often, a single family member harboring some sort of guilt, or too far removed from the situation to make difficult decisions, declines authorizing what would be in the best interest of the patient. Unable to truly represent their loved one's best interests, they typically default to the do-everything mode of medical management.

While seeing some patients live almost indefinitely despite any demonstrative will to do so, I have at other times been tormented by not being able to save the life of a young trauma patient who, if not for his mortal injuries, could have had so many more good years ahead of him. Joseph Brunner was one of my trauma patients clearly in the former category. He was an old, frail, and chronically ill, demented gentleman. Michael Mahon was one of my casualties who sadly fell into the latter group. He was a young, robust teenager who tragically aborted his own life, and took a piece of mine along with him.

Mr. Brunner was an eighty-six year-old-nursing home resident. His profoundly demented wife lived on a separate wing of the nursing facility, but neither one was aware of each other's proximity or existence. Joseph had been a sickly man for many years and his mind had experienced the ravages of advanced Alzheimer's disease. He had just recently been hospitalized at another facility with a case of severe pneumonia, where doctors had also discovered that Mr. Brunner's test results indicated the likelihood that his previously treated colon cancer may have recurred. In fact, they felt that Mr. Brunner's cancer might even be metastatic to other organs.

Mr. Brunner also had other chronic, medical problems, including emphysema, diabetes, painful arthritis, and a recent diagnosis of pulmonary embolism—a blood clot that had formed in his leg vein had dislodged and migrated into his lungs, further impairing his already limited ability to breathe. He had been hospitalized two additional times previously within the past twelve months with severe pneumonia, narrowly escaping being placed on the ventilator each time. To top things off, Mr. Brunner also suffered from advanced prostate cancer, the necessary treatment for which was to perform bilateral orchiectomies—removal of both testicles—eliminating any residual source of male hormones. The treatment did, in fact, quell the spread of his prostate cancer, but it also caused him to become androgynously feminized, causing the old man to look more like a little old lady than the former steelworker he apparently once was. Mr. Brunner had not walked in years. Crippled by his degenerative joint disease and extreme air hunger, he traveled around by wheelchair, pushed by nursing home attendants whose names he could never remember.

One day, Mr. Brunner fell forward and out of his wheelchair. He fell from a seated position, no more than a few feet from the ground. The impact of the fall caused a laceration to his head, and he was rushed to a local emergency room. The doctors sutured closed his small, bloody wound and, looking for evidence of additional injury, they performed a brain CT scan. The test unfortunately revealed a thin wisp of blood between his atrophied brain and his skull. Like so many other hospitals, that particular facility had no neurosurgeon able or willing to provide emergency on-call coverage. Without having available neurosurgical backup, no doctor was willing to admit Mr. Brunner to that hospital. Having no other choice, the hospital's emergency room physician initiated a call to me to transfer his patient to our trauma center, a good thirty miles away from the other facility. I listened to the referring emergency room doctor's request to transfer Mr. Brunner to me, and knowing that he was stuck between a rock and a hard place, I accepted Mr. Brunner as my patient.

Specialty transport paramedics, who work full-time shuttling patients from one hospital to another, picked up Mr. Brunner and brought him to me. I promptly evaluated him and determined that no brain surgery would ever be needed. I admitted Mr. Brunner to our hospital and asked our neurosurgeon to give his blessing that I transfer Mr. Brunner back to the nursing home after confirming with a repeat brain CT scan twenty-four hours later that the tiny bleed was indeed stable and too small to ever consider treating. I talked with Mr. Brunner's daughter, going over the sordid details of her father's medical conditions past and present. I informed her that although no special treatment was required of his trivial brain trauma, it would likely exacerbate her dad's already profound intellectual and physical dysfunction. I asked her to think about what she would like for us and other physicians to do should her dad's heart stop, or if he should be found unresponsive and not breathing. I asked her if she wanted us to perform the customary insertion of the breathing tube, place him on the ventilator, perform CPR chest compressions, and give him zaps of electrical energy to his dying heart. Or rather, should we just let him die peacefully and naturally and assign him the preemptive status of "Do Not Resuscitate."

My patient's daughter didn't seem to be interesteded in letting her dad die regardless of his advanced problems. She firmly stated that her dad should be aggressively treated with whatever was necessary should anything bad happen to him. Of course, we complied with her wishes, and two days after being transferred from the nursing home—to one hospital, and then to another—a paramedic crew shipped him back again to the old folks' nursing facility.

Less than one week later, I received a phone call from the same hospital that had sent Mr. Brunner to me before. The nature of the call was again about the very same patient, who again fell from his wheelchair, fracturing one of the bones in his brittle, osteoporotic neck. Again having no neurosurgical coverage, Mr. Brunner made yet another thirty-minute trip to our facility, where I again evaluated him, this time for his broken neck bone. Fortunately, Mr. Brunner's fracture was only a hairline break. There was no resultant injury to his spinal cord. His fracture would require that he wear a rigid, neck immobilizer for approximately two months. We fitted Mr. Brunner with his neck brace and he immediately resisted. His dementia prevented him from remembering from one minute to the next that he had fractured his cervical spine. He repeatedly pulled at the device firmly affixed to his upper chest, neck, and chin, frustrated by the cumbersome brace, and angry at having his head restrained.

For the next two weeks, Mr. Brunner suffered in our hospital from that neck immobilizer. His frustration over the wearing of the brace wore him out, and his ability to swallow had become impaired by being forced to keep his head in a fixed, upright position. He developed aspiration pneumonia after attempting to drink some water, which resulted in the liquid passing into his lungs rather than down his esophagus. We treated his recurrent pneumonia with antibiotics and breathing medications, and we fed him through a tube passed down his nose and into his stomach. We couldn't allow Mr. Brunner to eat or drink, knowing that another case of pneumonia could do him in. Trying to get Mr. Brunner's daughter to be reasonable about things, I asked her if she would like us to place a feeding tube through his abdominal wall into his stomach, or whether she would rather we just let him eat what he wanted, yet not subject him to the repeated treatments for what could possibly become yet another, possibly fatal pneumonia.

I again asked the daughter if perhaps she might reconsider converting her dad to a Do Not Resuscitate status, and she again firmly resisted the idea. Yet, she also hesitated on our necessary request to place the type of feeding tube that nearly all nursing homes require in such circumstances before they are permitted to return. I explained to her that the transabdominal, Percutaneous Endoscopic Gastrostomy feeding tube would help prevent her dad from aspirating his food and liquids, and would minimize his need to return to the hospital to treat the resultant pneumonia. She again refused.

She began to reconsider allowing the Do Not Resuscitate status for her dad after listening to her father's repeated, pitiful pleas for something to eat, begging her to get him some coffee and something sweet to chew on. She didn't want her father to have a feeding tube, but she also realized that when he did eat, he would again get sick. Finally, she acquiesced, and we changed Mr. Brunner's resuscitation status from full code, to DNR. We could finally allow him eat by mouth and enjoy one of his only pleasures left in life. We also would not be forced to put him on a ventilator should he develop aspiration pneumonia, which was highly likely.

We minimized Mr. Brunner's potential of aspirating by giving him pureed, thickened foods, which patients like Mr. Brunner often tolerate without any problem. Mr. Brunner did tolerate the pureed diet, fed to him by the nurses and technicians who also changed his diapers every time he wet or soiled himself. Mr. Brunner had become a sad sight, and I knew that it was just a matter of time until he developed some other serious problem. His frail life was finally starting to complete the unraveling process. Sooner or later he would again develop another case of pneumonia, perhaps from a resistant strain of a deadly organism, as his body became weaker and weaker. But now having orders to not perform intubation or cardiac resuscitation, he would finally be allowed to die naturally and peacefully—an event long overdue. Sadly however, although I knew that Mr. Brunner would soon meet a compassionate end, I also knew that his dignity had been taken from him a very long time ago.

Whereas Joseph Brunner had lived far too long, Michael Mahon did not live nearly long enough. Michael was a seventeen-year-old high school senior, an excellent student, and the son of two successful, professional parents who had been contemplating separation from each other. Although they allegedly lived together amicably, Michael became increasingly aware of his parents' plans to split up once he went off to college. Although he never made his parents aware of the growing sadness brewing within his heart, Michael apparently felt that he bore responsibility for not being able to keep his parents together. He began to slip into a deep depression. On the Friday morning on the last day of a busy workweek for his parents, Michael decided to end his torment by taking his own life.

Michael awoke that morning and asked his father if he would call his school and excuse him from attending classes. He told his father that he had a bad headache. Mike was never one to complain or to even sleep in, so his dad agreed to Michael's request and allowed him to stay home by himself as both parents busily went off to their respective jobs.

Shortly after his parents left, Michael reclined on his bed and began writing a three-page suicide note. He asked his parents for forgiveness, and he detailed his feelings of sadness and blame. After Michael had finished his note, he placed it on a dresser where it would be easily found. He then walked out into the living room and he picked up the crossbow that adorned the mantel of his parents' fireplace. It was a functional crossbow, and Michael had studied it for some time as he planned the details of his own death. He carried the crossbow back with him into his room and he pulled back on the bow string, locking it into the firing mechanism. He then loaded the bolt, pushed the crossbow into the dead center of his torso, and he pulled the trigger sending the heavy, metal projectile deep into his body. Michael writhed with pain and he began bleeding profusely around the remnant of steel protruding from his upper abdomen where both right and left rib cage margins came together. Michael felt confident that he had done what was necessary, and he knew that he would soon be dead. Wanting to die in a more comfortable position, he slumped onto his bed where he lay in wait of his own passing.

But Michael did not die as soon as he had anticipated, and he suffered agonizing pain from his self-inflicted injury. After writhing on his bed for over an hour, Michael decided that he needed relief. In a bold move, he grabbed the impaled crossbow bolt and he pulled it out of his upper abdomen. But Michael certainly did not feel any better. In fact, he began to feel terribly frightened and anxious. He grabbed the phone at his bedside and frantically dialed the 911 operator, who immediately dispatched an ambulance to his home.

When paramedics arrived, they found Michael in a pool of blood-soaked sheets, twisting and rolling on the bed, still awake and able to give them extensive details of what he was feeling inside and what he had done to himself as a result. Not wasting a moment's time, the paramedics scooped Michael onto a gurney and sped him to the ambulance just outside his home. One man raced the rig to the hospital as the second paramedic working in the back started Michael's IV line and attended to his bleeding wound. When the ambulance pulled up to our trauma center, I was already outside standing on the ramp awaiting their arrival, having been notified by the charge nurse of the details of the particularly grim and unusual occurrence.

Michael was still awake and was breathing on his own, but his color was almost gone, and he was starting to appear sleepy, as his body was progressing into the most advanced stage of hemorrhagic shock. I helped rush the paramedic gurney into trauma room number three, where I immediately began my resuscitative efforts while asking the emergency room charge nurse to have the operating room staff prepare a room for an emergency trauma exploration.

I instructed one of the emergency room doctors who came into the trauma room offering his assistance to insert a breathing tube. I simultaneously inserted a long, large bore, central venous catheter into the vessel just below Michael's collarbone, through which I began rapidly infusing O-negative blood to restore my patient's disturbingly low blood volume. I quickly grabbed the ultrasound machine and I examined Michael's heart, looking for any evidence of cardiac injury or blood accumulation in the sac surrounding his heart. There was no sign of such injury, which gave me some relief. I then had the radiology technicians staged in the trauma room quickly perform a portable chest X-ray to be sure that neither of his lungs had collapsed. After confirming no evidence of lung injury, we began rolling Michael toward the operating room.

The operating room nurses, technicians, and anesthesiologist were each disturbed by the dramatic nature of how my patient had harmed himself. Each mentioned how mortified they would be if something similar should happen to any of their own children. I, too, was bothered by thoughts of the possibility of my own son lying on that operating room table, with blood welling up inside of his body after such a brutal act of self-destruction. I pulled myself together—no one had seen my momentary lapse of focus—knowing that the only person able to keep the kid alive at that moment was me. I quickly ran out of the room to scrub, and after a lightning-fast cleansing, I reentered the room to gown and glove. Michael was already prepped and draped from head to toe, but the anesthesiologist yelled for me to get started immediately because Michael's blood pressure was becoming undetectably low. Knowing that Michael was dying, I needed to stop the bleeding quickly. I chose to open his chest and to clamp off Michael's aorta in an area I knew would not be obscured by a large pool of blood.

I cut from just below the left nipple straight down to the OR table, slicing through skin, fat, and layers of muscle in a matter of a few seconds. I then used the electrocautery device to cut through the thin layers of muscle between ribs four and five. I cranked open Michael's chest with a large rib spreader, giving me access to his left lung, heart, and the huge aortic vessel coursing downward just above the left side of his spinal column. I lifted the lung upward with my left hand as I bluntly dissected a window of space around the sole supply of blood to Michael's abdomen with the dissecting instrument in my right hand. Then, with a few clicks of a large vascular clamp placed completely across his aorta, I interrupted all flow to the rest of his body. The maneuver gave the anesthesiologist all the time he needed to pour in multiple units of packed red blood cells and plasma to correct Michael's blood pressure and heart rate to life-sustaining levels.

Next, I opened his belly in rapid, trauma fashion, gaining access to his insides in less than a minute. He was full of blood, and I shoved several lap sponges deeply into his belly, pushing them toward the area I suspected was bleeding. After suctioning out an entire collection bottle full of blood, I cut a three-inch, vertical hole through the thin layer of filmy material just to the right side of Michael's stomach. My cut gave me access to his pulseless aorta lying immediately behind my carefully placed incision. Configuring the index and middle fingers of my left hand in a V-shape, I bluntly swept away the filmy tissues from either side of Michael's aorta, working blindly deep within a substantial, residual pool of accumulated blood. Using my sense of touch more than anything else, I then directed and placed a second, large vascular clamp across the abdominal portion of his aorta, allowing me to release the vascular clamp in Michael's chest.

I then turned my attention to the left side of Michael's belly as I began dividing the tissues attaching Michael's spleen and the left side of his large intestine to the backside of his inner abdomen. After freeing up the organs overlying the area I needed access to, I rotated them all as a unit from left to right, fully exposing the large vascular structure the crossbow bolt had penetrated. For a moment, I was confused by what I was seeing.

Normally, the aorta runs down the center of the deepest part of the abdomen, and to the patient's *right* of that runs a large, parallel vein—the inferior vena cava. But my patient had a large, thin walled vascular structure paralleling the *left* side of his aorta, and it could be nothing other than a second vena cava. Whereas almost everyone is born with the same, basic anatomical structures, each of which are located in the same place every time, every once in a while surgeons encounter a developmental anomaly. These variations of anatomy can make surgery very confusing and difficult if encountered during an emergency procedure. But I was thankful for his anomaly in that particular situation, as the vena cava is a low flow vessel, as opposed to the aorta being a high flow vessel. I had a better chance of saving Michael from a vena cava injury than I would have had he speared his aorta.

I carefully placed vascular clamps above and below the hole in the left-sided vessel, definitively controlling the bleeding. I released the abdominal aortic clamp, returning the flow of blood through the uninjured, large artery. Taking my time carefully, I repaired one side of the injured vessel, and then rotated and repaired the opposite side where the crossbow bolt had gone through and through. After tying my last knot, I first released the upper clamp, followed next by releasing the lower clamp causing the anomalous, repaired vena cava to bulge back to its functional size. Blood oozed from a few of the suture holes in the repaired vessel to which I applied a thick layer of fibrin glue—a sticky substance synthesized from human blood products. I have often found fibrin glue to be very useful in similar circumstances.

After pressing a saline-moistened surgical sponge over the fibrin glue layer for about five minutes, I peeled away the pad and was pleased to see no evidence of any residual blood loss. I watched over the repaired vessel for a good five minutes before washing out Michael's abdominal cavity with about five li-

ters of warm solution and then suctioning the belly dry. I took one last look at
my repair site, and closed Michael's abdomen and thoracic cavity after inserting
a left-sided chest tube, which I would use to reexpand Michael's left lung and
drain any bloody fluid, which always oozes after performing chest surgery.

After cleaning off his skin, I applied a layer of gauze dressing to Michael's
abdominal and chest wounds, and I helped move him from the operating room
table onto the waiting intensive care unit bed on which Michael would be
transferred to his more permanent room in the ICU. Feeling almost elated at
the success of my work, I thought about how I would talk to Michael's parents
about what had happened. I felt good about being able to give them hope as I
felt confident that my repair was secure. I also thought about what I would
talk about with Michael when I eventually got him off the ventilator. I imagined
that I would give him words of encouragement, and counsel him as I would my
own child as to how to ask for help if he ever again felt as much darkness and
despair as he did earlier that day. I envisioned Michael smiling back at me days
later, and eventually shaking my hand as he left the hospital en route to the
psychiatric institution, where he would continue his mental healing process,
feeling great at having had someone who cared enough to rescue him from an
otherwise inevitable death. Of course, those were all figments of my own imagination, but I looked forward to the day when they would become a reality.

I walked over to the surgical waiting area looking for representatives from
Michael's family—hopefully his parents. As often happens after I perform emergency surgery, I walk into the family waiting area having absolutely no idea who
may be awaiting me or what the individuals might possibly look like. Obviously,
if I just operated on a Hispanic male, or someone of any distinctive, ethnic origin for that matter, I look for people of a similar race and ask if they might be
relatives of whomever I had just operated on. But often, especially on a busy day
when surgeons are working in all fifteen of our operating rooms, I walk out into
the waiting area bulging at its seams with visitors, and have no clue as to who
among the large crowd of individuals may or may not be representing the family of my trauma patient.

But on that day I immediately recognized two people who could be none
other than Michael's parents. There was a well-groomed, middle-aged man in
a business suit, and a similar-aged businesswoman. Both bore looks of painful
anguish, he with furrowed brows and jaws grinding, and she with makeup-
smeared eye sockets and tears rolling down her puffy cheeks. Both looked

toward me immediately, as if perhaps someone had described my features to them. I studied them for several moments before I openly asked if they might be relatives of Michael Mahon. Acknowledging their identities with an immediate expression of anxious relief, they quickly rose to their feet and they walked briskly toward me with pleading looks on their faces.

"Is he okay?" they both asked simultaneously. As I always do in similar situations, I instantaneously played back in my head all of the events that had taken place up to that point. I began by introducing myself, then asking if either of them was at all aware of what had happened to their son. The man clenched his mouth even tighter, closed his eyes, and while looking downward, he nodded affirmatively. The woman then blurted out in an explosion of tears that they were told that their son had shot himself with their crossbow and that he had been rushed into emergency surgery. I was glad that someone had already broken the most difficult part of the news to them. My job was to then focus on less of what had happened up until that point and talk to them about how well I thought he did during surgery. I would attempt to give them some solid hope, yet at the same time remain cautiously optimistic as I was well aware that numerous complications and setbacks could still take place.

I did tell them that despite their son having lost a great deal of blood and having injured a major vessel deep within his abdomen, I thought that the surgery went very well. I expressed hope that he would soon recover over a period of several days or weeks, but that he would remain on the breathing machine in the intensive care unit for an indeterminate period of time. I told them that their son was in critical condition, albeit stable. They seemed to latch on to that last word: "stable." As if I had just spoken the magic word, they both became weak by the somewhat reassuring news. Backing up to set down their terribly exhausted bodies, they thanked me for all I had done, and they thanked God for watching over their son.

Mr. and Mrs. Mahon and I spent the next fifteen minutes or so talking about Michael's mental state, about how he had been behaving up until that terrible day, and how his parents' talk of separation may have affected him. His parents gave no indication that Michael had been depressed, although they did comment that he seemed to be too busy with his schoolwork to have time for the extracurricular activities and sports he once participated in avidly. According to the Mahons, Michael was a very independent child destined to go on to college following high school graduation. They thought that he was nothing other than a very normal kid who they could never have predicted would have been capable of such a self-destructive act of violence. Of course, Mr. and Mrs. Mahon were mortified by how Michael must have been feeling about their marital issues, and they blamed themselves over and over for the tragedy that occurred. They clearly felt horribly guilty and entirely responsible for Michael's actions, barely able to maintain their composure as they described their personal pain. But despite their honest admissions of openly having discussed separation on several occasions, I saw nothing other than solidarity among the two parents. It almost seemed as if Michael's suicide attempt gave them resolve to deal with their own issues as a team and to consider Michael's feelings above all else.

I tried to give them whatever hope and comfort I could, and I hoped that perhaps in just a short while, both Michael's and his parents' problems would soon progress toward healing. After I concluded my discussion with them, I turned to depart and noticed the two, nearly estranged parents embrace in what appeared to be a genuine act of support and solidarity. I thought that perhaps as a result of Michael's tragedy, an entire family might soon heal.

The following day was a Saturday and was a scheduled military reserve, drill weekend for me. I did not work at the trauma center on either day. One of my partners remained in-house at the hospital overseeing and directing Michael's postoperative care. I thought about Michael that entire weekend and I looked forward to again seeing him and his parents after I returned from my weekend duty. But with great sadness to me, that would never happen.

When I returned to the trauma center the following Monday morning at 6:45, I logged into the hospital's computer system to pull up the trauma service's inpatient census list as I did at the start of each of my shifts. When I accessed my group's list of inpatients, I conspicuously noticed that Michael's name was not on my list. Mildly disturbed, I wondered why his name was absent, wondering if Michael had been transferred to another hospital—something very unlikely—or perhaps a computer error had accidentally deleted his name from our census, which would need to be corrected before I started morning rounds.

When my trauma group met up at 7 A.M. for our daily briefing, I was slapped with the devastating news that Michael had died over the weekend. The news was mind numbing, and I couldn't believe what I was hearing. The operation had gone so well for me and I had no inkling of any likely postoperative problems. I asked what exactly had happened to Michael over the weekend, and the explanation given to me was even more tragic than I could have imagined.

I was told that Michael had been completely stable in the immediate post-operative period. On the Saturday morning following my operation, Michael was awake on the ventilator and communicating nonverbally with my partner who had performed intensive care unit rounds that day. Michael was placed on a mode of mechanical ventilation, which allowed him to breathe on his own through the ventilator circuit—something we often do to determine if a person's lungs and body are strong enough to tolerate having the breathing tube removed. According to my partner, he planned on keeping Michael on that mode of ventilation for a few hours, and then obtain some objective measurements of his breathing, at which time it would be determined if Michael would or would not be extubated. Michael's blood count, kidney function tests, and vital signs had all been normal and stable, and the likelihood of coming off the machine seemed likely.

Apparently, a few hours into Michael's breathing trial, the teenager's condition precipitously crashed. His blood pressure plummeted and blood started leaking from between the staples approximating his midline, abdominal wound. My partner did a few rapid tests and concluded that Michael was again hemorrhaging internally and needed to be returned to the operating room immediately. But as the operating room staff was preparing to take Michael back to the OR, his heart stopped and Michael went into full-blown cardiopulmonary arrest.

A code blue was called and ICU nurses began performing chest compressions on my teenaged trauma patient. My partner raced back to Michael's bedside. Realizing that he had no better option, he reopened Michael's abdomen right there in the intensive care unit with the emergency surgical equipment kept in the area should such an emergency arise. Michael's abdomen was filled with blood and all my partner could do was reach deeply into his blood-filled abdominal cavity and blindly hold pressure over the area where he knew I had repaired the damaged vessel. His goal was to restore Michael's heartbeat and to stabilize him just long enough to get the teenager's back onto the operating room table to readdress the area of postoperative hemorrhage. But Michael never did stabilize. Despite an hour of aggressive cardiopulmonary resuscitation, blood transfusions, and pressure from my partner's hand, Michael's heartbeat was never restored, and he was pronounced dead in his intensive care unit bed.

The details of Michael's postoperative demise took my breath away. I replayed his operation in my head over and over and I couldn't think of where I might have gone wrong, or what additional injury I could have missed. The fact that Michael had been so stable for an entire twenty-four-hour period after surgery gave me no additional answers; rather, it perplexed me even more. I felt so terrible about what had happened—so terrible for Michael, for his parents . . . and for me. I had been feeling so good and so confident that Michael would do well. And now he was dead—dead at the youthful age of seventeen. It wasn't supposed to have turned out that way. My operation was a failure, and I took Michael's death very personally.

I never did get the opportunity to see or hear from Michael's parents again. I often wondered if Michael's death reunited their marital bond or whether it further drove a wedge between them. I often thought about how that young boy must have felt not only on the morning prior to his self-inflicted shooting, but during the hour he lay on his bed writhing in pain with the crossbow bolt lodged deep inside him. And I have often thought of how tragic Michael's death was, and how sad it was that a young boy with so much potential could feel so hopeless as to take his own life in such a dramatic fashion. I also wondered with great, personal anguish why it was that I lost my young patient despite all of my efforts.

Michael's death is one that leaves a scar on my soul to this very day. Each time I prolong the miserable lives of terminally ill patients like Joseph Brunner, I ask myself why it all seems so unfair that some people who seem as if they should not survive continue to do so, and why others like Michael Mahon die. It is a painful mystery that I will almost certainly never know the answer to. What I am convinced of, however, is that despite all of my efforts and despite having done everything correctly, the ultimate decision as whether a person is to live or die lies in the hands of an authority much greater than I—an authority I know better than to doubt or question.

19

Trauma and the Flesh-Eating Bacteria

The Brutal Disfigurement of a Woman's Body

Many physicians have well-organized, office-based practices where secretaries and nurses field patients' phone calls and schedule appointments for doctors who provide the largest volume of their care between the hours of 8 A.M. and 5 P.M. Most physicians have contractual relationships with large insurance carriers who provide a negotiated remittance to physicians for the care they provide to insured patients based on the disorder being managed. Whereas at one time, nearly all patients carried some sort of health insurance or managed to pay for medical care out of pocket, the percentage of insured patients seeking medical care these days is far smaller than in years past. To the chagrin of many physicians, despite an increasing complexity in patients' medical conditions in general, financial reimbursement paid to physicians from the insurance companies has decreased year after year, so much so that many doctors now take home far less income compared to what they used to earn over a decade ago.

What has become an even bigger problem than the decreased financial reimbursements paid by the insurance companies is the fact that more and more people have no health-care insurance at all. Whereas many doctors still do what they can to provide care to their patients who have no means to pay, a medical practice—like any other business—simply cannot survive if the cost of doing business exceeds reasonable profits. As a result, many office-based physicians simply choose not to care for uninsured patients, as the medical services provided go uncompensated, and despite providing pro bono care, a potential medical-legal liability situation becomes established.

But as many physicians choose to see fewer and fewer uninsured patients, some of us are in a completely different practice situation. Unlike most physicians, trauma surgeons are hospital based and, for the most part, the support we need is provided by the organization for whom we work. Unlike most of my private practice colleagues, I am an employee—a working stiff, if you will.

By the very nature of my specialty, doctors like me provide emergency treatment to those wounded and injured—people with whom we have absolutely no prior financial, professional, or contractual relationship—whose injuries are often the result of their own destructive behaviors. Drunk drivers, drug addicts, gang members, barroom warriors, criminals, homeless individuals, reckless thrill seekers, and mentally ill people who refuse to take their medications make up a large majority of our trauma patient population. Trauma surgeons take on all comers. Sometime, well after we have initiated our trauma workup, a hospital administrative official looks into whether or not the patients we have already accepted responsibility to care for have any health insurance. In the long run, it really doesn't matter to us because we continue to practice regardless—that is, as long as our medical centers remain committed to the trauma mission and keep trauma surgeons like me employed.

Physicians choose to specialize in and practice trauma surgery for various reasons. I continue doing what I do because I believe that caring for trauma patients makes me a better surgeon. I also believe that it makes me a better person in general. I have met people who live some of the craziest and saddest lives—people who make me feel so fortunate for all that I have been blessed with having. Although I have found that some of my trauma patients can be painfully unsavory characters to care for, I have also found out that many have been some of the most rewarding patients I have ever treated. Patients such as Mary Cosgrove.

Mary Cosgrove was a twenty-eight-year-old lady with a very complicated past. As I would later learn from her mother, she was previously married and had two children from that marriage, both of whom were placed in the exclusive custody of their biological father. Apparently, Mary had some serious drug problems and had a lifelong affliction with unstable bipolar disorder. She apparently became heavily addicted to snorting heroin during one of her manic phases and later began using crack cocaine. Seeking sustainable sources to support her drug habit became an obsession. She often stayed away from her home for days at a time and occasionally left her two infant children unattended while her husband was away at work. Mary's addiction resulted in her eventual divorce and left her with a bad drug habit and no source of income to feed it. She apparently turned to prostitution, and she walked the streets for several years before getting badly beaten by a pimp or one of her johns.

After spending a period of time in a community hospital's critical care unit, Mary left town and settled somewhere in Texas where she somehow became involved with a pretty rough motorcycle gang. According to her mother, Mary rode with the group for almost a year. They kept her drug habit well satisfied, but in return she was repeatedly subjected to what sounded to me like gang rape or sexual abuse at the very least. No longer wanting to be treated like the group whore, Mary ran away from this Texas crowd and migrated to a rural area in the county adjacent to ours. There, she met a young guy who was a recovering drug addict himself. They decided to move in together just a few days after meeting. They quickly became codependent on one another.

Just two weeks after they met, Mary and her new boyfriend decided to take his four-wheeled vehicles out riding in the rural mud pits. Inexperienced at driving an all-terrain vehicle, Mary flipped the four-wheeler, catapulting her over the handlebars into a stagnant, putrid mud hole. The vehicle then caused her additional harm as its momentum carried it on top of Mary's abdomen, crushing her insides. Mary was taken by paramedics to our trauma center for what would start out to be a fairly routine case of severe, blunt trauma. But Mary's situation would soon evolve into one of the most complicated and difficult trauma cases I have ever had to deal with.

Mary was brought in to me awake and alert, breathing well on her own, but in severe distress from excruciating abdominal pain. She was in shock, with her blood pressure very low. I immediately determined her shock to be secondary to uncontrolled bleeding from within her abdomen. Her left wrist was broken and she had a small cut on her left thigh, but other than those two fairly innocuous additional injuries, her abdomen was the clear source of her immediately life-threatening problems.

Mary was covered from head to toe in a thick layer of mud. As if she had been hand-dipped in a bath of rancid chocolate, the gooey, foul-smelling, earthen liquid saturated every inch of her, including her ears, nose, and between her legs. Before I could even apply my handheld ultrasound probe to her abdomen, nurses and technicians literally poured bottles of warm fluid over her naked body, crudely attempting to clean her up. The washing caused lakes of brown water to pool on the trauma room floor under Ms. Cosgrove's emergency room bed. I confirmed my suspicions of intra-abdominal bleeding with the ultrasound, and I quickly rushed her back to the operating room to find and control her source of hemorrhagic shock.

The operating room staff was none too happy that we brought Mary back still rather dirty. Compared to how she presented to our trauma room, she looked quite clean. But we didn't have any more time to waste attempting to make her pretty. Mary's blood pressure was responding only temporarily to the blood and intravenous fluids we were infusing, and I knew that the bleeding in her abdomen was not going to stop without expeditious surgical intervention.

Once the anesthesiologist had Mary deeply asleep and the OR nurses had prepped her abdomen to a reasonable standard, I began my surgical exploration. Her abdomen was full of blood and I immediately presumed that she had shattered her spleen or her liver. As I always do in emergency trauma explorations, I packed her bloody, abdominal cavity with a dozen or more surgical sponges, sucked out as much of the sanguineous fluid as I could, and began my rapid but meticulous exploration. To my surprise, her spleen, liver, and her other solid organs for that matter were not injured at all. I identified her source of ongoing blood loss as an avulsed artery from within the fan of blood vessels that feed the small intestine. Unfortunately however, despite seeing exactly from where she was bleeding, I could not safely control her blood loss before doing a few surgical maneuvers to cut and mobilize a portion of her small intestines. I knew that if I blindly clamped the bleeding area, I could easily cut off all blood supply to her entire small bowel and to the right side of her colon. If that occurred, the consequences would be disastrous, as most of her insides would rot and die. Mary's demise would then soon follow.

Choosing to be cautious, I took a few extra minutes to divide the ligament of Treitz—a fixed layer of intra-abdominal tissue suspending the first portion of Mary's small intestine. Cutting the structure allowed me to sweep her small intestine away from the source of her ongoing blood loss, allowing me perfect visualization of the streaming, vascular injury. I was glad I had decided to take the few extra moments that I did because the torn vessel had been ripped directly off her main intestinal artery, the superior mesenteric artery. Clamping and tying off that particular vessel would have killed her. By carefully repairing the torn eighth-of-an-inch-thick vessel with tiny sutures, I was able to stop the bleeding and at the same time preserve the needed blood flow to her entire digestive tract.

Once the bleeding was definitively controlled, I washed out her abdomen, looked for any other injuries, and closed her up. Instead of stapling closed her skin as I usually do, I decided to place just a few staples spaced several centimeters apart, between which I placed gauze wicks—a maneuver intended to minimize her risk of postoperative wound infection. Having been thrown into mud and presenting covered with God only knows what, I felt that Mary was at a greater risk than most for developing wound problems after surgery.

I then looked at the small cut on her left thigh. It was only an inch long, through the skin, but did not extend into the muscle compartment. I thoroughly washed her small wound with sterile saline. Once satisfied that it was clean, I placed a few staples between which I placed a single gauze wick. I wrapped her entire thigh with rolled, surgical dressings, and I ended my surgical procedure. Looking up at the anesthesia monitors, I saw that her blood pressure was normal and that her heart rate was coming down nicely. I felt that all that needed to be done had been accomplished. I then left Mary in the capable hands of the operating room crew, who would soon take her to the intensive care unit.

Mary did very well after surgery. Although she was kept on the ventilator overnight, by the following morning she was breathing well enough to have the tube removed. For three solid days, her vital signs had all remained stable, and all of her blood tests were normal. Mary was awake, alert, and thankful for all everyone had done to help her. She was complaining of a fair amount of pain, but she also admitted that because of her previous drug abuse history, she always needed more than the usual dose of narcotics to take away her pain. I thought nothing of the amounts of narcotics that were being given to her. Drug addicts unfortunately need a lot more pain medication than most, and Mary had a legitimate source of pain. After all, I had just opened up her belly. Just because she was a drug abuser was certainly no excuse to not treat her pain.

I really couldn't have been more pleased with Mary's progress. However, late in the evening of her third postoperative day, Mary's developed a fever and her heart rate went up dramatically. I did a few routine tests and saw that her white blood cell count had also dramatically risen. I checked her lungs, looking for evidence of pneumonia and examined her abdominal incision, looking for any evidence of a postoperative infection. I checked her for a urinary tract infection, and I examined her leg wound. I found nothing that explained Mary's fever, increased heart rate, and increased white blood cell count other than maybe a hint of inflammation from around the edges of her thigh where I had washed and loosely closed her small cut. But Mary was starting to look sick, and that fact troubled me. Experienced doctors and nurses—and parents for that matter—know the look of when someone they are caring for is starting to become ill, regardless of what the specific findings support. Mary was also starting to ask for more and more narcotics to control pain that she could not describe.

The following day I became even more troubled by Mary's condition. Her fever had been persistently elevated all night despite frequent doses of Tylenol, and her heart rate was beating at over 130 beats per minute. Her white blood cell count continued to rise, and I still didn't have a great explanation for any of it. I became worried that her thigh wound might be getting infected. It had become bit red and was quite painful to the touch. Worried that pus might be accumulating underneath the injured tissues, I removed the loosely placed staples and I widely separated the healing wound edges. That was a very painful experience for Mary, and she screamed as I worked despite the extra dose of morphine the nurse had administered. But there was no pus, and I saw nothing that alarmed me in the depths of her wound. I decided to prescribe antibiotics that would treat what I thought was probably an evolving cellulitis—a skin infection on Mary's thigh.

By the following day, Mary's situation was getting critical. Her blood pressure was dropping and she was making less and less urine. She continued to have fevers, her white blood cell count was at an alarmingly high level, and she was complaining of pain everywhere, including her abdomen. She was hurting more than I would ever expect, even in a drug-addicted individual.

Mary was getting septic—a situation where inflammation from an infectious source generalizes throughout the entire body. I needed to identify the source of Mary's sepsis, but it wasn't obvious. Knowing that I had performed a delicate repair on her superior mesenteric artery, I was well aware that if a clot had formed at my repair site, preventing blood from flowing through to her intestines, her entire small bowel could be dying. Certainly that would cause her dramatic findings, and I really needed to take another look inside her abdomen. I decided to take her back the OR just as soon as a room was available. I told Mary what I planned on doing that day, and I also told her that I had also decided to cut deeper into her thigh wound to look for a pocket of pus, which might have eluded my previous day's limited bedside procedure. Mary didn't care at all what I did. Her attention was wandering and her level of consciousness was fading from both the excessive amounts of narcotics being given to treat her pain and withdrawal symptoms, as well as from the sepsis itself.

Knowing that Mary was not in an appropriate state of mind to give me authorized consent to take her back to the operating room, I placed a long distance call to her mother who one of the hospital chaplains had located in Mary's home state. Our phone conversation was the first I had had with Mary's mother, who I perceived to be a very caring person whose relationship with her daughter had become one of a parent's worst nightmares. She remained calm during our entire conversation and thanked me repeatedly for taking care of her daughter. She told me extensive details of Mary's dark past, hoping that I would understand why the two had become so estranged. She gave me unlimited permission to perform any treatment or procedure necessary to help her daughter, adding that she would make arrangements just as soon as she could to come out and sign whatever legal documents were needed. I assured the mother that her verbal permission was all that I needed. But Mary's mom wanted to see her daughter, and I knew that I would soon be meeting the woman.

About two hours after my conversation with my patient's mother, I was scrubbing my hands outside the operating room, contemplating the potential badness I might soon be encountering as I prepared to dive back into Mary's belly. I envisioned reopening her abdomen and finding her entire length of intestine black and necrotic. I have operated on patients with dead bowel a few dozen or so times previously and it's a terrible problem to deal with. Typically, an older person with an irregular heartbeat flips a small piece of clot from one of his cardiac chambers down the circulatory stream until it lodges in one of his abdominal arteries. Blood flow beyond the obstruction is abruptly interrupted and the intestine that follows becomes strangulated, producing agonizing abdominal pain not too different from that experienced by individuals suffering a massive heart attack.

There is absolutely no mistaking dead bowel once the abdomen is opened. The rotten entrails emit the unforgettable odor of death, powerful enough to make the heartiest of operating room team members retch and occasionally vomit. Surgeons have only one option in such situations to prevent the individuals' otherwise, inevitable demise—complete removal of *all* rotting intestine. But cutting away one's entire intestinal tract leaves the postoperative patient no natural means to absorb any nutrients, and death is often the end result regardless.

By the time my mind had finished wandering, I was already gowned and gloved with surgical scissors in hand, ready to face whatever disaster awaited me deep inside Ms. Cosgrove's abdomen. I exhaled an exasperating sigh, then cut through the sutures holding together the fascia—the densest of the deep layers of my patient's abdominal wall. To my surprise, there was no horrific odor, there was no rancid fluid, and there was no black intestine. In fact, as I quickly rummaged my hands around the abdomen, pushing aside loops of small bowel to better visualize the large intestine, it quickly became apparent to me that Mary's abdomen was just fine. I took a close look at the small section of artery I had previously repaired. It looked pristine, and I felt the distinct, pulsatile vibration of blood flowing through the vessel beyond the level of my sutures. I looked everywhere in her abdomen and I couldn't find anything to account for Mary's sepsis. I was quite relieved knowing that everything was fine in her belly and quickly reclosed her fascia, leaving her abdomen back in the condition I had left it after my initial operation.

Not quite finished with my work, I reminded the OR team that I still needed to open up her thigh wound and perhaps remove a little pus. Most of those in the room forgot that I had said before the case even started that I would also be taking another peek at the thigh, and a few responded with a sarcastic groan. With a few creative cuts with scissors through the layers of the surgical drapes, Mary's thigh wound was exposed and ready to be opened. Hopefully, my little add-on procedure would take me no more than just a few minutes. I decided to cut fairly long and deep, extending the original wound at least an inch on each end and deep to the level of exposed muscle. I wanted to leave no stone unturned. If there was a hidden pocket of pus, I would soon find it.

I opened Mary's thigh wound just as I had planned and found no pus as I thought I might. However, cutting a little further and exposing the deeper layer of tissues released a noxious plume of horrendous odors that could not be mistaken for anything other than death. The odor was the smell of a rotting corpse, and the smell sent a chill up my spine. I knew that the horrible odor indicated that festering under the skin of Mary's thigh was a rotten layer of fascia, teaming with numerous flesh-eating bacteria. From my experience and training, I knew that the deadly bacteria were digesting Mary's fat, fascia, and muscle at an overwhelming speed, all of which would soon kill her.

Flesh-eating bacteria and its by-products consume the tendinous layer of tissue which blankets all muscles—a layer known as the fascia—which separates the muscles from the overlying layers of fat and skin. The flesh eaters destroy everything in their path, digesting muscle, fat, skin, and even blood vessels, leaving a slimy trail of putrefaction and death. The horrible problem, called necrotizing fasciitis, spreads like a match set to gasoline once it takes hold. Unlike most infectious disease processes, antibiotics are of almost no use in the treatment of flesh-eating disease. The only hope for cure is complete surgical removal of any and all human tissue potentially infected with the aggressive organism.

Quite horrified by my finding, I had no choice but to make a long incision down the entire length of Mary's thigh exposing all of her thigh muscles in order to determine how far the flesh-eating infection had possibly spread. As I cut through the swollen skin and fat covering Mary's thigh muscles, I knew what I would find below by the feel of how my knife cut through the tissues. I can't describe what I felt in words, but my muscle memory knew as I was cutting that I had felt that particular type of resistance while removing the fetid tissues of necrotizing fasciitis several times previously. Once I had objective evidence that the muscle coverings were in fact putrid and dead from her left groin crease to just above her knee, I was forced to be aggressive. I sliced away and removed all skin, fat, and dead fascia covering the muscles of Mary's entire left thigh. Even after I removed that huge amount of flesh, leaving all of her muscles exposed and without any protection from the elements, I realized that the flesh-eating colonies had spread even farther upward, extending onto Mary's lower abdominal wall. With additional bold swipes of my scalpel, I removed even more of the infected, rotting tissue, leaving the lower left portion of Mary's abdominal muscles completely bare.

Convinced that I had been at least as aggressive as I had needed to be, I dressed Mary's huge tissue defects with numerous twenty-foot rolls of sterile gauze. I soaked each roll of dressing material in sterile saline solution and layered the wet gauze on top of Mary's thigh and lower abdominal muscles. After layering about a dozen rolls of the gauze into the wound, I covered everything with large, dry, burn dressings.

By the time I had completed both abdominal and thigh operations, Mary had become very unstable, and the anesthesiologist had started a Levophed infusion—a medication used to artificially raise a patient's blood pressure when dangerously low due to generalized sepsis or infection. Levophed is one of those medications most of us don't like to see our patients receive. Many of us still quote the saying told to us over and over during our residency years: "Use Levophed, you leave 'em dead." Basically, people often died while on Levophed, and many of us were never really sure if the death was due to the underlying disease process or the medication itself.

Mary survived the night but she remained in critical condition. Her entire body had become grotesquely swollen from the liters of intravenous fluids needed to keep her circulatory system from collapsing. Her heart rate was too fast, her blood pressure was too low, and her body was making barely enough urine to avoid going into kidney failure. Being all too familiar with the ravages of necrotizing fasciitis, I knew that despite my having cut away every bit of bacteria-laden, dead tissue the evening before, Mary's body was probably still infected. I needed to take her back to the OR again for another look at her wounds. I knew from previous experience that I would almost certainly be cutting away more tissue at my next operation that day.

As I unveiled Mary's wounds in the operating room, removing the gauze packing layer by layer, I again caught a heavy whiff of the distinctive odor of death. Once all dressings were off, I was able to see that, in fact, the necrosis from the flesh-eating bacteria had spread rather extensively. Knowing what I had to do, I started by cutting away additional tissue from the lowest portion of her left thigh wound, now denuding everything to the level of her midcalf. As I usually did in take-back, flesh-eating, necrotizing fasciitis cases, I slid my gloved hand on top of the already defatted and skinned muscles, poking my fingers into the edges of the fatty tissues which remained. What I have found is that if my fingers easily poke through the dissolving, slimy tissues, it all needs to be removed. However, if the tissue feels firm and rubbery and my fingers don't easily poke through, then it can remain. For the most part, everything I poked into gave way as the decaying flesh literally fell apart as I touched it.

Exposing additional areas of dead tissue released more of that overwhelming smell. The odor was so bad that the anesthesiologist pulled out a bottle of mint oil from his anesthesia cart and rubbed it onto his mask. The mint oil overwhelmed the olfactory senses so that the putrid smell couldn't be noticed. He passed the bottle around the room, and the circulating nurse graciously applied some of the oil to my mask.

I did a lot more cutting. By the time I was done with the second tissue-removal procedure, I had collectively removed all skin, fat, and fascia covering the muscles of Mary's left calf, thigh, buttock, flank, abdomen, and lower chest. I was forced to remove some of the tissues in her genital region, completely removing her left labia. The upper limit of my tissue removal ended just below her left breast crease, and her back was exposed all the way to her spine. I had left Mary in a horrifying condition—one which was necessary, but one which I was having difficulty dealing with. She looked like a butchered animal laying there on my operating room table. I had no idea how I, or anyone else for that matter, would ever be able to close her wounds and make her whole again. I wondered if she might be better off dead at that point. But that wasn't for me to ponder. I just hoped that I had finally removed all of the flesh-eating infection, and that Mary would start to get better.

By that time, Mary's mom had arrived from out of town, and I had the most unpleasant task of breaking the news of Mary's infection and the disfiguring operations I had needed to perform to keep her alive. Expectedly, Mary's mother was saddened, but she had obviously had her heart broken many times before and had become rather stoic in dealing with her grief. She asked me how it all happened. I explained to her how the overwhelming, flesh-eating disease is not exclusively due to a particular bacteria or organism per se, but caused by a perfect storm of simultaneous events, including bacterial contamination and temporary immune system failure. In her daughter's case, her thigh wound had obviously been contaminated by something from the mud hole, and the years of drug abuse, lack of sleep, and malnutrition had established the foundation for the second requirement. Her ATV accident, which caused the shock and massive internal hemorrhage, further suppressed Mary's immune system, and the numerous units of blood products necessary to fix the situation added the icing to the immunosuppressive cake. Most people don't realize that blood transfusions cause short-term, immune system suppression. The phenomenon was actually learned decades before in the early years of kidney transplant surgery, as blood transfusions were sometimes used to blunt a patient's immune response, delaying rejection of a transplanted organ.

By the following day, Mary looked just as bad as ever. I really thought that she was going to die, but she kept hanging in there despite her swollen, mutilated, septic state of being. Since I had found so much additional dead tissue the day before, I was obligated to take Mary back to the OR for yet another look. I had really hoped to not find any more dead tissue, but I, of course, did. This time the flesh-eating organisms had extended all the way up Mary's back, and all the way up her chest to the level of the collarbone. The muscles of her chest wall were necrotic, and I needed to peel off everything, leaving just a bony rib cage. I cleaned the infected skin, fat, and fascia off her back, leaving just muscles, and I removed a lot of additional tissue on Mary's chest. Even though I probably should have, I didn't have the heart to remove her breast entirely. Instead, I dissected it off her chest wall and I cut away all of the dead tissues on the back of her breast, leaving the majority of it attached to an infection-free flap of tissue connected to the right side of Mary's chest.

After my third, take-back operation, I needed a full hour just to dress Mary's enormous wounds, which now comprised more than 50 percent of her body. I was really starting to become demoralized, and I was beginning to feel inhuman—like a sick torturer. I was starting to feel anxious about even looking at Mary's wounds, for fear that I would find more and more infection, forcing me to carve away even more than I had already been able to stomach. I knew, of course, that I needed to come back to the OR again the following day, and I absolutely dreaded the thought of it.

Before I took Mary back for her fourth, take-back operation, I sat down with her mother to discuss just how aggressive she wanted me to be. I told her that despite multiple strong antibiotics, excellent critical care management, and aggressive removal of the infected tissues, Mary was not getting any better. I told her mom that I was starting to feel uncomfortable with how badly I was disfiguring her daughter, but at the same time I stated very clearly that the only way to stop the disease process was to do exactly what I had been doing. If I hadn't been so aggressive, there is no question that Mary would have been dead days before. Mary's mom again thanked me for all that I had done and she asked me to take her daughter back to the operating room one more time. She told me to do whatever I needed to do, but she stated that she probably would not consent to her daughter having anything more cut away after this time. She told me that she would pray that whatever God had planned for her daughter's future would be decided at that day's operation. Feeling that there might soon be an end to all of our suffering, I took Mary back for what was probably going to be our final tissue-removal operation.

Once back in the OR, I removed the numerous layers of dressings filling the enormous cavitary defects, which covered more than half of Mary's body. I sheepishly peered at each of the skin edges and muscle layers, again poking my hand as I had done on each of the days prior, looking for new areas of necrotizing fasciitis. Her leg, thigh, and torso all looked pretty good. I didn't see, feel, or smell any more dead tissue. But when I stuck my hand up under Mary's skinned and defatted collarbone, my stomach sank. The tissue was dead! Releasing my hand brought with it the hidden, rotting fumes, and the liquefied human products of bacterial digestion. I was heartbroken, knowing that the flesh-eating disease just couldn't be stopped. Deciding to perform one more reasonable tissue removal, I asked the OR technician for my scalpel and once again I began carving away.

I cut away more tissue above and over the collarbone and slightly over the shoulder area. The dead tissue below her collarbone was a bit more difficult to safely remove. Bit by bit, I picked away the decomposing flesh until I was left with a huge defect containing only the large, skeletonized blood vessels coursing between Mary's heart and her left arm. I saw traces of necrotic material on the outer layer of the vessels, but removing that final bit of diseased tissue would require my removing a large piece of the vessels themselves. By removing the vessels, her arm would certainly die. I really couldn't reconstruct the vessels in a situation like that for a variety of reasons. If the disease was to progress naturally, it would either eat through the artery and vein causing a horrible, bloody end to Mary, or clot would form throughout the vessels causing her arm to die regardless. I was stuck between a rock and a hard place. Considering the discussion Mary's mother and I had just prior to the operation, and considering all that Mary had been through the past week, I decided to cut no more. Perhaps Mary would continue to get better; perhaps she wouldn't. We would just have to let nature take its course at that point and see which way Mary's condition turned.

For the next week, the intensive care unit nurses, my trauma partners, Mary's mother, and I engaged in watchful waiting over Mary. We continued with all of the usual critical care treatment regimens—aggressive antibiotic therapy, ventilator management, kidney dialysis, and intravenous nutrition therapy—as well as daily bedside dressing changes. We did not take Mary back to remove any more tissue. On several occasions, we thought that Mary's death was imminent, but something always seemed to breathe life back into her, and she continued to maintain the status quo.

Another week passed and Mary was still with us. She was getting better, and I became certain that Mary had beaten the flesh-eating disorder. She was stable, off life-supportive medications, and was waking up enough to maintain eye contact with her mother. I took advantage of that window of relative stability and converted Mary's breathing tube to a tracheostomy in the operating room.

We consulted a plastic surgeon to help us figure out how to deal with Mary's huge wounds. Despite my having described her wounds to him in great detail, the plastic surgeon was a bit stunned when I actually took down all of her dressings. He decided that at that point the tissue defects were just too large to cover with any reconstructive, surgical rotation flap, or even skin grafts. So together, we filled Mary's cavities with specialized, sponge material and we covered everything with numerous layers of clear, adhesive drapes. Several vacuum devices applied to the spongy dressings completed the assembly. It was the largest vacuum-assisted closure device I had ever configured.

Vacuum-assisted closure devices (VAC) apply constant suction on wound edges, and significantly accelerate wound healing. They also create a more hygienic situation for the patient as well as the nurses. Every two to three days, we changed the vacuum device, and we noted small buds of healthy tissues forming in the depths of the massive wounds on each occasion. The plastic surgeon felt that we might have to wait a few months before the vacuum device would shrink the wounds small enough to facilitate a reconstructive procedure. Knowing that Mary would be in a stable holding pattern for a long while, we asked our social workers to begin looking into skilled nursing facilities where she could reside as she awaited her ultimate surgical procedure.

Apparently, Mary's mother had also been looking into outside facilities for her daughter. Mary's mother was from out of state, and having Mary transferred to a facility closer to her mom's home would be very helpful for all parties. As it turned out, Mary's mother was an employee of a prestigious university medical center. She had already asked a number of physicians and surgeons to consider accepting her daughter in transfer, and they apparently were interested enough in Mary's case to call me. I discussed the case with a plastic and reconstructive surgeon, who arranged for a surgical intensivist to accept Mary as soon as a bed could be made available for her. Two days later, Mary was loaded up into the back of an ambulance and she ventured off with her mother back to her home state and to a brand-new medical team.

Almost a year passed after Mary and her mother left us. Intensive care unit nurses had received periodic updates from Mary's mother by way of cards and brief phone calls, but neither my partners nor I ever heard any news of Mary's progress. One morning, while my partner was seeing patients in the intensive care unit, Mary returned for a surprise visit. I wish that I had been there to see her. From what I was told, she was happy, energetic, and was so grateful to be alive that she felt that she had to return to thank as many people as possible. She had received several reconstructive surgical procedures at the facility in her home state, and she apparently looked absolutely normal when covered by clothing.

I'm sure that Mary was nothing close to normal—scarred extensively both outside and in, from misadventures both recent and remote. I know that she had a very problematic past, and I hoped that just maybe the tragic events of the past year would cause her to see life from a brand-new perspective. Mary had made it through her period of rock bottom, and perhaps left with great hope and opportunity for a better life. But I also knew that Mary could fall back so easily into the abyss from where she came, using her scars as excuses to drink, to abuse drugs, and to again live recklessly. None of us ever again heard from Mary. I pray she is still doing well.

20

Parking Lot Murder

A Senseless Killing

For as long as there has been man walking upon this earth, there has been another man trying to pick a fight with him. I really don't know what makes us so biologically aggressive and so stupidly territorial over the most trivial of things, causing my gender to repeatedly get itself into so much trouble. Fighting seems to be instinctive and often culturally acceptable. It's even encouraged among some groups. The entire city of Rome used to gather at the Colosseum to watch gladiators battle one another and wild animals, often to the death. A little less than two thousand years later, we still watch men duel in the ring in no-holds-barred fighting competitions, where both participants often end up with broken bones, bloody faces, and serious concussions.

Although those who express their manhood engaged in violent fisticuffs rarely want to cause their opponent life-threatening harm, that all too often is the case. When victims of violent assaults end up in hospital intensive care units in critical condition, more than one person suffers. The loser of the battle often suffers significant disability, and sometimes even death. And the winner of the scuffle often finds himself in a second battle, defending himself in the courtroom as a judge and jury deliberate the attacker's fate. Jail time and life-long criminal records often mar the lives of the young, urban warriors, long after they have lost their fighting spirit.

On a warm, summer's evening, when the humidity was as high as the ambient temperature, two cars of grossly inebriated, young men pulled into the crowded parking lot of a fast-food Mexican restaurant. Only one parking spot was vacant on that night and the drivers of both cars were dead set on occupying that space. Both sped to claim their spot, abruptly braking to avoid a collision as the front ends of both cars nearly breached the narrow opening between the parallel, yellow lines. Steven Gladstone was the only occupant of his car, but the other was brimming with people all wanting to punish him for challenging their right to park their automobile. The cars emptied and angry men with swelled-up chests confronted each other, preparing to square off in physical defense of their little piece of asphalt turf.

Steven was terribly outnumbered and was destined to lose that fight from the very beginning. And lose he did, getting punched repeatedly, primarily by the driver of the other vehicle. Steven's brother happened to be at the restaurant when the confrontation took place, and he saw the fight in evolution. As any good brother should, he went to the aid of his sibling but armed himself along the way with a heavy, industrial-sized, metal flashlight, hoping to gain the advantage over his brother's attackers. However, the larger group was a seasoned cadre of street fighters, and they quickly wrestled away the flashlight and proceeded to club the two brothers into submission. Whereas Steven's brother had retained the physical strength and agility to run away from the losing battle, Steven was knocked senseless from the blows. Unable to extract himself from the uncontrolled rage of his violent attacker, Steven lay obtunded as flashlight blows repeatedly landed on his skull, smashing the hard bones and damaging his brain within.

Steven's attacker only stopped his senseless beating when people eating at the restaurant piled out onto the sidewalk and urged the assailant to stop. The perpetrators then all sped away and Steven's brother returned from hiding to tend to his brother. In what would later become a very controversial point of contention from the main attacker's defense attorneys, the brother attempted to drag Steven back into his car and shouted at bystanders to leave them alone and not call the police or an ambulance crew. Finally after about twenty minutes time, a disgusted restaurant patron ignored the illogical requests of Steven's brother and dialed the 911 operator requesting help.

A few minutes later, the distant wail of police and ambulance sirens chased away many of the remaining rubberneckers. Steven was badly injured and desperately needed the emergency, resuscitative care of the paramedics who pulled up just behind the police vehicles. The emergency medical services personnel found Steven deeply comatose and they quickly inserted a breathing tube and ventilated his lungs hoping to oxygenate the man's injured brain. Steven had not been breathing normally for at least twenty minutes prior to the paramedics' arrival, and his brain was starving for oxygen. Blood poured from a large, deep gash in his scalp, which paramedics tightly wrapped with gauze dressings before they started infusing intravenous fluids. They then rushed their patient off to our trauma center.

When I received Steven, he was completely unresponsive. Respiratory therapists connected Steven's endotracheal breathing tube to the ventilator circuit and the machine took over control of his breathing function. His blood pressure was moderately high and his heart rate was inappropriately slow, beating at only sixty beats per minute—one of the findings often observed when a person's brain pressure is abnormally elevated. I removed the bloody scalp dressing and I found the large, bleeding wound, which I expeditiously whipped closed with heavy, nylon sutures. Steven never even flinched or opened his eyes when I pushed the suture needle through the frayed edges of his bloody scalp. I assigned him a Glasgow Coma Score of three—the lowest coma score possible in a brain-injured patient.

I examined Steven's eyes by shining a flashlight onto his corneas. Dilated, nonreactive pupils stared blankly back at me and gave me further evidence of the seriousness of Steven's injuries. Having heard the details of all that had happened, I suspected that Steven's brain had suffered damage well beyond his physical wounds, a result of diminished oxygen to Steven's brain during the twenty-minute interval prior to the call to the paramedics. I examined the rest of my patient's body from head to toe. Other than a bloody nose, I found no other physical evidence of injury. I X-rayed his chest and pelvis before heading over to the CT scanner, confirming no hidden injuries of significance. I then ordered a stat dose of the drug Mannitol to empirically begin shrinking Steven's swollen brain, despite not yet having any radiographic confirmation of such.

The CT scan did, however, confirm my clinical suspicion of severe traumatic brain injury, demonstrating multiple breaks in the back of Steven's skull, a thin layer of blood between the left side of his skull and his brain, and multiple tiny spots of hemorrhage deep within his swollen cerebral hemispheres.

The findings were troubling as I saw evidence of generalized brain injury but nothing of a discrete size or configuration that would be amendable to surgical treatment. To rule out anything else of significance, I scanned Steven's neck bones, chest, and abdomen, all of which were negative for injury.

Shortly after the Mannitol had completely infused into Steven, I saw a bit of improvement in his neurological condition. Whereas he had previously not moved a muscle, Steven was starting to gag on his breathing tube and he began extending his arms and rotating his legs inward as brain-stem reflexes were starting to become evident. In general, it was not a great sign, but better than no movement at all. After I gave orders to admit Steven to the intensive care unit, I called the neurosurgeon to discuss the case. The neurosurgeon reviewed the scans and we agreed that Steven's injuries were troubling. We also agreed that nothing on the CT scan gave any indication that surgery would be of any benefit. We decided to continue administering frequent doses of the Mannitol, and to repeat Steven's brain scan later in the middle of the night.

The repeat CT scan performed hours later showed no change in Steven's brain. Despite receiving the medication to decrease Steven's brain swelling, he did not improve clinically. By morning, what little arm and leg movement Steven had demonstrated during his resuscitation period was gone. Steven was showing few clinical signs of any brain activity, and he had lost most of his brain-stem reflexes.

Areas of the brain can be categorized in many ways, but the most basic system classification separates the organ into two functional areas—the higher brain and the brain stem. The higher brain includes the cerebral hemispheres, with its frontal, parietal, temporal, and occipital lobes. The higher brain initiates conscious movements and forms thoughts and emotions. It also receives input from the rest of the body including all of its sensory organs. It interprets and integrates all information received. The higher brain is the central processing unit of the body, without which the body's activities resemble that of a corpse with a heartbeat. The brain stem, however, controls reflexive and automatic functions. The initiation of breathing, the regulation of the body's blood pressure, and how the pupils constrict or dilate in the presence of light are all controlled by the brain stem, which is the most primitive of our brain's subsegments.

By mid-afternoon of the day following Steven's attack, Steven no longer demonstrated any higher brain or brain-stem function. Steven's blood pressure was controlled entirely at that time by continuously infusing intravenous medications. If we would have stopped the ventilator, he would not have been able to initiate a breath. Steven appeared to be brain dead, which occurs when ongoing swelling within the brain squeezes down on the blood vessels supplying oxygenated blood flow to its tissues, eventually cutting off all incoming blood supply. A brain without blood flow or a brain without oxygen eventually dies an irreversible death. That seemed to be what had occurred to Steven.

To confirm my clinical suspicions, I started by again examining Steven for any signs of brain activity. At no time had I administered any sedatives or narcotics, so I could definitively exclude medication as a source for Steven's comatose state. I shined a light into Steven's eyes, which again revealed widely dilated, nonreactive pupils. I pushed Steven's breathing tube deep within his throat looking for evidence of a reflexive gag, but I saw none. I squirted iced water into his ear canals, looking for the reflexive eye movements that normally occur when the bedside test is done. But again, I saw no response. I then stood behind Steven's head, and while holding his eyelids open with my index fingers, I rocked his head left and right watching for eye movements usually seen when the brain stem is still alive. Ordinarily, that type of movement causes the eyes to follow the head position slowly, rather than remain in a fixed, rigid position, moving at the same rate as the quickly turned head. Steven's eyes remained fixed like the eyes of a doll, giving me additional evidence that Steven's brain stem was dead.

I waited another day to repeat my clinical tests. They all again confirmed what I had seen the afternoon prior. I then performed one additional clinical test to see if Steven could initiate any spontaneous breathing. I performed a bedside apnea test, where I temporarily disconnected his breathing tube from the ventilator circuit and closely observed him for any reflexive chest movement. Our bodies continuously generate carbon dioxide, eliminated almost exclusively by our lungs as we exhale. When carbon dioxide levels build up in our bodies even slightly, a functional brain stem senses the accumulation of the gas and it involuntarily initiates deep breaths, not to take in more oxygen, but to eliminate the carbon dioxide waste product. I pumped oxygen down Steven's disconnected endotracheal breathing tube by way of a suction catheter connected to the wall oxygen outlet. I continuously monitored Steven's oxygen levels reflected as a percentage of how much of his blood hemoglobin was saturated with oxygen molecules. I then placed my hand on his chest and, with Steven no longer attached to the breathing machine, I watched and waited for him to take a breath.

After six minutes by my watch, Steven had not initiated even a tiny breath. I quickly drew a sample of arterial blood from Steven's wrist artery and sent it to the respiratory lab to analyze the gases in Steven's blood. I then reconnected Steven to the ventilator circuit and I waited for my results.

Not five minutes later, the respiratory therapist brought me Steven's arterial blood gas tests. The crucial value was Steven's arterial carbon dioxide level. Normally, our body keeps the level at around forty, and if it rises even slightly to say forty-five, and certainly by sixty, our brain stem reflexively initiates a very vigorous breathing reflex even in the most comatose of patients—that is, in comatose patients who aren't brain dead. But Steven did not take a breath and his carbon dioxide level had risen to seventy-eight. By definition, if it had risen to at least sixty and he had not started to breathe, his brain stem was considered dead. Steven's level was seventy-eight, and I knew with certainty that he was, in fact, brain dead.

The implications of declaring someone brain dead are enormous. To a lay individual, a brain-dead patient on a ventilator looks identical in appearance to a brain-injured patient, and even to that of a patient under general anesthesia. The physical exam tests I had performed, in addition to the apnea test, confirmed to me that Steven was brain dead. I was soon going to have to explain it all to Steven's already mortified family. Trying to explain brain-stem reflexes and respiratory physiology to a grieving family is usually an impossible endeavor. I knew that I needed to perform one additional, confirmatory test that could objectively demonstrate to his family that Steven's brain was no longer working. I ordered a nuclear brain flow study.

A nuclear brain flow study uses minute amounts of radioactively labeled material injected into the body. A nuclear scanner then images the patient's head and prints a picture of all areas where the radioactive-containing blood is circulating. In patients who are not brain dead, the entire head and neck emit a radioactive signal and scalp, brain, facial, and neck structures can all be visualized. When a person is brain dead, and no blood is flowing to any part of the contents within the skull, the resultant image is that of a hollow shell with no evidence of radioactivity within, surrounded by a halo of glowing scalp tissue, from the radiotracer particles, which continue to circulate through the skin vessels. That is exactly what Steven's nuclear scan showed, and I would use it as a piece of visual imagery to explain the terribly sad news to his family.

By that time, the neurosurgeon and I had prepared Steven's family for the possibility of the terrible outcome. We had suspected from the beginning that Steven's injuries could certainly progress to brain death. I went back to Steven in the intensive care unit, armed with a printed image of the nuclear brain-flow scan, and I asked the bedside nurse to summon Steven's family. Within minutes, Steven's parents, siblings, and a few close relatives all entered Steven's room, each bearing the looks of pain and sadness loving family members always show at such times.

I began my conversation by rehashing many of the details of Steven's initial findings when he arrived to our trauma center, and I detailed the lack of progress Steven had made over the past day and a half. I then told them that I suspected that Steven had progressed to a state of brain death. After taking a short pause to let the thought momentarily sink in, I continued by telling them I had performed several tests confirming that, in fact, Steven was brain dead.

His mother fell to her knees, and tears streamed down his father's cheeks as he tried to support his wife from falling over completely. His siblings cried and they hugged each other, and the brother who was at the scene of the attack looked as if he was going to pass out. I told him to sit, and helped physically ease him into a chair. I then told them all how sorry I was for their loss of Steven, assuring them that we had done all that we possibly could.

I waited a good five minutes before I showed them the nuclear scan, and upon viewing the picture of the hollow tomb of Steven's skull, they each nodded with understanding and acceptance that Steven's brain was gone, and that he was indeed brain dead. I then told them as of that moment, Steven was pronounced dead, and that his body was being maintained by the machines and the chemicals attached to it. I informed them that they had two options at that point: they could elect to have me turn off the machines and disconnect the medications, after which Steven's body would stop working entirely, or they could have me keep his body going by artificial means and arrange for his organs to be removed and transplanted to many different people with terminal organ failure in need of healthy body parts like Steven's.

It is often a painfully difficult decision for a family member to make. Often, grieving parents just want to bury their child and get on with things as quickly as possible. But at other times, they are consoled by the understanding that by donating their child's organs, perhaps something good can come of such a tragic situation. I did explain to the family that if they chose to donate his organs, an organ transplant team from a different hospital would come out and perform extensive tests on Steven's body. I also explained that the actual organ procurement operation might not take place for one to two days, as the transplant team would have to locate suitable organ recipients before they could actually begin the final, surgical procedure.

The family was reeling with the difficulty of their decision, so I told them to spend some time together, to talk about everything, and to let me know when they had made their decision. After concluding our difficult discussion, I gave them one more expression of condolence, and left the intensive care unit.

It took Steven's family the rest of the day to make their decision. As the sun was setting, they decided that they just could not deal with the situation any longer, and they decided to have me withdraw all support and let Steven's body go. I understood their decision, but I also felt that it was a tragic shame. Steven's organs were no longer of any use to him, and there were so many others out there who desperately could have used them. But their decision was what it was, and at that time, there were no laws or provisions to do what Steven might have wanted, rather than what his grieving family chose to do to ease their own suffering. Thus, in accordance with the wishes of Steven's family, I had the breathing machine and the medication pumps turned off, and Steven's heart slowed down to a complete stop.

Steven's legal status then changed from assault victim to murder victim. In accordance with state laws, Steven's body had to be turned over to the county coroner. I contacted the official personally, as I do in all violent death cases, to discuss the details with him. I was told that one of the coroner's deputies would be sent to the hospital to collect Steven's remains, and that an autopsy would be scheduled for the following day.

Several months passed and Steven's body had long since been buried. News articles of the upcoming, murder trial dominated the local papers. I fully expected to be summoned to testify in court since I had been Steven's treating physician. I received my subpoena as I had anticipated and on the second day of the murder trial, I entered the courtroom as I had done during several other such trials to answer any and all questions posed to me by the prosecuting and defense attorney teams. Taking my seat on the witness stand, I glanced about the room to take in a full view of my audience.

I recognized Steven's parents, his brother, and several others who had stood vigil by his bedside during those terrible days and nights. I then looked at the prosecutor's table and sized up the state's attorney's legal staff—a fairly young group of three lawyers whose average age I guessed was no more than about thirty. I looked over at the defense table where I saw the young man on trial for murder, looking well groomed and sharply dressed, hardly like any violent criminal I could have imagined. I felt sorry for him, despite knowing all that had happened. I could only imagine that the man on trial—no older than his mid-twenties—had regretted every moment of that fateful day as much as did the victim's family seated several rows behind him. But the defendant was flanked by four, well-seasoned attorneys, each likely in his fifties. I felt that he would likely get the best deal money could possibly obtain.

Finally, I looked over at the jury box where the twelve jurors and several alternates sat. It was early in the trial, and each still seemed quite interested in the details of the case. I usually notice a few heavy eyelids if I'm asked to testify later in the trail. But on that day, each of the defendant's supposed peers seemed wide awake.

The judge welcomed me to his courtroom and directed me to the court officer who asked me to raise my right hand and swear to tell the truth, the whole truth, and so on. I affirmed the oath resoundingly and took my seat. I then spent the next several hours answering questions from the attorney groups representing both sides of the trial. The prosecutors were most interested in the details of Steven's physical injuries, and how I went about making my various diagnoses. The defense attorneys, meanwhile, were clearly more focused on areas of minutia, most specifically whether or not a lack of oxygen to Steven's brain contributed to his ultimate demise. I recognized the defense strategy, which claimed that Steven's brother's interference with the restaurant patrons attempting to get the victim prompt medical attention may have contributed to Steven's ultimate demise. They argued that perhaps Steven's injuries could have been easily treated if it hadn't been for the brother's doings.

But I was just a treating witness and I was not responsible for deciding any degree of guilt or innocence. I answered every question factually. Whenever I was asked to give my opinion to either side, the attorney representing the opposite team promptly interjected with a loud "I object—speculation" comment. The judge always responded with directions as to how the jury should handle my answers and we continued on. When the state and the defense were both through with me, the judge thanked me for my testimony and I departed the courtroom. As I walked out, I looked at Steven's family and then at the man on trial. I gave them each a subtle nod, hoping that each understood that I was wishing that each of them be well.

About a month later, I heard that the jury had reached a decision and that they had found Steven's assailant not guilty of murder, but guilty of some lesser crime. I had also heard that he was sentenced to only a few years in prison, and that he would likely serve only a portion of his sentence. Not really knowing how I felt about the jury's decision, I chose to not think about it any longer. Steven was dead—killed at the hands of another. But there were other factors involved as well. Not having heard all of the details, I chose to not judge the man who beat Steven to death, aware that he would certainly not be enjoying his upcoming stay in prison, regardless of how much time he would be serving.

Knowing that I occasionally get subpoenaed by various legal jurisdictions to testify in front of lawyers, judges, and juries to detail the care I've provided to the criminals and to their victims in our trauma region, doctors often ask me if I mind getting "commanded" to show up to courtrooms on one of my rare days off, to receive no compensation for my time, and to provide testimony, which could easily be read to the jury from my extensively detailed trauma notes. Whereas my participation in our legal process is a nuisance and an imposition that I would rather avoid, I do try my best to support our legal professionals who altruistically strive to preserve fairness and accountability. When my physician colleagues tell me that I'm crazy for playing nice with the legal professionals, I simply smile back at them and retort half mockingly, "It's all part of the life of a trauma surgeon, my friends—a life I don't expect you to understand," and I casually move on.

21

The Sniper's Rifle

The Benevolence of a SWAT Team Member

My trauma surgeon duties cause me to spend a significant portion of my days and nights in the emergency department where I often interact with the numerous paramedics and law enforcement officers in our area. I have developed a sincere respect for the individuals—professionals whose work is dictated by the bad luck and poor choices made by citizens needing their services. Like me, they are public servants, working for the people who need them, which often tend to be at the most inconvenient of times. Every one of our police and fire professionals works his or her annual share of weekends, holidays, days, and nights. They are people who receive few if any accolades for having to miss family birthdays, special events, and even federal holidays despite the fact that most individuals enjoy the days relaxing and enjoying each other's company. Unlike teachers, postal workers, and countless others who are virtually guaranteed days off on Christmas, Thanksgiving, New Year's Day, and each and every Sunday, it is a foreign concept and a luxury not afforded to our policemen and firefighter-paramedics.

I have witnessed hundreds of interactions between the police and the individuals in their custody brought in to our emergency room for evaluation of some medical or mental condition. I can't even begin to estimate the large number of people I have seen, already in legal trouble, who can't seem to help but make matters worse for themselves. I have seen scofflaws argue with, make verbal and physical threats toward, and even spit at the officers who have placed them under arrest. Although I know that alcohol, drugs, and mental instability often impairs the judgment of many people under arrest in our emergency room and in our trauma bays, I am always surprised when a pair of handcuffs doesn't immediately tame the wildness out of most of those in custody. I am convinced that whenever I hear someone badmouthing police officers in general, it must be because of some adverse experience in their past when they or when someone close to them broke the law and were unhappy that the police had treated them like the lawbreakers they were.

I give so much credit to the city cops, county sheriffs, and state police officials who go above and beyond tolerating what I consider absolutely inappropriate behavior from their arrestees. I have seen officers of the law demonstrate extreme acts of restraint toward the very individuals whose actions would make me want to beat them senseless. I don't know if it is their special training or what which keeps the officers so calm. I truly think that our police deserve much more credit than they ever receive for putting up with some of the most arrogant, righteous, and nastiest people I've ever seen. Fortunately for me, most of my trauma patients are usually too badly injured to give me any trouble. However, sometimes after they've recovered from their surgeries and their period of critical illness, they reveal the ugliness and unpleasantness of their true personalities.

On a late spring day, a man named Dale Woodridge kept both the police officials and our trauma service very busy. Dale was distraught over something in his life, and like so many times before, he decided to drown his problems in a bottle of booze. He was frustrated, angry, and thinking through the cloudiness of his intoxication, which created havoc for several city blocks surrounding his home. Dale had barricaded himself in his house, holding his wife and himself hostage with a hunting rifle he owned. The local police had already been on the scene keeping neighbors and bystanders a safe distance away from Dale's home, not knowing if he might start shooting randomly. On several occasions, Dale opened his door, screaming obscenities and waving his weapon wildly in random directions, which gave police good reason not to rush the building and risk getting shot in the process.

The regional SWAT team was called to the scene and snipers positioned themselves on the roofs of adjacent homes should their expertise be needed.

For six hours, a hostage negotiator tried to get Dale to lay down his weapon and exit his home peacefully, but to no avail. Contact had been made with Dale's wife and she seemed frightened but unharmed. The tense situation was at a standstill and my partner, who was the in-house trauma surgeon that day, was put on notice as to the events that were proceeding.

Without warning, Dale exited his home and he raised his rifle to his right shoulder and took careful aim in the direction of a group of police officers taking cover behind squad cars. Dale was sternly ordered to drop his weapon but it was clear that he was not interested in complying with the SWAT team officers. And then a loud report from one of the strategically positioned AR-15 sniper rifles ended the standoff before any innocent individuals could get hurt. Dale collapsed as the military round, traveling at nearly 2,400 feet per second, exploded just left of the midline through Dale's left, lower rib cage. SWAT team members and paramedics immediately descended on Dale, cleared him of all weapons, and began performing life-saving, emergency medical treatment.

Dale had been immediately rendered unconscious by the supersonic round, as his left lung collapsed and blood and gastrointestinal contents poured into his wounded body cavity causing instant, hemorrhagic shock. Paramedics began breathing for Dale through a skillfully placed endotracheal tube. Intravenous lines were placed and pressure dressings were held over his gaping wound. Dale was then rushed into the back of the awaiting mobile intensive care unit ambulance and sped to the trauma center, where my partner was waiting to receive him.

Throughout all of the excitement, I was at home after having worked all night in the hospital caring for other trauma patients. But I was on backup call that day, available should I be needed in case multiple patients requiring emergency surgery were brought in simultaneously, or in cases like on that day when an extra pair of educated hands were desired. I received a page from the trauma room notifying me that my partner requested my assistance, and within minutes I was in my car and driving to the trauma center to help in whatever way I could.

By the time I had arrived, Dale was already in the operating room undergoing emergency surgery at the hands of my partner. I went directly to the operating room after changing into surgical scrubs. I saw my partner with his hands elbow deep inside Dale's abdomen. Moments later, he withdrew his hands and pulled out Dale's shattered spleen, dripping with blood, with clamps still attached to the vessels my partner had divided. Seeing that the spleen was out, I wondered if my partner still needed my help. Chuckling at my inquiry, my partner asked me to take a look inside Dale's abdomen, and I saw that there was a lot of damage still needing repair. Without saying another word, I went out to the scrub sink and prepared myself for some exciting surgery.

Once gloved and gowned, I took my position at the patient's right side while my partner stood at his left. He then told me the crazy circumstances of our patient's injuries. I asked what had already been done, and my partner told me that he had placed a drainage tube into Dale's left chest cavity. Because of the trajectory of the bullet, he had assumed correctly that the majority of the injuries were in the patient's abdomen, prompting the abdominal exploration where he found the shattered, bleeding spleen.

Dale's abdomen looked like a bomb had gone off, mangling his insides. Within moments, I saw that most of his stomach had been blown away, and the pancreas gland—located behind the stomach and coursing up into the inner surface of where the spleen once was—had also been badly damaged. A large cavity within the muscles along Dale's spine was oozing blood, and we packed it tightly with surgical sponges, allowing us to address his more alarming injuries first.

The stomach was unsalvageable, and we decided to remove nearly all of it, leaving only the uppermost remnant of the healthy organ connected to the abdominal portion of his esophagus. Once the majority of the stomach was removed, we suctioned out the partially undigested meal our barricaded subject had recently eaten, which was now contaminating his abdominal cavity. We then washed out Dale's insides with a few liters of fluid, allowing us to fully inspect the badly damaged pancreas gland more accurately.

The long, narrow gland's main portion looked pretty healthy, but the tail end of his pancreas was destroyed and needed removing. We gently dissected the delicate organ off the back wall of Dale's abdomen and fired a surgical stapling device across the midbody of the pancreas, removing everything beyond the level of our carefully placed staple line. But several pancreatic vessels continued to bleed, requiring us to suture-close each of the bleeding points. We then placed two surgical drains next to the edge of the surgically divided pancreas, knowing that the injured gland would continue to ooze digestive juices for many days after surgery.

We continued to explore the rest of Dale's abdomen and found four holes in the small intestine. The injured bowel was too badly damaged from the blast energy of the high-powered rifle to repair. We removed the injured portions of bowel and reconnected the healthy ends together using both surgical staplers and hand-sewn techniques.

Next, we examined the left side of Dale's diaphragm, knowing that the bullet had to have passed through it. Having already removed the spleen, stomach, and the left half of the pancreas, we had more than enough room in the gaping, residual space to clearly see the badly frayed, thin leafy muscle, which separated Dale's chest and abdominal cavities. Fortunately, the diaphragm is very flexible, and even after cutting away the dead edges of the injured muscle, we were able to pull together the gaping wound without tension and hand-sew everything back together using several layers of well-placed suture.

Finally, we had to definitively restore continuity of Dale's gastrointestinal tract. At that juncture in our operation, Dale's tiny, remaining stomach was not connected to the rest of his intestine. After debating how best to complete our repair, we decided to pull up a loop of healthy bowel and sew it to the gastric remnant reestablishing unobstructed flow throughout. We sewed everything together with meticulous precision, knowing that a leak in the area would not be tolerated by Dale's body. By the time we were done, we were quite happy with our completed work.

We removed the packing from the hole in the muscles adjacent to Dale's spine and saw that the wound was still oozing. Knowing that the packing had done a lot of good, we decided to repack the hole with a dissolving, clot-forming surgical material, which we could leave in place and not worry about having to come back and remove. We packed the hole tightly, again washed out and suctioned dry Dale's abdomen, and then tightly closed his abdominal wall. We concluded the operation by applying layers of gauze dressing over the abdominal and chest wounds, and connected the two drains we had placed through the abdominal wall to suction bulbs, which we taped to Dale's skin. The OR crew then moved Dale onto a transport cart and we delivered him to the intensive care unit nurses.

Although I was more than pleased with the work my partner and I had done on our patient, I knew that he would have a potentially stormy, postoperative course. What worried me most was Dale's pancreatic injury. Pancreatic injuries are notorious for giving surgeons grief and more than their desired share of gray hair. Everyone who operates on the abdomen knows this well. In fact, there is a saying among surgical residents going through their training that helps them survive their years of educational torture. As the simple, all-inclusive saying goes, "Eat when you can, sleep when you can, and if at all possible, *don't* mess with the pancreas."

The pancreas is the most unforgiving of all of the body's organs. It resides deep within the abdominal cavity, making access to it difficult. It has a soft, but crumbly consistency, and is easily damaged even by the gentlest touch of a surgeon's fingers. Numerous small and sizable blood vessels course through it, causing it to bleed easily. The pancreas produces multiple hormones and digestive enzymes, which can ooze from its damaged tissues. The enzymes ordinarily digest the fats and proteins we ingest on a daily basis. When those same enzymes leak inside the abdomen, they begin digesting the abdominal fat and protein structures, creating intense pain and chemical damage not unlike an internal, caustic burn.

The two drains we placed near the end of the surgically resected pancreas would be key to preventing complications in our postoperative patient. Any leaking enzymes would be collected by the drains minimizing any internal damage. We placed two drains because as the old Special Forces saying goes, "Two are like one, and one is like none." In essence, collection of any leaking pancreatic juice was so important to our patient's overall well-being, that we just couldn't trust that one drain would be sufficient.

Knowing that I had done all that was needed of me, I decided to head for home. Mr. Woodridge would be under the very able care of my partner and the intensive care unit nurses. I also knew that in about twelve hours, I would again have to come back to the hospital and assume all responsibility for the trauma service, which included our new patient. I was also still on backup call and still very tired from my last period of in-house duty. I could still get called back that night and getting some sleep was a priority of mine. So I left the hospital and managed to get some much needed rest in preparation for the next day's events.

As I had predicted, Dale did develop some problems after surgery. His pancreas leaked large amounts of enzyme-containing fluids, which were all fortunately gathered up and cleared by the two drains we had placed during surgery. He also had some postoperative respiratory problems, which necessitated us leaving Mr. Woodridge on the ventilator for more than a week. Fearing that we might not be able to remove his breathing tube in a reasonable amount of time, we obtained permission from our patient's extremely forgiving wife to perform a tracheostomy if needed. She asked that we delay the procedure for as long as possible to allow her husband every last chance to improve without the additional procedure. We accommodated her request.

We were faced with the extra challenge of providing enough nutrition to Mr. Woodridge without using his gastrointestinal tract. As we often do after performing complicated stomach or intestinal surgery, we like to delay feeding our patients by conventional means, allowing the bowel to heal and return to normal activity first. It ordinarily takes only a few days, but in Dale's case, the pancreatic enzyme leak delayed our ability to feed him for a much longer time. Pancreatic enzymes are stimulated by the presence of food in the stomach, and by dripping liquid nutrition through a tube passed down his nose or mouth, we would only further increase the pancreatic leak, and delay healing even more.

To meet Dale's nutritional needs, we began feeding him total parenteral nutrition, or TPN. TPN is a concoction of amino acids, carbohydrates, and lipids, added to a carefully created electrolyte- and vitamin-enriched solution, which gets slowly infused through an intravenous catheter inserted deep inside a patient's central circulatory system. Like chemists, we analyzed each day's lab values, determining exactly how much material to add or remove from the daily mix of nutrients in order to provide enough sustenance to heal our patient, yet not too much to cause any one of the myriad of problems often encountered when administering TPN. We also began injecting Mr. Woodridge daily with a hormone that inhibits the secretion of pancreatic enzymes. The combination of therapies—TPN and inhibitory hormone injections—continued for two weeks until the fluid in the drainage tubes we placed during surgery began to slow down to only a scant amount each day.

Healthier from the absence of the caustic, pancreatic juices and from just the right amount of intravenous nutrients, Dale became strong enough to be removed from the ventilator. However, wound problems became an issue. The bullet entrance wound in his left lower chest was healing slowly as was the exit wound in his back. We changed his wound dressing twice daily, each time packing the cavities with a saline-dampened layer of gauze. Slow progress was being made and the wounds were not becoming infected, but Mr. Woodridge was largely intolerant of the painful dressing changes as we rolled him onto his side to access both wounds. Once the breathing tube had been removed, he obsessively requested more and more narcotic, pain medications, which made him weak and prevented him from participating in physical therapy.

We eventually felt comfortable enough to begin feeding Dale by mouth, but his tiny stomach remnant could not hold more than a few swallows of food and he vomited repeatedly after each meal. We finally found the right combination and volume of food, which prevented him from vomiting and which maintained his nutritional requirements. Dietitians brought Dale tiny meals every three hours, each packed with protein, and each of which he consumed over about an hour's time. The regimen seemed to work well, but he still remained very weak.

Due to the events of the day that caused Mr. Woodridge, the SWAT team, and the trauma service to become acquainted, psychiatrists were consulted to assess his mental state and to determine how best to help him once we were ready to discharge our patient from the hospital. Dale was technically under arrest, but he was in no condition to run from the law even if he had somehow managed to leave the hospital. An agreement was reached between Dale and the law enforcement officials, giving him freedom of movement. Dale would have his legal proceedings begin after he had recuperated. The psychiatrists felt that Dale would benefit from a few weeks of inpatient psychiatric care after we were through with him. Dale agreed to the plan, knowing that spending time on the psychiatric ward could only help extend his freedom and keep the police and the state's attorneys from bothering him for an extended period of time.

After one more week in our hospital, we discharged Mr. Woodridge to the psychiatric facility. As it turned out, Dale ended up spending not two weeks but four weeks confined on the psych ward, as he repeatedly expressed the desire to hurt himself and possibly others. When the psychiatrists finally felt that Dale was no longer a threat to himself or others, they released him to the care of the woman who he held hostage at gunpoint in their own home nearly two months previously. As ironic as that may seem, the psychiatrists felt that Dale never really had any intentions of harming his wife, and his wife chose not to press any charges against her husband. And so, Mr. Woodridge was released on bond for some relatively minor charges, and he was eventually discharged to his home.

About a week later, Mr. Woodridge followed up in our trauma clinic for us to evaluate his nearly healed wounds, and for us to remove his pancreatic drains. I was the surgeon running the clinic that day when Dale returned to us.

He was accompanied by his wife. The three of us talked at great length of the events that had taken place since the day of his shooting. Mr. Woodridge was a very different man on that day compared to how he was when we transferred him to the psychiatric ward. Whereas he had previously been a sniveling, broken man, Dale had become overly energetic, very arrogant, and completely devoid of any responsibility of his getting shot by the SWAT team sniper. I listened as Dale rambled on and on, while I inspected his residual wounds, removed his drains, and reapplied small dressings. I wondered what diagnosis the psychiatrists had missed because Dale seemed more like a narcissistic than a depressed, suicidal victim. I sensed that Mr. Woodridge's wife was under his control, thoroughly manipulated, and convinced of his innocence of all matters causing his physical disability.

Then Mr. Woodridge started discussing his lawsuit against the local police department and the SWAT team that fired the single bullet. He arrogantly boasted of how his attorney was going to make him a rich man, and how he would soon own the city that put him in the terrible situation. With my tolerance for Dale's drivel growing excessively thin, I looked him in the eye and asked him why he was so angry at the police for doing their job and why he couldn't just be thankful for being alive. He looked at me as if I was crazy, and then began telling me how he would never have died from his one gunshot wound. Realizing that Dale needed a serious reality check, I began telling him in great detail how the bullet had blown through his lower chest, cut through the lowest portion of his lung, tore through his diaphragm, and shattered his spleen, stomach, and pancreas. I told Dale how his intestines were pouring liquid stool throughout his abdomen, and just how close he had come to meeting his Maker. I explained to Dale the details of the surgery my partner and I had performed on him, and how lucky he was to be alive despite his serious injuries.

But Dale had neither the interest nor the desire to hear what I was saying. His wife was listening quite attentively, however, and I knew that all that I had said was getting through to her. I then asked Dale if he knew what he had been shot with, and if he knew anything about weapons. Dale did not know that he had been shot with a military sniper's rifle, and he seemed to momentarily come to his senses when I compared it to the power of one of his deer-hunting weapons. Still, he was convinced that the police had used what he called "excessive force" against him, so I responded by telling him that he was lucky the sniper had intentionally missed. His attention suddenly captured attention, Dale jeered, telling me that if the sniper had missed he wouldn't have had to have so much surgery and spend so many months in the hospital.

I then explained to Dale what I meant when I said that the sniper intentionally missed. I told him that back when I was in the military, we were taught to shoot for certain areas of the body to guarantee a fast kill. I drew a human target on the paper of the examining room table and I penned a circle within the head area with a two-inch swath of ink extending directly down the center of the chest and abdomen. I told Dale that if we could hit anywhere within the area I drew, that our bullet would guarantee death for our target. I informed him that I could hit an object dead center from three hundred meters with iron sights— that is, without the use of a high-powered scope. But I wasn't a sniper. I was a military doctor who just happened to shoot well, but nowhere near as well as the elite snipers. I assured Mr. Woodridge that the snipers, who had been sitting up on those roofs less than two hundred feet away from him, had him perfectly sighted through their high-powered scopes and could have taken the wing off a mosquito if they had wanted to. I told Dale that technically, the sniper had screwed up, and Dale should have been a dead man lying on his front lawn. But obviously, the sniper who took the shot that day felt just a little bit sorry for Dale and wanted to give him a chance to live. So he must have intentionally missed, causing Dale to drop his weapon but not necessarily die.

I continued by saying that he was lucky to have had the sniper who shot him, because most men wouldn't have been so kind. I then told him that if I had been up there on that roof that I wouldn't have missed. But as fate would have it, I do surgery for a living and the sniper who fired the rifle shoots people for a living. I restated that Dale was indeed lucky that day, and I again told him to be thankful for being alive.

My last bit of commentary seemed to get through to Dale, and suddenly his arrogant and confident disposition turned into passive sheepishness. He was no longer talking a mile a minute but was quietly thinking about what I had told him. I smiled at Dale and I shook his hand, telling him to keep working hard at getting better. I told him that his wounds were healing so well that he no longer needed to come back to our clinic unless he had additional concerns or problems. With that, Dale and his wife quietly thanked me and together they left the office.

Dale never returned to our clinic, and I was never asked or subpoenaed to testify on Mr. Woodridge's behalf or on the behalf of the police department as the treating physician who cared for Dale Woodridge. That would all ordinarily be a routine occurrence in a lawsuit involving something as dramatic as was the situation with Mr. Woodridge. But I never heard anything, and I can only presume that perhaps I got through to Dale and convinced either him or his wife to come to their senses and to drop their ridiculous lawsuit against the police.

22

The Alcoholic Trauma Patient

One of Many Ways to Ruin One's Life

S ubstance abuse is one of society's most pervasive problems these days. I have treated hundreds—no, make that thousands—of people who have injured themselves or who have been the victims of violent crime as a result of substance abuse. And I have managed countless individuals who have suffered one or more of the many complications of excessive drug or alcohol consumption, in one form or another. My trauma patients frequently pop positive for one or more of the illicit substances tested for on the routine, trauma toxicology screen, or they present to our trauma bay grossly intoxicated from alcohol, well beyond a reasonable or acceptable level. I have seen people across the entire social spectrum who use and abuse substances to excess. I have seen people of all ages—grade-school children through octogenarians—brought into our trauma room physically and mentally impaired from one or more substances, or from a combination of liquor and hard drug use. Substance abuse, without question, has no financial, social, or cultural boundaries.

In years past, cocaine was the illegal drug most commonly abused by the trauma patients I have treated. It was not unusual for paramedics to bring casualties to our trauma center after the cokeheads careened several stories over balcony ledges, having suddenly fallen asleep while standing, following a multiple-day, continuous drug binge. But cocaine is now just one of a multitude of common illegal drugs of abuse. The long list includes heroin, ecstasy, LSD, crystal methamphetamine, and, of course, marijuana. A huge percentage of the drugs abused, however, are not illegal in and of themselves. They are often prescribed by doctors for therapeutic treatments of one malady or another. Many people seem to have turned prescription drug use into a recreational phenomenon. The most commonly abused prescription drugs my patients seem to use in excess include the anxiety-relieving agents Ativan and Xanax, as well as the narcotic, pain relievers oxycodone, hydrocodone, and Dilaudid. I can't even begin to estimate how many of patients I see brought in to me after a serious accident or injury were already addicted to these prescription medications or various street drugs.

Some patients actually believe that they have genuine medical conditions requiring multiple doses of antianxiety pills or painkillers daily for years on end. Most patients do not realize that the conditions for which they are being treated, by the licensed physicians who endlessly rewrite their prescriptions, are often nothing more than common addictions to the medications they continuously refill. These patients go back to their doctors on a monthly basis for years to obtain refills of the drugs that should have been stopped long ago. The addictions develop insidiously, and neither patient nor doctor may realize that a serious chemical dependency is developing. After a while, however, both parties realize that if the patients go without their drugs, the chronic abusers will inevitably develop painfully miserable withdrawal symptoms.

It can be almost impossible to relieve patients addicted to pain pills, who subsequently suffer traumatic injuries, of their new pains. Bodies addicted to narcotics become hypersensitive to noxious stimuli, requiring huge doses— often dangerously large amounts—of narcotics to ease their suffering. Patients addicted to sedatives and anxiety pills become hyperagitated when their pills are withheld. Their bodies' central nervous systems rebound without their usual doses of medication to slow them down, often leading to paranoia, hallucinations, and occasionally even seizures.

Substance abuse is clearly a terrible problem. But that doesn't necessarily make the people who abuse drugs bad people. I believe that some people are genetically predisposed to be more likely than others to become addicted to various substances. I also suspect that a genetic marker that codes for drug and alcohol addiction is probably closely linked to various mental illness genes, as I have noticed a strong correlation between the two problems. Obviously, those people biologically predisposed to chemical dependency need to expose their bodies to the substances to which they become addicted, but exposure can easily occur under fairly benign circumstances. Hospitalized patients undergoing elective, outpatient surgical procedures are routinely discharged with at least one prescription for narcotic pain relievers. And people suffering the loss of a family member, or any other emotionally traumatic event, often get prescribed medications to relieve short-term anxiety. Both groups of people prescribed potentially addictive medications for legitimate reasons may unknowingly soon become hooked on the drugs originally intended to abate suffering of one form or another.

It's easy to understand how both examples can evolve into substance abuse and substance addiction if neither physician nor patient pays close enough attention to how much medication is being prescribed, refilled, or consumed. Even those individuals who become addicted to street drugs may never have intended to consume more than just one experimental dose of whatever it is they get hooked on. But if biologically predisposed—genetically hardwired to become addicted—the otherwise decent individuals lose control over everything else in their lives as they become physically and psychologically overtaken by the sole need to obtain and consume more of the mood-altering drugs.

By far and without question, the substance of abuse that damages more bodies, destroys more relationships, and ruins more lives than any other legal or illegal drug is none other than ethyl alcohol—the popular and intoxicating component of beer, wine, and hard liquor. Most people recognize the destructive potential of alcohol, as everyone has known town drunks or have seen homeless bums who drink booze from bottles shrouded in paper bags. But far more numerous than the destitute, street alcoholics are our society's functional drunks and closet drunks.

Functional alcoholics often hold down productive jobs and lead respectable lives, yet work alcohol into their daily routine as if it were as essential as breakfast, lunch, and dinner. They may have a few beers or cocktails at lunch, or they may stop by a bar or restaurant after work to throw back a few among friends. They often wind down their days and workweeks with scheduled binges, yet always know how to appear sober when necessary or appropriate. Functional alcoholics rarely get themselves into trouble, but can become medical disasters when admitted to a hospital for long periods of time. Depending on the level of an alcoholic's addiction, physical withdrawal can begin after just one day, or it can take several days to manifest itself. When alcohol withdrawal does happen, it is an extremely unpleasant and physiologically dangerous situation.

Unlike functional drunks who openly drink alcohol yet seem to responsibly imbibe, closet alcoholics drink and get drunk in secrecy. It always amazes me how spouses and live-in family members can have absolutely no idea that a person living among them is an alcoholic. Closet drunks often have a previous history of admitted problems with alcoholism, and many have spent one or several periods of time in an alcohol rehabilitation program. However, having again fallen off the wagon, many of these people can no longer admit to their friends and family that they are drinking for fear that they may get thrown out of their home or disowned. Often humiliated and embarrassed by their repeated failures, they work diligently at keeping their addictive habit to themselves, and secretly drink only when they feel confident that they won't get caught. However, our paths often cross during unusual times of the day, such as in the midmorning when a grossly intoxicated individual crashes the family car after he or she drops the children off at school and downs a secretly stashed bottle of liquor. Paramedics bring the drunk, injured patients in for me to treat, and family members eventually learn of their dirty, little, addictive secrets.

I could have chosen any one of an abundance of the substance-abusing trauma patients I have managed over the years to share the trials, tribulations, and pains we all endured caring for them. But one individual stands out among my cluster of memories. One particular individual truly exemplified all of the unique aspects of a substance abusing trauma patient. His name was Ronald Davis.

Mr. Davis was a fifty-something, out-of-work alcoholic. He was not a closet alcoholic, but I don't believe that he was a very functional drunk, either. He and his wife had been married for thirty years and his spouse worked for most of those years as a registered nurse. At the time, she had been working full-time in the emergency room of a small-town community hospital. Mr. Davis had been out—several counties away from where he and his wife lived—apparently looking for work. He was driving around on his job search while drunk. The exact details of exactly how the accident occurred are unclear, but regardless, Ron's car impacted another automobile at a very high rate of speed, causing significant damage to both vehicles and to Ron.

When paramedics arrived at the scene, Mr. Davis was in very bad shape, requiring endotracheal intubation, and emergency evacuation to the closest hospital emergency room, which just happened to be a Level II Trauma Center—a trauma facility capable of handling some of the more common, but less complicated trauma patients.

Unfortunately, by the time Mr. Davis had arrived at the closest hospital, his heart had stopped beating. He presented to the facility in full cardiac arrest. The emergency room team performed chest compressions, flooded his veins with epinephrine and other emergency cardiac drugs, and transfused numerous units of blood into Mr. Davis's body aggressively, attempting to save his life. Needles and tubes were placed into both sides of Ron's chest cavity to empirically treat the possibility that one or both of his lungs may have collapsed—a common cause of cardiac arrest in trauma patients. Various bedside diagnostic tests were performed, attempting to determine the cause of Ron's moribund condition. After almost thirty minutes of aggressive efforts, the emergency room doctors had successfully resuscitated Mr. Davis. He once again had a heartbeat, a pulse, and a blood pressure, but he was still very unstable. The doctors determined that Mr. Davis was bleeding internally, but their surgeons, for whatever reason, didn't feel comfortable operating on him. They requested that he be transferred to a higher level of care, and a medical evacuation helicopter, which had been sitting on standby at their hospital, airlifted Mr. Davis emergently to our Level I Trauma Center.

Mr. Davis arrived to our facility unstable and in profound shock. There was little time to do anything other than to take him straight back to the operating room to determine from exactly where his internal hemorrhage was originating. As he was getting packaged for the move to the OR, I quickly checked over the lab and X-ray reports of the studies, which had been performed at the other hospital. The one lab value which stood out was Mr. Davis's alcohol level—the level was 315!

Having treated more intoxicated trauma patients than I care to remember, I frequently brief family members as to the interpretation and understanding of an elevated blood alcohol level. They often ask me for an explanation, based on their family member's alcohol measurement, how drunk the family member actually was at the time of the accident or injury. I try to keep things as simple as possible and explain that for the average person, consuming one alcoholic beverage—one beer, one shot of liquor, or one glass of wine—usually elevates a person's blood alcohol by approximately 25 points. But the body also burns off about 25 points of alcohol each hour. So, say in Mr. Davis's case, having a measured ethanol level of 315 implies that he must have consumed *at least* twelve drinks, assuming that he drank everything in just one hour. More likely, however, he drank more than twelve drinks that day over a much longer period of time. I always tell people that driving with an alcohol level greater than 80 is considered drunk driving. And as I know I told Mr. Davis's wife, Ron had enough alcohol in his system to get nearly four people drunk enough to get ticketed for driving under the influence.

Once in the operating room, I moved pretty quickly to get Mr. Davis's abdomen opened, knowing that his heart had already arrested once. If continuous blood loss was the cause of his cardiac standstill, I wanted to stop his hemorrhaging as soon as possible. My partner happened to be in the hospital and available at the time. Knowing that it might be a difficult surgical case, I asked him to join me in the operating room and to provide me the assistance only another trauma surgeon could. When we cut through the deepest layer of our patient's abdominal wall, blood gushed out faster than we could neatly remove it with two suction devices dialed up to their maximal levels. Blood flowed over the sides of the operating room table and spilled over onto the floor beneath our feet. My partner and I packed Ron's open abdomen as fast as we could and we held pressure on the twenty or so surgical sponges we jammed into his open belly, hoping to compress the source of the tremendous blood loss in order to keep Mr. Davis alive.

Anesthesiologists poured blood into Mr. Davis's veins as fast as it seemed to spill out from his belly. My partner and I held pressure on our patient's internal organs for at least fifteen minutes before the anesthesiologist had enough of the various and different blood products transfused into our casualty to make us all feel comfortable enough to continue operating. As we carefully removed our sponges, it became obvious that our patient was bleeding more than is typical. He was clearly coagulopathic, meaning that his blood was thin and did not form clot as normal blood should. There could be any number of reasons why his blood was so thin. Perhaps he had been taking blood-thinning medications. Perhaps his body had already bled out the majority of its available clotting factors, leaving little more than red blood cells and intravenous fluids circulating throughout his bloodstream. Or maybe his body was just a bit too cold, causing whatever clotting factors that were left in his system to not work properly.

Any or all of these possibilities could have been causing the excessive hemorrhage, and our anesthesiologists did a great job doing whatever they could to remedy the situation. In addition to administering multiple bags of red blood cells to increase our patient's ability to transport oxygen throughout his body, the anesthesiologists also infused numerous bags of platelets and clotting-factor-containing plasma products. All of their efforts helped, but ongoing bleeding made it difficult for us to see exactly which of our patient's organs had actually been damaged.

His primary source of bleeding seemed to be coming from an area in the center of his abdomen. Carefully focusing our suction devices in that region, and via creative repositioning of surgical packs, I saw that our patient was hemorrhaging from an area I call the snake pit—that is, the region of the head of the pancreas. Bleeding from any portion of the pancreas is bad, but bleeding from the head of the pancreas is particularly problematic. Several, large blood vessels, natural drainage ducts originating from the liver region, and the most delicate part of the small intestine are all intimately attached to the head of the pancreas. Damage to the pancreatic head can be notoriously bloody and difficult to control. Fortunately for my partner and me, we were able to visualize a tear in the side of a large vein coursing directly behind the pancreatic head. With nothing less than significant difficulty, we were finally able to repair the bleeding vessel. We might never have even seen the unusually large vein if it wasn't for the major crack in the pancreas itself, which splayed itself open, giving us a perfect view of the damaged, exsanguinating vessel.

Having the major source of bleeding controlled, we were then able to evacuate our patient's abdomen of enough blood to actually see what we were doing. Mr. Davis was still oozing from all over, but our suckers and the multiple sponges kept our operative field clean enough for us to be able to perform a thorough exploration. It seemed that no other organs had been injured from the car crash, but we did find a big problem completely unrelated to his traumatic injuries. Mr. Davis's liver was markedly abnormal. It was firm, shrunken, and nodular. Without question, Mr. Davis had cirrhosis of the liver, almost certainly due to all of his years of excessive drinking. Cirrhosis is a terrible problem and always complicates patients who have just had surgery or who are trying to recover from traumatic wounds. Mr. Davis fell into both categories, and as a result, I expected the whole gamut of complications to follow our operation.

The liver is ordinarily a very robust and self-sufficient organ. Most of it is protected by the rib cage and although often injured, the liver has the remarkable ability to repair itself in most ordinary circumstances. A healthy liver serves many purposes. It produces many proteins, including the numerous, natural clotting factors that circulate throughout our bloodstream, preventing us from bleeding to death after minor wounds and surgical procedures. The liver also produces digestive juices, which when routed into our intestinal tract, allow our bodies to absorb the food products we consume. The liver also chemically modifies the blood carried away from the small bowel before passing into the heart and circulating throughout the rest of the body. The liver thus acts as a detoxifying organ, preventing or minimizing the amount of substances, which adversely affect brain function and other organ systems.

A healthy liver works very efficiently, but a liver damaged by cirrhosis has many limitations. Internal scar tissue replaces much of what was once previously functional liver tissue. The diseased organ no longer generates clotting factors or any other protein for that matter, at the rates and quantities which the body needs. As a result, patients with cirrhosis bleed terribly. Cirrhotic patients can easily bleed to death from relatively trivial injuries and minor operations because their body just can't form clot. In addition, patients with cirrhosis are often intolerant of the various medications and tube-feeding solutions we prescribe to critical care patients in the intensive care unit. In short, patients with cirrhosis are very brittle and the slightest complication or problem often results in their bloody, dramatic death. We often tell our medical students jokingly that patients with cirrhosis can barely tolerate a haircut let alone major surgery.

Knowing that we were lucky to have been able to control our cirrhotic patient's bleeding as well as we had been able to, we knew better than to press our luck any further. It was clearly a time for damage control surgery. So we left all remaining packs in place and we tightly placed a few others over the cracked pancreatic head. We then placed a vacuum-assisted closure device over our patient's open abdomen and moved his chemically paralyzed body off the operating room table and onto an ICU bed. Mr. Davis was wheeled back to the intensive care unit, where we hoped to be able to stabilize him over the next few days before taking him back to the operating room to complete the rest of our surgical procedures.

Over the next several weeks, Mr. Davis remained quite sick and unstable. We took him back to the operating room a half dozen or so times, where we eventually removed all of the internal packs, closed his abdomen, and performed our customary tracheostomy and feeding-tube procedures, preparing him for a long, recovery phase in a skilled nursing facility somewhere remote from our hospital. But even though each of our surgeries was tedious and difficult, nothing we did in the operating room was as frustrating or painful as what we had to deal with every day at our patient's bedside—Mr. Davis's well-intentioned, but incredibly difficult wife.

For starters, it took days for us to convince her that her husband had cirrhosis of the liver. She admitted that her husband drank, but she couldn't believe that his liver was as damaged as we said it was. She kept insisting that her husband had had a needle biopsy of his liver three years before, which had only revealed minimal cirrhosis. She couldn't understand how his liver could have worsened as much over the years as we said it had. For days, she insisted that we obtain the records from the other hospital where her husband's needle biopsy had been performed. She hoped to somehow convince us that her husband couldn't possibly have the problems we knew that he had. Exasperated by the wife's unreasonable requests and her illogical thought process, we finally told her that having seen his hard, shrunken, and nodular liver with our own eyes, we had all the clinical evidence that we needed to make our diagnosis. We would no longer debate or discuss her husband's alcoholic cirrhosis. However, she remained stubbornly unconvinced of our assessment. To resolve matters once and for all, I took photographs of her husband's diseased liver during one of our scheduled, take-back operations and I showed the wife the ugly images afterward. Seeing the pictures with her own eyes finally convinced her to stop arguing with us about her husband's condition as the images clearly revealed the unequivocally diseased and damaged state of Mr. Davis's alcoholic liver.

Mr. Davis went through all of the phases of florid, alcohol withdrawal, as we had expected he might. Despite our having used huge doses of several different medications to minimize or prevent his delirium tremens, Mr. Davis still progressed to full-blown seizures—the extreme at the end of the spectrum of alcohol withdrawal syndrome. Yet, despite seeing her husband restless and agitated while on excessive doses of sedative medications, as well as having seen the intraoperative photos of his diseased liver, Mrs. Davis still couldn't get herself to admit that alcoholism was entirely responsible for her husband's problems. She even watched her husband convulse, but still seemed to deny that her husband had a serious alcohol problem. I became convinced that Mrs. Davis must in some way have enabled her husband's behavior and, for whatever reason, she must never have opened her eyes wide enough to convince herself or her husband that he indeed did have a severe drinking problem.

Mrs. Davis made it perfectly clear on numerous occasions during her lengthy bedside visits that she was a nurse, and as such, she stated that she was perfectly able to understand everything going on with her husband. The odd thing, however, was that Mrs. Davis seemed to want to be involved more as a nurse caretaker rather than as a wife. As a result, Mrs. Davis micromanaged everything our nurses did and she picked the doctors' brains to the extreme point of alienating everyone around her. She politely criticized the way the nurses inserted IV catheters, the manner in which they changed her husband's dressings, and even the way they shaved her husband's face. As far as I could tell, each nurse did a stellar job caring for Mr. Davis, and I thought that Mrs. Davis was doing nothing other than creating trouble.

When we made daily rounds on Mr. Davis in the ICU, his wife always presented us with a long, written list of questions. She expected that one of the trauma surgeons would answer each and every one of them to her satisfaction before we would be allowed to move on. Mr. Davis was complicated, and it often took nearly an hour of my time to perform a thorough physical examination, as well as to review all of the laboratory, X-ray, and nursing data. Taking an additional hour, each and every day, to answer all of Mrs. Davis's questions was getting to be a ridiculous and unreasonable burden.

As Mr. Davis became more stable, we began to mention to Mrs. Davis that her husband would soon be getting to the point where he would be transferred to a skilled nursing facility where nurses would manage her husband's long-term medical problems for many months until he became strong enough to participate in aggressive, physical rehabilitation. My comments obviously made Mrs. Davis uncomfortable. She clearly did not want her husband to leave us, but we could never get a straight answer as to why she was so resistant about letting her husband be moved from our hospital. One of our social workers finally started to unpeel the complicated layers of the Davis family, ultimately giving us a better understanding of just how profoundly Mr. Davis's alcoholism had adversely affected the lives of his entire family.

Mr. Davis had apparently not held a stable job for a very long time. Undoubtedly, his alcoholism played a role in his lack of successful employment, but Mrs. Davis repeatedly downplayed the extent of her husband's drinking. Because her husband had no reliable source of income, Mrs. Davis was the one who worked to support the family. She was also the one whose job provided health insurance for both of them, and she knew better than to work less than full-time lest she lose her health insurance benefits. She also had no place to live. As it turned out, the reason Mrs. Davis spent nearly all of her time at her husband's bedside was because she had no home to go back to. Apparently, something happened to the Davis family, causing them to lose their house. Mr. and Mrs. Davis had been living with one of their children, but it was a rather tenuous relationship. I hadn't realized that the couple even had children, as none had ever visited as far as I knew. As it turned out, when Mr. Davis crashed his car while drunk, the child with whom the Davis parents had been staying threw them both out. Obviously, the ramifications of Mr. Davis's alcoholism extended much further than his wife ever wanted to admit, which alienated most, if not all, of Mrs. Davis's family and support system from her.

The day did finally come when Mr. Davis was stable enough to leave our hospital and begin the next phase of his recovery and rehabilitation process. I spent a full two hours with Mrs. Davis on the day her husband was transferred out, answering every question and hypothetical scenario imaginable. I knew that spending a few hours prior to his leaving might potentially save me countless phone calls over the next several weeks. After Mrs. Davis and I had gone over everything to her satisfaction, I asked her how she was doing. She looked puzzled and she didn't answer my question right away. I told her that her whole life was again going to change, and I asked her if she felt strong enough to move on. She then looked at me and she broke down in tears. I wondered if I had said something inappropriate, but Mrs. Davis assured me that she wasn't crying because she was upset at me. Instead, she was crying because she was scared. She admitted that her husband had put her through hell over the years, and that she was angry for having been put in such a terrible situation. She also said that she had worried herself sick when she thought that her husband might die, but once knowing that he would live, she worried even more that he would again start drinking just as soon as he completed his rehabilitation.

Clearly, Mrs. Davis had a lot more on her mind than she talked about when her husband was in our intensive care unit. Her miniature, emotional catharsis probably released no more than the very top layer of a massive pile of psychological baggage, which had undoubtedly accumulated for years. Mrs. Davis had spent the past two months in our ICU receiving more attention than she had probably ever received in her entire life. But Mrs. Davis was not my pa-

tient, and her husband had spent enough time with us. It was time for him—
and time for her—to go.

Like a few of our trauma patients do, Mr. Davis came back to visit us in the
intensive care unit several months after we discharged him from our care. His
wife brought him back, and I saw the two of them walking slowly in the ICU
corridor—my former patient ambulating with the assistance of a walker. With
some reservation I walked up to the couple and greeted them both. Mrs. Davis
obviously wanted a hug, to which I awkwardly acquiesced. I took a good look at
the man standing behind the walker. I really did think that Mr. Davis looked
great, considering all that he had been through. He, of course, didn't even remember me. Despite the fact that we spent the better part of two months together, Mr. Davis had not even the slightest inkling of what I had done for
him. He had heard my name mentioned by his wife and by people at the rehabilitation facility, but he didn't even really seem all that interested in meeting
the guy who had spent so much time inside his abdomen and at his bedside.

I told Mr. Davis that he was a pretty lucky guy, having died once at the other
hospital, and then almost dying at our hospital. I briefly summarized all that we
had been through together, including details of some of the operations. I told
him about his liver, and how the alcohol had caused irreversible damage. I
told him that with his cirrhosis being as bad as it was, choosing to drink again
could certainly kill him. I encouraged him to stay away from alcohol for the rest
of his life, but I didn't get a good feeling that he felt sobriety was a viable option.
Mrs. Davis, on the other hand, seemed very happy when I told her husband to
keep away from the liquor. I'm sure that she had spoken to her husband countless times before about his drinking without success. She seemed grateful that I
said what she had obviously hoped I would say.

I know that nothing I could possibly say has much if any bearing on whether
or not an alcoholic or a drug abuser stops using. I know that most addicts need
to hit their own personal rock bottom before they ever choose to make changes
substantial enough to overcome their powerful addictions. One person's rock
bottom may not be far enough down for another. And what may seem like the
lowest possible place imaginable for one individual might not even be close to
low enough for another to force him to change his ways. Rock bottom is a very
personal point only recognizable to the individual who has found himself down
that hole. Mr. Davis certainly had hit a bottom, but only he himself knows if
that particular bottom was his rock bottom.

23

Back to the Combat Zone
Deployment to Iraq

I choked on a lung full of dust as I followed the sea of human movement toward the trauma receiving area. I entered a room very unfamiliar to me in which dozens of people began assembling at their assigned stations, awaiting the arrival of the casualties. In the treatment area, I inhaled the stench of blood and sweat my olfactory memory was quite familiar with. It was the foul smell of unclean individuals—dirty, wounded men. It was also the identical smell of homeless men who had been brought in to my trauma bays, recently beaten to a bloody pulp, and it was the smell of migrant workers living in barns who had knifed each other over the loss of an unpaid bet. It was a wretched, unpleasant smell, which, being in the trauma business, I was all too familiar with.

Being unfamiliar with how matters were conducted at that facility, I assumed a position out of the way and I watched as the emergency medicine physicians took charge of the three patients wheeled in on the rickshaw gurneys. I watched with great interest as a half dozen health-care personnel swarmed the three casualties, each member of the team performing his or her duties in a manner that had obviously been rehearsed many times before.

I was particularly interested in a man covered in bloody gauze that was wrapped crudely over his entire left arm and leg. He was groaning loudly and incoherently. The patient's yelling contributed to the cacophony of screaming and high volume shouting, which coalesced into a deafening roar of indecipherable noise. The emergency medicine doc skillfully placed an endotracheal tube into the respiratory orifice of the patient I was visually fixated on. I marveled as this all happened within a minute or two of the casualty's arrival. Nurses hung intravenous fluids and administered pain medications as numerous assistants cut off clothing and dressings.

Once disrobed and unbandaged, the nature of the man's pain was made readily apparent. Both his arm and his leg were torn and riddled with holes, each about a half inch in diameter. The markedly swollen, bloody, and grossly disfigured limbs were not actively hemorrhaging as each had been fitted with an appropriately tightened tourniquet, preventing any additional loss of the life sustaining, precious body fluid. Surgeons I had met less than twenty-four hours earlier pounced on the badly injured man and they directed the anesthesiologist to move the patient into the operating room as quickly as possible. Having an obvious personal interest in the subject matter, I followed the patient as he was wheeled around the corner less than five minutes later into the crude yet adequate operating suite.

I followed the operating crew into the room after placing a surgical cap on my head and a mask on my face. I watched as the anesthesiologist rapidly connected the bloody, mutilated patient to the complex machine, which delivered the sleeping gas. Two crudely dressed men scrubbed the patient's body from head to toe with soapy, brown antiseptic. They painted his body with a thin, brown liquid, after which they declared him clean. Technicians then draped numerous blue, disposable linens over the patient leaving the two limbs punched with holes exposed. Two general surgeons and one orthopedic surgeon walked away from the single hand-washing station with arms held up and extended, dripping with water. Scrub technicians handed each of them a sterile paper towel with which they dried off before pushing their arms into surgical gowns and gloves.

"We could use a hand if you're interested," one of the gowned surgeons said to me. More than eager to get involved, I hopped toward the scrub sink and washed my hands before donning attire identical to the rest of the team. I was gestured by the sole surgeon who chose to work on the patient's arm to join him as the other two worked on the bloody leg. I assumed a comfortable stance, pushing my abdomen into the operating room table. I then lifted the patient's mangled arm into my hands feeling his unstable, broken bones grind under his swollen, multiply pierced skin.

"Looks like a brachial artery injury," the seasoned veteran muttered. I nodded in agreement as we positioned the arm into the exact position we both knew was necessary to facilitate optimal opportunity to access the damaged artery. I counted eight holes, most of which were clustered about the elbow region. A portion of the limb was gaping wide open, as if a strong, blast wave had passed directly through. Bloodstained fat billowed through all open areas, causing the wounds to appear even more gruesome than they already were. His forearm was nearly twice its normal girth as the projectiles that had cut clean through his flesh had bled significantly into the tissues underneath.

The lead surgeon created a six-inch, linear incision in the junction between the biceps and triceps muscles on the inner aspect of our patient's upper arm area. He sliced through uninjured tissues well above the major site of injury. He terminated the cut as his knife struck the surgically prepped tourniquet placed prior to the casualty's arrival. I instinctively sponged away the blood created by the surgeon's incision.

"Kelly," he shouted. The scrub technician slapped a surgical instrument into his hand and the surgeon began separating the fatty tissues, which obscured the artery we were seeking. Once a glimpse of the vascular structure came into view, he slowed his movements and he carefully dissected out the upper portion of the brachial artery. I asked for a right-angled clamp, which I received instantly. Knowing what I needed to do, I passed the instrument under the healthy portion of the distally injured vessel and I gently opened its jaws as the lead man passed a thin, rubber strip into its opening. I clamped down and pulled the vessel loop under the artery. I then passed my instrument once again under the vessel and the surgeon again fed my right-angled instrument the free end of the narrow piece of rubber. As a result of my maneuvers, the strip of rubber was now wrapped circumferentially around the brachial artery. I clamped the free ends of the looped material to a piece of the surgical drape. I then placed a vascular clamp across the surgically exposed vessel, which shut down all circulation to our casualty's arm. The vessel loop was our safety net if we needed to arrest blood flow in an emergency. If my clamp sprung loose, all I needed to do was pull snugly on the rubber tubing, and all blood flow beyond the loop would cease.

We then released the tourniquet. The skin below the device was contaminated and an operating room nurse painted the dirty skin with a sponge stick soaked in iodine to preserve the sterility of our operative field. The surgeon then used his scalpel to create a hockey stick–shaped incision over the crease in our patient's arm, where we suspected the penetrating object had violated the solitary arm vessel. Careful dissection revealed the shredded artery. Several centimeters of the vessel were missing, and the ends of the retracted portions of the vessel were in tatters. As if torn by the teeth of a feral dog, the injury to the artery was so severe that a meticulous reconstruction would be necessary to restore blood flow to the rest of our casualty's arm. But we had no time for such a procedure; it would take us several hours to perform. The tissues of his arm were so badly damaged from the numerous holes and the blast of the weapon, which fired the projectiles, that extensive bony and soft tissue reconstruction would be necessary to heal the man. But without adequate blood flow to the rest of his arm, it would all surely die and he would lose the arm entirely.

To combat the problem, we decided to place a shunt across the damaged segment of artery. We threaded one end of a sterile, rigid tube into one end of the damaged artery, and we fed the other end into the damaged vessel below the injury. We secured the shunt in place with a few, snugly tied sutures, and I released my previously placed vascular clamp. Blood instantly flowed through the clear plastic tube, providing healthy flow to the arm below the level of the horrible injury. Our casualty's previously mottled hand pinked up, and I palpated a brisk pulse in his radial artery at the wrist. Satisfied that we had given our patient's arm the necessary blood flow to remain alive, we washed out the wounds and we packed the multiple open areas of his injured elbow area with saline-moistened gauze. We then sutured closed the upper arm wound.

Not yet done with our limb-sparing, meatball operation, we knew that we needed to address the uninjured lower portion of his forearm. Unfortunately, the numerous delicate strips of tissue that flex and extend each of our digits are exquisitely sensitive to periods of time devoid of vascular flow. Once circulation had been reestablished below the elbow, it would only be a matter of hours until the swelling in our patient's forearm compartments became so great that it would compress the arteries deep with the multiple muscles enshrouded by its dense, unyielding coverings of fibrous, fascial tissue. To not do what we knew was necessary would be to subject our patient to losing his arm despite the work we had already done. We needed to perform prophylactic fasciotomies.

Prophylactic fasciotomies look fairly gruesome but are necessary in such cases of penetrating vascular trauma to the arm. We created long slices through the front and back of our patient's forearm, cutting through the outer rigid coverings of the muscle. Muscle bulged through on both sides confirming that our decision was indeed the correct thing to do. We left the wounds open to allow more muscle to bulge free over the ensuing hours, and we covered our work with a thick layer of sterile gauze.

We fashioned a long arm splint from plaster we wet in a bucket of water next to the operating room table. We held the slimy white material onto the underlying, gauze covered arm until it hardened, and we were through.

We finished our work at about the same time that the leg team finished their part of the simultaneous operation. Knowing that our facility did not have the capabilities needed to manage the complexities of our casualty's wounds, we called for a helicopter to fly our patient to a more robust medical environment. Within twenty minutes, the blades of the helo were turning—our patient situated on a stretcher in its rear cargo hold—and heading to a larger place where more definitive care would be provided.

The very nature of having done all that had just taken place was my first stark reminder that I was no longer in the friendly confines of my Level I Trauma Center back home. No, I was not home. I was in Iraq. It was my first real day on the job, and the previous group of doctors and nurses had not yet even left.

Almost two and a half years after returning home from Afghanistan, I received another set of military, deployment orders. It was two days prior to my forty-third birthday, and the news enclosed in the thick manila envelope sent to me from the Department of the Navy was both surprising and rather distressing. I wasn't angry about having to go back to war, but I was upset about having to leave so quickly, and for so long. My orders gave me less than three weeks time to get my affairs in order before having to leave everything behind and report to Camp Lejeune, North Carolina. I really thought that I should have been entitled to more notice than I had received, but I was in no position at the time to argue. What killed me was the line on my orders, indicating that I could potentially be gone for a year or longer. At the time, I just couldn't imagine leaving my wife and children for such a very long period. Even though I knew that my wife and kids were strong and independent, I became flooded with mental images of situations in which my family might need me but I would be too far away to be of any help to them.

I made a few phone calls to see where the military would be taking me. I soon learned that I was to deploy with the marines of the Second Marine Expeditionary Force to Al Anbar Province, Iraq, in support of the military surge. The news channels made me well aware of the military surge, in which President Bush ordered about thirty thousand additional troops to be sent to Iraq to regain control of the war that seemed to be at a stalemate. With the increase in troop strength there would, of course, be more fighting, and more fighting would lead to additional combat casualties. The additional war fighters sent to engage in battle would need more surgeons to care for their injuries, and I was one of the extra military physicians chosen by somebody unknown in Washington to again go forward.

One thing that bothered me about having to deploy again was that I wouldn't be going with anyone in my unit or with anyone I had ever worked with as far as I knew. Despite still being assigned to a reserve Navy SEAL team, the needs of Uncle Sam superseded my desires to remain with my old unit. Knowing that the marines and soldiers of our conventional armed forces needed experienced surgeons to take care of them in battle, the Navy Bureau of Personnel tagged me as one of the desired assets to join up with an East Coast, active duty contingent of marines in support of the Iraq Surge.

I had not served with a Marine Corps unit for thirteen years, and I had no friends or acquaintances at Camp Lejeune. The thought of going off to war for a year with a complete group of strangers made it hard for me to focus on all that I needed to do over the next few weeks to prepare myself for a journey to a land where plenty of Americans had already died and countless more had been wounded. Although I knew that I was being sent to Iraq to treat the wounded, I couldn't help but think that perhaps my luck was running out and that I might become a casualty myself. I couldn't help but wonder what the chances could be that I might be so unlucky as to be hit by a stray rocket or mortar round, and die far from home. I realized that I was a little frightened. The unknown has always frightened me some, and although I had been to war before, my upcoming deployment had plenty of aspects which were very unknown to me.

After spending more than a full calendar day in transit, our plane finally landed in Kuwait City sometime near midnight. Kuwait was the last stop for all U.S. service members before they were sent off to the various combat zone areas. It was also the last place where we could feel relatively safe. Kuwait was the hottest place I had ever been to, peaking in the 120-degree range the following day outside our canvas tents staked into the bleached, desert sand. I waited in Kuwait with the rest of our group for three days before the plane taking me to my ultimate destination departed. On the evening of my flight back into the combat zone, I donned my fifty-pound body armor vest, firmly affixed my helmet to my head, grabbed my rucksack, and I boarded the C-130 en route to Al Taqaddum, Iraq.

Once in Iraq, I was assigned to the surgical hospital aboard Camp Taqaddum, which we affectionately called TQ Surgical. TQ Surgical was a makeshift hospital assembled within a large Quonset hutlike building. About one hundred navy personnel were assigned to the medical facility aboard the expeditionary marine base. Included among the one hundred people were thirty-three officers, about half of which were physicians. About half of the physicians assigned to TQ Surgical were surgeons. Nurses completed the complement of the officers, and enlisted corpsmen comprised the bulk of the health-care providers in our military hospital.

TQ Surgical was, in fact, a surgical facility, but we were not a robust, medical hospital like the ones in Baghdad or Balad. We were a larger version of the medical facility I operated out of when I was at Camp Salerno, Afghanistan. We were one of several expeditionary, surgical facilities established close to the combat areas. Casualties too unstable to make the long flight to Baghdad or Balad would be taken to facilities like ours where we would provide life-saving emergency care, and emergency surgical treatment if necessary. TQ Surgical had a large emergency medical receiving area, four operating rooms, a pharmacy area, and a few storage rooms. All were housed within the large, tin-covered, half cylinder of a building. We had very limited lab and X-ray capabilities, no CT scanner, a very limited blood bank, and no intensive care unit. Unfortunately, because we had no critical care holding capability, anyone hurt badly enough to require emergency surgical treatment at our facility needed to be shipped out by Medevac helicopter to a higher level of care. The larger, well-established U.S. military hospitals in Baghdad and Balad took most of our patients, but occasionally the hospital in Al Asad took some of our casualties after we had done all which we were capable of doing.

At TQ Surgical, we treated U.S. and foreign casualties. Most of our foreign casualties were Iraqis, some of whom were friendly, and some of whom were insurgents wanting to kill us. We treated all of the injured equally and we went to great lengths at all times to preserve both life and limb of every one of our patients, be they friend or foe. Because so many of the casualties we treated suffered injuries from improvised explosive devices, or IEDs, we often operated on multiple body parts simultaneously. The insurgent bomb makers went to great lengths to make their IEDs as destructive as possible, often packing their bombs

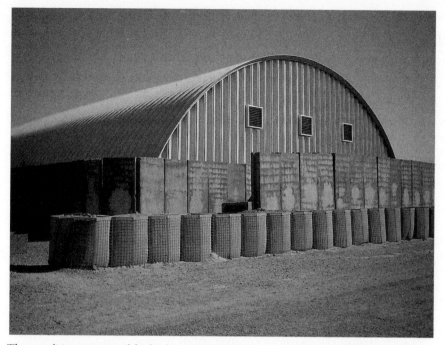

The expeditionary, surgical facility known as TQ Surgical, aboard Camp Taqaddum, Iraq.

with nails, screws, washers, and ball bearings—anything which would cause greater harm to their victims when the lethal, flying debris cut through their bodies like hot knives through butter.

It was not uncommon for our casualties to have been peppered by twenty or even thirty pieces of flying metal, suffering penetrating wounds to their head, neck, groin, and extremities. Most U.S. service members did not suffer wounds to their chest or abdomen, as the thickly plated body armor protected most people in those areas. However, flying debris had a way of seeking out vulnerable areas, such as the armpit, or in the crotch region. A piece of shrapnel entering a person's underarm could cut right through both sides of the chest. An upward explosion from a ground-based IED could send dozens of pieces of flying metal under the body armor and up into the abdomen. We saw patients with those patterns of injury fairly often, and those who made it to us alive often required emergency surgery.

One such casualty was a young Marine Second Lieutenant, who was leading a small group of war fighters on a cordon and knock mission. On cordon and knock missions, large groups of military personnel encircle a community

of buildings and homes, and go house to house, knocking on doors and looking for suspected terrorists or persons of interest. At one particular home, a
small squad of marines led by that particular lieutenant knocked on the front
door as they always did. An Iraqi translator announced in Arabic the intentions
of the Americans, and he ordered the home owners to open their door. When
there was no response, the lieutenant kicked open the front door of the small
home, where a woman was awaiting him not three feet from the door's thresh-
old. The woman was waiting for that very moment, and with her intruder's leg
still kicked up high in the air, she plunged the handheld detonator wired to her
suicide vest, blowing herself up in a blaze of jihadist glory.

The young marine was showered with explosive debris, most of which penetrated his inner thighs, scrotal area, and buttocks. Because his leg was kicked
upward, the blast energy pierced his abdominal cavity through his groin, causing him extensive internal injuries despite his wearing his body armor. He was
brought into TQ Surgical by helicopter, where several teams of medical and
surgical personnel awaited his arrival. When our young lieutenant arrived, he
was shocky but talking. His head, neck, and chest all seemed to be injury free.
He must have had at least two dozen holes in his thighs, scrotum, and in the
area between his buttocks, from objects approximately one half centimeter in
diameter, which I had presumed were ball bearings. We started infusing intravenous fluids, and I called for blood. Recognizing the pattern of the young
man's injuries, I knew that he was certain to have metal fragments in his belly,
and an emergency exploratory laparotomy was definitely indicated.

We rushed him down the TQ Surgical corridor to one of the makeshift operating rooms where the navy anesthesiologist put our young casualty to sleep.
The navy nurses and corpsmen then prepped his fragment-riddled body with
antiseptic solution, and covered him with surgical drapes. Two of us scrubbed
to perform the actual surgery. I started working on the abdomen, and the other
surgeon started working on the thigh and groin wounds. Being a healthy and
physically fit specimen, my trauma patient's abdomen had very little fat to cut
through, making entry into the belly cavity rather easy. Once inside, I encountered a fair amount of blood. He wasn't actively hemorrhaging, but he had
nearly a half liter of blood from his injuries. That kind of blood loss wouldn't
kill a young, otherwise healthy person. But missing a hole in a piece of intestine certainly could. Knowing that fact, I performed a diligent search looking
for what I knew would be multiple small holes in the bowel.

I checked every inch of small intestine, large intestine, stomach, bladder, and every other organ within the abdomen. As it turned out, my patient had a total of thirty holes through loops of small intestine, colon, bladder, and stomach. I repaired the injuries in his stomach and bladder with simple sutures, but the wounds in the intestines were too ratty to safely repair. Stool had leaked from the holes, further increasing the likelihood that suturing the wounds would be unsatisfactory, and so I decided to surgically remove several small sections of the injured bowel to optimize my patient's outcome.

I removed four or five small sections of small bowel, and one segment of the left colon, leaving the entire length of intestine in multiple, disconnected sections necessitating what would be a second-look operation in a day or so after arriving at the next hospital in either Baghdad or Balad. I concluded my portion of the operation by covering his open abdominal cavity with a blue surgical towel and a sticky surgical drape. My partner finished his portion of the operation on parts below, and we called for a Medevac chopper to take our intubated patient off to a higher level of care. We did all which we needed to do, and all that we could do at our medical facility. Perhaps we saved his life. Perhaps he would have made it if he had been flown directly to the larger hospital bypassing us entirely. But for all anyone could have known, the surgeons in Balad or Baghdad might have all been tied up in the operating room at the time, and perhaps without us, the young marine may have waited hours before getting the surgery he certainly needed. Maybe he would have died if he hadn't been brought to us first. But regardless, we did a good job and we took care of him.

Another guy I'll never forget was a young marine corporal brought to us as he was preparing to go out on a combat mission with his unit. Apparently, he had been gathering the various ammunition magazines, grenades, and flares he felt he would need when sent outside the wire. He strapped smoke grenades, fragmentation grenades, and concussion grenades to his body armor so that they would always be within an arm's reach should he need any of them in an emergency situation. Somehow, while affixing one of the concussion grenades to his suit, he accidentally released the detonating mechanism, setting off the explosion. The concussion grenade was still in his hand when it detonated, and it blew his limb off at the mid-forearm level.

Despite being in a lot of pain, my one-handed casualty was in fairly good spirits. His left arm was mangled, and hoping that he was right-handed like most people, I asked the corporal which hand he used to write. Unfortunately, he told me that he was left-handed. He apparently didn't know that his arm was injured as badly as it was, because he asked me if he was going to have to lose it. A little surprised by the question, I told him as kindly as I could that I did not think that there was any way to save his badly injured arm. He didn't know it at the time but the remnant of his left upper extremity was in tatters. Both forearm bones were sticking out, broken off at oblique angles leaving sharp edges. Strips of muscle hung limply in space, anchored by the thick, healthy, upper forearm tissues near the elbow. The ends of the meaty little pieces once attached to individual hand bones and fingers now dangled freely like untied shoelaces. I needed to do something with his bloody limb, and I took him to the operating room to make it a bit more presentable.

Unfortunately, there wasn't much I could do for my patient's arm. I cut the bones down to a level where I would be able to cover the rough edges with remaining muscle tissue. Pieces of burned, dead, or dying muscle and skin needed to be trimmed away. Crevices between muscle flaps and skin edges needed careful probing and washing as bits of gunpowder and other pieces of debris had become lodged in difficult-to-see places, creating potential sources of future infection. I tried to leave as many pieces of healthy muscle, no matter how small and insignificant they seemed. Despite the hand and fingers being completely gone, I knew that down the line, a limb prosthetics specialist at the U.S. Army Institute of Surgical Research at Fort Sam Houston, Texas, would likely be able to electrically locate the tiny muscle remnants under the healed skin. The prosthetics specialist could then use the neurological signals generated by each of the residual muscle portions to create a cosmetically acceptable and fairly functional, myoelectric arm. I knew that the more I could preserve, the more sophisticated the prosthesis my patient would ultimately be able to receive.

The emergency treatment area at TQ Surgical was busy every single day. Many of our daily patients were not the victims of the traumatic injuries of war, but were simply sick with common, everyday maladies such as gastrointestinal diarrhea, upper respiratory tract infections, and skin rashes. Our family physicians and corpsmen managed most of the people who walked in with the common, ambulatory illnesses, but they also participated heavily in the management of the combat-wounded casualties. As we often received multiple casualties simultaneously, everyone had to help out in whatever capacity they could. Emergency medicine physicians often assumed responsibility for the overall

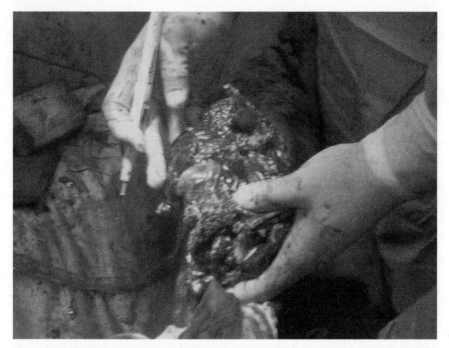

The author holding the bloody, mangled stump of what was left of a marine's arm after being blown away by a grenade. *(Courtesy Commander Jerry Dotson, NC, USN)*

management of individual trauma casualties, while teams of nurses and corpsmen assisted them at each of the numerous trauma resuscitation stations in the TQ Surgical emergency treatment area. For the most part, surgeons like myself stood near the feet of the resuscitation stations, waiting to be directed to a particular casualty in need of a surgeon's skills.

Despite a continuous stream of patients going in and out of our medical treatment facility, I was always a little bored. Back home, I was responsible for managing the critical care patients in the intensive care unit as well as the emergency trauma casualties and patients needing urgent surgery. At TQ Surgical, I was much less busy than I was back home and I felt the constant need to do more. I did have a collateral duty assigned to me, but I wasn't able to do much with it during my first two months in Iraq. My added assignment was that of Officer in Charge of the mobile Forward Resuscitative Surgical System. To use military jargon, I was the OIC of the mobile FRSS (pronounced *friss*).

The mobile FRSS was nothing more than a crude emergency surgical suite, which we could set up or break down in less than an hour. A FRSS team usually includes two surgeons, two operating room corpsmen, one anesthesiologist, one critical care nurse, one field corpsman, and one chief hospital corpsman. We did all of our work out of two fifteen-by-eighteen-foot tents. One was used exclusively as an operating room, and the other was used as an emergency casualty receiving area and postoperative holding area. All of our equipment was modular and was contained in boxes or hanging bags. Everything fit into storage containers, which could be easily loaded up onto a truck and transported to wherever needed—which was always some forward, combat hot spot.

Our operating table and nearly all of our modular equipment was identical to the materials I worked with when I was assigned to the USSOCOM unit in the past. Being a full-time civilian trauma surgeon with past military experience on mobile surgical teams, I felt quite comfortable accepting my collateral assignment as OIC of the mobile FRSS. I looked forward to the opportunity to take my team outside the wire. I did, however, make a few modifications to my small unit. I added an emergency medicine physician and an extra corpsman to the group. In addition, I handpicked each of the members on my team, using past military experience, physical strength and field hardiness, and medical skill sets as the main criteria for joining my team. We trained at least once each week, setting up and taking down the tents, assembling and disassembling the equipment, and going through all the boxes and hanging bags. We each became familiar with a particular piece of specialty equipment—one becoming the expert at running the portable oxygen generator system (a.k.a., the POGS); one knowing the ins and outs of the portable ventilators, suction machines, and cardiac monitors; and myself assuming authority over the two electrical generators.

We had two generators, each of which produced three kilowatts of electrical energy. When all of our equipment and lighting was in use, we needed almost six kilowatts of energy. However, when we turned on the portable oxygen generator system, it momentarily drew nearly a full three kilowatts of power before settling down to a baseline energy consumption level of about one and a half kilowatts. If most of our electrical equipment was drawing power from the two generators and we subsequently turned on the POGS, the temporary, additional draw of electrical energy blew the generators. That was a critical problem if it happened at the wrong time, or if it happened in the dark of night. Realizing just how important those six kilowatts of power were to my team and me, I assumed full responsibility for the management and maintenance of the FRSS generators.

Being outside the wire had its pluses and its minuses. For the most part, I enjoyed being out on my own, away from the micromanagement, leadership style aboard Camp Taqaddum. But there certainly was a bad side to being away from the largest military encampment in all of western Iraq. Being outside the wire meant that we were pretty much responsible for securing our own shelter, water, food, and, at times, our own security.

We set up camp on piles of thick dust—the ultrafine remnants of what was once the drifting sand of the Middle East. Each of us lived in our own personal tent, perhaps six feet long and three feet wide, inside of which we kept our sleeping bags, rucksacks, and any personal equipment or gear we chose to carry with us. We were always armed, and our weapons were always at the ready. Latrines crudely constructed from plywood balanced over burn barrels served as our public toilets. Chow often came from the cases of cold MREs—military Meals Ready to Eat—which we brought with us on each of the convoys. Trucks, Humvees, and even enormous military tanks barreled by our medical tents by both day and night. With each pass, huge clouds of Iraqi dust rose from the passing vehicles, choking us as we inhaled the ubiquitous pollution. There was little if any opportunity to wash, and for the most part we remained filthy while outside the wire.

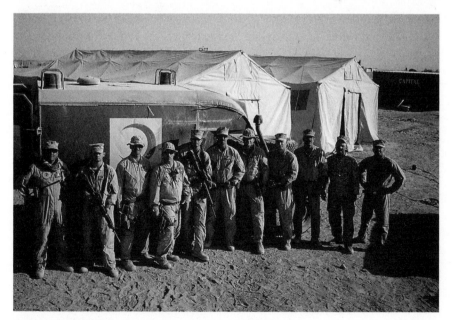

Cole's mobile FRSS team, in Al Anbar Province, Iraq.

I rarely showered or changed my clothing more often than once per week. Although some people might imagine my Iraq field-living conditions as terrible or unacceptable, when thrust into a survival situation, little things that might ordinarily seem bothersome barely ascend to the level of even trivial concern.

Several aspects of my adventures into the combat zones were particularly noteworthy. First of all, I never realized just how cold the Iraqi desert gets at night during the winter months. The temperature dropped below freezing each evening, and without any source of heat, we shivered in our tiny tents at night, hoping that the sun would soon rise and give us a break from the freezing cold. We often awoke to find icicles hanging from our water containers and frost covering the tops of our living areas.

Having experienced both extremes of weather in Iraq, I believe with conviction that extreme heat is more tolerable than extreme cold. I didn't much enjoy the 120-degree weather when I first landed in Kuwait, but I never suffered so much as I did during those subfreezing nights in that bitterly cold, thin-skinned tent.

I finally left the field about three weeks into January of the new year and headed back to the main base aboard Camp Taqaddum. Everyone in my party

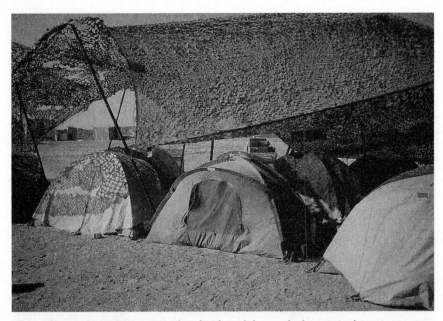

The small tents the FRSS team members lived in while outside the wire in the various combat zones.

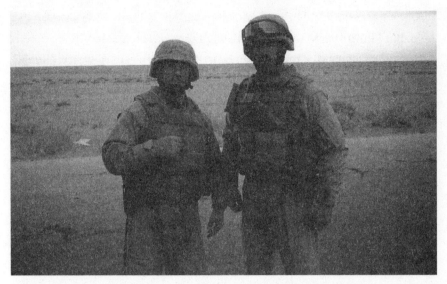

A chief corpsman and CDR Cole outside the wire in Al Anbar Province, Iraq.

had lost weight and we were all physically and emotionally spent from suffering for so long in the cold and filthy desert. I had been in Iraq for more than six months, but it felt as if I had been there forever. I was really starting to despise that country.

The war was clearly winding down, at least in Al Anbar Province. When my group had first arrived to Iraq, the surge had been underway for only a few months. Fighting in our area was brutal and casualty rates were exceedingly high. But as the surge tactics began to work, pockets of insurgent resistance became fewer and farther between. Local Iraqis began turning over Al Qaeda sympathizers to the coalition, and fighting in general seemed to occur less frequently. Whereas TQ Surgical had once been a very busy, expeditionary, medical treatment facility, it became fairly quiet. Fighting in Fallujah—once an epicenter for great battles—became such a rarity that the military surgical hospital in the city actually shut down. Even with all of Fallujah's injured people being redirected to TQ Surgical, we were still very slow and very bored. But by that point in my deployment, I was fine with being bored. I had spent enough time outside the wire and I treated enough casualties to call it quits. I was ready to go home, and in just a few months time, I would be doing just that.

When I left Iraq with the rest of my unit in March, I found it difficult to identify anything positive that had come out of my experience in Iraq. Of course, I had operated on a number of trauma patients and some of them would have undoubtedly died had a surgeon not been there to immediately help. But I think that beyond my duties as a surgeon, I found it difficult to want to remember any part of my experience in that nasty place. However, after getting home and reuniting with my wife, children, and extended family, I began to realize that I did have some positive experiences out there in the desert.

I learned that I had developed a better understanding for how homeless people lived. Living for long periods of time in my tiny tent gave me a better appreciation for what "home" really is. For me, while living out there in the filthy dirt and powdery sand, my tent was all I had. My tent was my home, and with nothing else I could claim as mine, I became strangely protective of my little cloth space. I also learned that food, water, and any form of comfort for that matter are never guaranteed. I developed a completely different understanding of what food really meant to me. Food was a luxury to be consumed wisely, as there was no guarantee that there may be enough of it tomorrow or the next day. The same was true for water. My group ran out of water for almost an entire day and we missed meals on multiple occasions. And, of course, my experience outside the wire taught me that shelter from rain and cold were as precious as just about anything else I could imagine.

Once settled back home and back into my civilian job, I realized that all my miserable experiences in the Iraqi desert were actually very important training evolutions for me as a human being tasked with having to integrate among the entire spectrum of society. As a trauma surgeon, I have treated so many social derelicts, deviants, and bums. What I had never been able to do prior to that deployment, however, was have any genuine understanding for how they lived and for why they lived as they did. But that all changed after my deployment. I felt humbled by my entire experience. Certainly, even if I had learned nothing else, my experience in Iraq taught me more about human compassion and understanding—all good things for any human being to truly comprehend.

24

Guns, Knives, and Drugs

Urban Violence

Setting foot back on American soil was wonderful. I was overjoyed to see my family again, all of whom actually drove over a thousand miles to North Carolina to greet me as my military group finally pulled back into Camp Lejeune after our across the globe journey. That was an incredible day that I'll never forget. I was overwhelmed with happiness yet at the same time a bit sad, knowing that I had missed out on so many of my children's sports games, family gatherings, holidays, and other important events. The Marine Corps kept me in North Carolina for almost a week after returning to the States. As soon as I was released from active duty, my family and I left Camp Lejeune, hoping none of us would ever see the place again.

Once we had all made it safely home, I slowly reinserted myself back into my former everyday life. Going back to life as usual wasn't as easy for me, as it had been several years before when I returned from Afghanistan. I wasn't feeling very social, and other than being with my wife and kids, I had very little desire to get together with my old friends and neighbors. It's not that I disliked any of them; in fact, I felt very grateful for how kindly they all had treated my family in my absence. But I felt different. I just didn't feel the desire or the need to relive my Iraq experiences, which is what I knew would inevitably have to happen when I finally decided I was ready to get back with my social group.

I wasn't yet eager to retell the stories over and over to people who would certainly ask about my time spent overseas.

I couldn't help but notice the conspicuous absence of good news being reported on the television and radio networks regarding progress made by the surge in Iraq. In fact, if I had not actually just been there I would never have known that the fighting was down and casualty rates were at an all-time low in the formerly most violent part of the Middle East. People I chose to speak with about my recent experiences all seemed to want to eventually digress into political discussions regarding whether or not we—as if any of them had ever been there themselves—really had the right to be in Iraq, fighting a war many Americans clearly did not support.

I heard multiple talking points thrown at me, obviously initiated by some political commentator who had a large following of listeners or readers. The comments were all clearly well thought out, but just weren't factually accurate based on my recent journey throughout all of western Iraq. No one seemed to have any idea that most Iraqis really appreciated all that the Americans had done for them. No one seemed to have any knowledge of all the humanitarian work—the medical care, the rebuilding, the educating and training—that American service members had been doing for the Iraqis. It was all pretty demoralizing, and I didn't appreciate engaging in the discussions. So, I simply avoided most people and stayed clear of the television and the radio for a while.

When I started to again listen to the news, I realized that most of the stories all had a bleak, negative tone in general. Stories of crime, death, and suffering all seemed to be popular news topics, and I couldn't help but notice that an excessive number of murders seemed to be happening at that time in Chicago, Illinois. It seemed that someone was being killed every day in the Windy City. On some days, several people were killed or badly injured in gun or gang violence, and of those killed, many were young teenagers. I started to wonder where I would rather be at that time if optimal safety was my goal—Iraq or Chicago.

I did a little research looking into the number of violent deaths in Chicago and I compared the data to the number of hostile deaths of U.S. service personnel in all of Iraq during the same periods of time. I queried a variety of official Web sites to access the data I needed to make my comparisons. My findings supported my suspicions. I was quite shocked to actually see the official numbers showing that although during the early part of the surge the number of American deaths in Iraq far outnumbered those killed in Chicago, during the last three months of the surge, the number of killings in Chicago actually surpassed the number of GIs killed in the war zone. I had uncovered amazing news that the war zones in Iraq had actually become safer than some areas of one of our nation's largest cities, yet it was not worthy of mentioning by our news professionals. I suddenly realized that although the American party line was to support the troops, there was, in truth, very little enthusiasm to support the actual mission or the work accomplished by the troops allegedly supported by the people of our nation.

Getting back to work at the trauma center was both easy and—at the same time—very difficult. So many people wanted to talk with me about all I had experienced in Iraq that for nearly a month I could hardly get through intensive care unit rounds without stopping a half dozen times to share short vignettes of my time in the combat zone with the dozens of nurses, technicians, and doctors who had kindly kept me in their thoughts during my absence. But I had absolutely no difficulty getting back to actual work as a trauma surgeon. For the most part, compared to my combat casualties, my civilian trauma patients were less injured, were more stable, and the surgeries needed to fix their problems were less complicated.

There were a few challenging trauma patients that brought me back to the war zone and challenged my skills as a surgeon. Two of my earliest trauma patients after coming back home were Dantrell and Lamarcus Johnson. Although they shared the same last name, they weren't brothers but were first cousins who apparently lived in the same home together, along with at least one woman and several schoolaged children. Dantrell, Lamarcus, and the woman apparently ran a fairly successful, illicit, home business, from which they sold low-end marijuana laced with the hallucinogenic drug phencyclidine—street named PCP—to area customers. Those involved in the drug trade often get themselves mixed up with trouble they wished they could have avoided from the very beginning. That was the case for the Johnson family.

To complicate matters, there was another cousin at the home that day. He, too, was somehow involved in the business, but he may very well have been a buyer. Regardless, something very bad happened that morning causing serious havoc in the Johnson home. Something set off this unidentified cousin and sent him into a violent frenzy of carnage and murderous butchery. He shot the woman to death at point-blank range, pumping numerous rounds into her chest and abdomen, right in front of her own children. The assailant then started shooting Lamarcus and Dantrell, hitting Lamarcus in the buttocks, flank, and left hand. As Lamarcus lay on the ground, rendered helpless from his gunshot injuries, Dantrell was assaulted with the assailant's handgun as well as his very large knife. Dantrell received multiple gunshot wounds to his arms and legs, but he was also stabbed multiple times in the chest, shoulder, and arms with a knife that must have been several inches wide. I thought that perhaps he might have been stabbed with a hunting knife or a huge carving blade, as something very large was needed to have created the injuries Dantrell had sustained.

According to the collective stories from all parties involved, the children escaped from the home during the bloodbath and ran to a neighbor's house. Someone unknown called the police. Inside the home, the woman was killed instantly and she continued to bleed out as the two cousins continued to be assaulted. Lamarcus was injured too badly to move and he lay wounded in the home. But Dantrell had somehow mustered the energy to run from the house, leaving a bloody trail behind him, and eventually ending up on the steps of one of the city's nearby public buildings, where police and paramedics eventually found him. The assailant managed to flee and remained on the run for three days before police tracked him down far from where he had committed his heinous acts.

The entire business interaction that turned sour at the Johnson house took place in the early morning, when I was still in the hospital rounding on the floor patients after having worked all night. One of my partners had assumed primary trauma surgeon responsibilities already, and together we tried to complete hospital rounds before the daily traumas started to roll in. Not yet done with rounds, our trauma alert pagers went off, informing us of the impending arrival of the two cousins whom we would soon meet.

Having both my partner and me still in-house that morning made managing simultaneous trauma patients fairly easy. I took Dantrell and my partner took Lamarcus. Dantrell was a huge man, with the habitus of a bodybuilder and nightclub bouncer all rolled into one. His muscles were unusually large, and he reminded me of some of the football players I met while I was in college, whose biceps were larger than my thighs. Dantrell had been assaulted in a very violent manner. What struck me as most disturbing were the sizes and depths of his stab wounds, one of which went through and through Dantrell's right bicep. The length of the wound was nearly a foot long from the knife that pierced his arm at an oblique angle; the width was several inches across.

Through his right pectoral muscle, an equally wide gash had filleted open the meat of his athletic chest wall. I could see within the depths of the wound that the knife had been stopped by the bony junction of where his rib cage met his breastbone. Probing the injury with my gloved finger, I felt the divot in the bone where the knife thrust had been abruptly halted. The sheer power needed to create such wounds must have been remarkable, and the man who overpowered my huge patient must have been an impressive physical specimen or, more likely, a crazed individual, out of control from PCP.

Penetrating trauma patients require very little workup in the emergency room. I knew that my patient needed his wounds explored, washed out, and repaired in the operating room. I felt that any delay in moving from the trauma room was merely a waste of time. I told my partner that I was taking Dantrell to the OR, and that I would catch up with him when I was done with my patient. He told me that he, too, would be heading back to the operating room shortly because his patient had several gunshot wounds and a firm, tender abdomen in need of exploratory surgery.

Once I had Dantrell in the operating room and my patient was anesthetized, I was able to fully explore his numerous wounds. I counted two gunshot cavitations in his right triceps area, two bullet holes in his left forearm area, and four more in his right calf. All were paired wounds, each with entrance and exit areas connected by a narrow, permanent blast cavity. I also saw the huge stab wounds in his right biceps area and his chest, and I counted several additional, small slash marks in both his right and left forearms. I imagined that Dantrell had been defending himself against his attacker blocking his face and torso with his arms, only to have them carved into by the merciless and brutal attacker. It was a wonder to me how my patient ran away to safety with as many injuries he had received to his right leg. Obviously, his ability to flee was what had saved his life.

I carefully explored each of the wounds. Some of them required carefully placed sutures to stop bleeding vessels deep within the muscles. I trimmed away areas of dusky tissue where the blast from the gunshots had caused irreversible damage. Doing anything less would set my patient up for delayed infections and abscess formation. I placed a chest tube through Dantrell's ribs as I suspected that at least a part of the knife had penetrated the chest cavity. Indeed it had, and I evacuated almost a half liter of blood from the inside of my patient's right hemithorax. Quite amazingly, no major structures of importance had been wounded by any of the gunshot wounds or stab wounds. I looked for evidence of arterial injury, major venous injury, and nerve injury, but everything I checked out was perfectly intact. I concluded my operation by thoroughly washing out each of the wounds and packing each of the gunshot cavities with thin strips of gauze. I closed the stab wounds with surgical, skin staples, and I dressed everything with heavy layers of surgical, dressing material. My operation was fairly simple yet tedious, but it was completed. As soon as I could write out an operative note and a full set of orders, I would go and check up on Dantrell's cousin, who my partner was almost certainly operating on by that time.

As I took off my bloody gloves and gown, a nurse from the adjacent operating room burst into our room with an anxious disposition and informed me that as soon as I could break away from my case, my partner needed my help. She then looked at me with very wide eyes and told me that the sooner I could get in there, the better things would be. Realizing that something must be seriously wrong next door, I abandoned writing any notes or orders and went into the room where my partner was operating.

I walked in to find my partner standing calmly with his left arm buried deep into his patient's abdomen. He told me that he was holding his finger over a hole in the aorta, and he needed my help to get things repaired in a controlled manner. I told him that I was more than happy to join his adventure, and I actually enjoyed the opportunity to fix another complex, abdominal vascular injury.

Once scrubbed, gowned, and gloved, I plunged my hands into Lamarcus Johnson's belly while my partner still held pressure over the bleeder. I saw that several sections of small intestine had already been surgically resected, obviously done by my partner before discovering the more serious abdominal aortic injury. I asked him what had happened and he told me that at first, the only injuries he identified were several through and through gunshot wounds to the small bowel. Feeling that the intestine was too severely injured to tolerate suture repair, my partner decided to remove the damaged bowel segments. Just prior to reconnecting the surgically stapled, healthy segments of intestine, my partner noticed a large area of blood welling up from under the deepest layer of filmy tissue covering the bottom of the abdominal cavity, high up near where the abdomen transitions into the chest. It was then that he realized that he had not accounted for the bullet that struck Lamarcus in his buttocks. Realizing that it must have entered the man's body tangentially, penetrating the structures in the deepest part of his abdomen, the bullet must have injured something in the vicinity of the blood pool.

My partner suspected that the bullet may have injured Lamarcus's left kidney. To gain rapid access of the area, he released the deep layer of tissue covering his left kidney and realized that the bullet had not damaged the suspected organ but had taken a medial path and had lodged directly into the highest portion of the abdominal aorta. He discovered the injury by blindly palpating the damaged, relatively nonbleeding tissues, with his finger. He realized that the hard, metal object lodged within the rubbery, pulsating tubular organ could be nothing other than a bullet within the aorta. The problem, however, was that when he gave the injured area a good feel, he pushed the bullet farther into the aorta, causing torrential bleeding. My partner's carefully placed finger managed to keep Lamarcus from bleeding to death right there on the OR table, but he was completely unable to perform any surgical repair with one hand committed to plugging the hole.

Feeling strangely excited, as if again back in the operating tents of Al Anbar Province, I quickly performed a few surgical maneuvers, which enabled me to place a noncrushing, vascular clamp across the aorta. I placed the clamp across the massive artery within the lowest part of the chest cavity, which I accessed through the abdomen by cutting through a section of diaphragm. I knew that the approach would give me perfect access to the desired segment of the largest vessel with the greatest amount of blood flow in the body.

I controlled back-bleeding by placing a second clamp across the aorta below the area of injury near the level of the kidneys. Finally, my partner was able to remove his finger from the hole, allowing us to work together to better expose the area of damaged aorta. It was not an easy region to work on. The uppermost segment of abdominal aorta is covered with a densely adherent layer of tissue, which requires careful snips with a heavy scissors before clear access to the vessel can be achieved. Once skeletonized from its adjacent tissues, we saw that the bullet had pierced the front of the aorta and had lodged through the back of the large vessel. Thin shards of metal attached to the bullet had created tiny slices adjacent to the front and back holes. I had never seen a bullet quite like that one, and I suspected that it might be some sort of illegal ammunition created to cause harm above and beyond that of a normal round.

My partner and I carefully removed the bullet and we repaired both the front and the back of the damaged aorta. It was tedious work but it seemed to go perfectly, with no leaking after we had released our aortic clamps and again permitted blood to flow past our repair site. Realizing that it would be wisest to convert the operation to a damage control case, we decided to not hook up the unattached bowel segments at that time. We temporarily closed the abdominal wall with a vacuum sponge, and we continued resuscitating the patient in the intensive care unit. We decided to take him back to the OR the following day to reinspect our arterial repair, and to reattach the divided but stapled bowel ends.

As it turned out, morning did not come soon enough. In the late hours of that night, Lamarcus started to again bleed from his abdomen. My partner, still in-house from the morning, called me and asked that I help him once more as he took our patient back to the operating room trying to again control the hemorrhage. I, of course, drove back to the hospital where I found my partner already back in the operating room with Lamarcus's abdomen reopened and packed off. My partner told me that he saw an area of bleeding at one of the suture lines and felt that if we just threw an additional stitch or two in the aorta, that the bleeding patient should be fine.

After reexamining the repair that we had performed earlier that day, I saw nothing wrong, other than a narrow stream of blood spurting from between our previously placed sutures. I carefully placed a stitch and tied it tight. It slowed down the bleeding almost completely. But that was a take-back operation, and we didn't want to be unexpectedly fixing the area a third time. So we placed a few more sutures for good measure. My partner and I each placed at least three additional security stitches in Lamarcus's aorta, hoping that each one would further guarantee us not having to again return to the OR. We did, however, know that we still needed to hook the intestine back up, and that night was not the right time. We decided to cover our repair sight with some clot-forming, fibrin glue. We repacked the area with surgical sponges, and replaced the temporary abdominal wall vacuum-assisted closure device.

We waited an additional thirty-six hours before taking Lamarcus back to the operating room. At that third operation, we removed the abdominal packing from around his upper aorta where we happily found our vascular repair to be healing perfectly well, without a single drop of blood oozing from our suture line. We also hooked up all previously discontinuous intestine, after which we gave our patient's abdomen a thorough washing. We closed his abdominal wall and then took him back to the intensive care unit.

Meanwhile, Dantrell had recovered quickly from his injuries. We removed his chest tube on his third hospital day, and by day four, we couldn't keep him in the hospital even if we had wanted to. We discharged him to home, but in fact, Dantrell was under arrest and on police hold. When the law enforcement officials heard that we were ready to discharge our patient, a uniformed officer escorted Dantrell from the hospital to continue their murder investigation.

Lamarcus, on the other hand, did not recover quickly. He developed nearly every complication in the book, including liver failure, kidney failure, respiratory failure, and several infectious problems. He required dialysis nearly every day following that third surgery, which continued on a three-times-per-week basis for the next two months. His liver failure caused him to have a cloudy mental state, and necessitated our feeding him with specialized nutritional formulas through a feeding tube. We could not wean him from the ventilator, and we were forced to perform our ever-so-common tracheostomy and feeding tube procedures. We treated Lamarcus for pneumonia, as well as for an abdominal abscess, which required several trips back to the operating room to enable us to completely drain the accumulation of pus.

His hand injury alone required several operations: one of the bullets took off the ends of his index and middle fingers. A plastic surgeon who specializes in hand reconstruction worked to salvage as much of Lamarcus's remaining hand and to preserve as much function as possible.

Lamarcus petered along in our intensive care unit for what seemed like an eternity. Ordinarily, we would have been able to get patients like Lamarcus into a long-term, acute care nursing facility or a rehabilitation center by that time. We had completed all of Lamarcus's necessary inpatient treatment at that point, but he clearly needed several additional months of specialized nursing care and reconditioning before he would again be independent enough to be able to return to home. Often, several different facilities compete for patients like Lamarcus: young, previously healthy patients with good rehabilitation potential. But no one wanted our patient. He, too, was under arrest, as someone was murdered in his presence while actively dealing illegal drugs. Although Lamarcus was a victim, he was definitely involved in a nefarious narcotics business, which made him undesirable to the nursing and rehabilitation centers.

But a facility did finally accept Lamarcus, and we sent him there almost two months after he was first brought to us with his cousin. He continued to have several setbacks, which required short periods of readmission to our hospital, but he ultimately became well and independent enough to be discharged back to his home.

The cousin—the one who killed the woman, shot and stabbed Dantrell, nearly killed Lamarcus, and terrorized the deceased woman's kids—was eventually apprehended. News stories reported the details of his alleged victims' death and injuries, news we had all been made privy to by that point. Dantrell never followed up with us in our trauma clinic, and I have no idea how his staples or sutures were removed. Cousin Lamarcus came back to visit us several times. The poor guy had lost so much weight. He hardly looked like someone I would suspect as being a drug dealer or a community troublemaker. But apparently he was. I have no idea if Lamarcus was ever convicted of any particular crime, or how much, if any, time he was sentenced to serve in prison. Whatever eventually happened to him, hopefully his time spent with us was sobering enough to change him for the better. After all, we had operated on him no fewer than eight times and we snatched him from the jaws of death—parroting a commonly used trauma cliché—more than once. Perhaps he and his cousin would, from that point forward, follow a nobler path in life. But who knows? Trauma does seem to be a chronic disease with an unusually high rate of recurrence. Like many forms of cancer, you can treat it, but you often can't completely cure it.

25

Poor Roger

A Painful, Bitter Ending

Everything eventually comes to an end. In terms of human relationships, the final end to every interaction between people—simple acquaintances, lifelong friendships, professional relationships, and even solid marriages—comes with the passing from life to death. Sometimes, the end comes very suddenly, but at times its arrival lingers painfully for months or even years, torturing those who await its grim materialization. Sometimes, death brings gut-wrenching agony to those left behind, and for the fortunate, it brings serenity and peace. For those awaiting their own end, some fear their final moments, wondering what if anything is to happen to their soul. Others wonder if a soul even exists. For some, the end is a time yearned for, when with great confidence they believe their spirit will be escorted into heaven where bliss awaits. I have experienced a lot of death, and thus I have been a firsthand participant in the irrevocable severance of many relationships, as in mine with my patients. I have seen the end many, many times.

I have to admit that even though most of my trauma patients get admitted to our service under fairly dramatic circumstances, I tend to forget most of them. The majority of my trauma patients spend a portion of their time in the intensive care unit, on one form of life support or another for a period of time, and often undergo at least one surgical procedure or trauma operation, so it becomes easy for me to confuse the details of one patient with another. Over time, so many patients come through our trauma system that most of them become nothing more to me than a mental blur. The incredible and horrific nature of their injuries is the very aspect of what lumps them all into the same category. Whereas any one of my trauma patients undoubtedly etches permanent, painful memories into the minds of those close to the casualties, to those of us who manage the gravely wounded on a daily basis they as individuals are easily forgotten. Health-care workers not used to dealing with gunshot wounds, stabbings, and massive blunt trauma usually remember with vivid details when one of their established patients suffers significant traumatic injury. But to those of us in the trade, we often forget which patients had which injuries within a week or two of discharge.

Of course, I remember every one of the patients I have treated if in the future I review the notes my partners and I generated on each casualty throughout the time they were admitted to our service. But often, if I were not to pore over a patient's discharge summary, I might forget just how difficult even some of our most complicated and tricky patients had been, despite unique combinations of posttraumatic surgeries, complications, or protracted illnesses. That's just how it is in my business. When every one of the people my partners and I admit is the most acutely ill of all those receiving care in our hospital, how can we be expected to remember one from another unless some very unique aspect of a patient's situation sets him apart from the others?

Family members often ask me if I believe that their loved one, who I just admitted to my service or on whom I recently performed emergency surgery, might likely die as a result of his or her injuries. I, of course, do my best to give the family members my educated estimation as to the likeliness of my new patient's chances of dying. I always include the caveat, however, that despite my training and experience, neither I nor any other physician is truly capable of accurately predicting survival or death with 100 percent certainty. But when I predict that a trauma patient will almost without doubt survive and then he or she dies unexpectedly, the entire memory lingers and remains a part of me. I do not forget them. Endings like that are tragic for the surviving family members, and endings like that are tragic for me as well. Regardless of whether people believe it or not, trauma surgeons—like anyone else in this world—are entitled to experiencing their share of human emotions, despite our usual tendencies to keep many of those thoughts and feelings to ourselves.

Roger and Ella Morgan were an elderly couple who suffered multiple, blunt traumatic injuries on an early spring day. Both were presented to us in pretty serious conditions, and we had our doubts from the very beginning whether even one of the two would survive the ordeal. We worked hard to save them and as a result, my partners and I developed fairly close relationships with the Morgan couple as we treated them through thick and thin. One of the two eventually became well despite serious setbacks, but one gradually slipped to the point of no return, dying a slow and miserable death. But matters didn't evolve as any of us might have predicted, which is what made it so difficult for everyone when the end eventually came.

On March 21, seventy-one-year-old Roger was driving the family sedan and his sixty-seven-year-old wife, Ella, was in the passenger seat next to him. Tragedy struck when a minivan sped through an intersection and smashed into the passenger side of Roger and Ella's vehicle. The Morgans were trapped within the badly crushed and deformed automobile; it took fire and rescue personnel nearly an hour to cut the vehicle apart and to extricate the two. Both occupants were anxious and confused at the scene but were alert enough for paramedics to not suspect that either of the two had suffered a serious brain injury. Mrs. Morgan's right leg was badly broken and both bones of her shin poked through the fat bulging from the bloody edges of a large laceration. Both patients were taken to the closest hospital, which was accredited as a Level II Trauma Center, certainly capable of handling most traumatic injuries.

Roger was a thin and muscular man. He tried to maintain a healthy lifestyle but his seven decades of life and some unlucky genetics resulted in a previous open-heart operation where surgeons bypassed two occluded coronary arteries and replaced an abnormally tight aortic valve. Prior to the car accident, Roger generally felt well, but his past heart problems made it necessary that he take the blood thinner Coumadin daily. Without it, a clot could form on Roger's artificial heart valve which might then cause him to suffer a stroke or some other serious medical catastrophe. Wanting to extend his life as long as possible, Roger ate well, walked a little on the treadmill every day, and dutifully took his medication as his cardiologist had prescribed. Roger looked healthy and he felt strong and robust.

On the other hand, Ella was morbidly obese and over the years she required increasing amounts of insulin to obtain marginal control of her diabetes. She also had longstanding high blood pressure and she was miserable from years of chronic back pain. She took multiple medications on a daily basis and visits to various doctor's offices seemed to be a recurring theme for the corpulent, old lady who always seemed to be sick. Unlike Roger, whose mental attitude made him feel younger than his stated age, Ella looked and felt much older than her partner of so many years.

Upon arrival at the initial hospital, Roger's blood pressure, heart rate, and oxygen levels were stable. Ella, though, was not doing as well. Her blood pressure was running low, her heart rate was fast, and she was having difficulty breathing. Doctors and nurses infused multiple liters of intravenous fluids into Ella, attempting to combat her low blood pressure, the cause of which had not been initially determined. Apparently, Mrs. Morgan's condition was so worrisome to the doctors at the other facility that they performed only a few diagnostic tests before calling our hospital requesting that we take her off their hands. Ella's chest X-ray revealed several right-sided rib fractures and a broken right scapula. A pelvis X-ray demonstrated fractures of her sacrum as well as her right hemi-pelvis. A right leg X-ray confirmed her obvious tibia and fibula fractures, and X-rays of her right arm demonstrated a complete break through the midportion of Ella's humerus.

A helicopter was sent to the transferring hospital to emergently transport the unstable and badly injured Ella Morgan to our trauma center. Meanwhile, the emergency room doctors and nurses at the other facility continued evaluating Mr. Morgan, who at all times remained stable and seemingly well. They performed CT scans of his brain, neck, chest, abdomen, and pelvis, all of which were reportedly negative for any evidence of traumatic injury. An apparently incidental abnormality was noted, however, in Mr. Morgan's liver. The radiologists noted what they felt could have been a liver mass—perhaps a tumor—which would need further workup at some time in the future. Being stable and without any apparent injuries of significance, Roger was admitted to their hospital for observation, as his past cardiac history certainly warranted at least an overnight stay on the general medical ward.

When Ella arrived to our trauma room, her blood pressure was low and she was far from stable. She was in hemorrhagic shock from blood loss as a result of her pelvic, arm, and leg fractures. Despite several liters of rapidly infused, intravenous fluid, her blood pressure only corrected partially. We transfused three units of packed red blood cells before we could even stabilize Ella long enough to perform the myriad of CT scans necessary to determine exactly what had been injured. She was having difficulty breathing due to severe chest pain, which we knew was likely from her multiple rib and scapula fractures. She required 100 percent O_2 delivered through a face mask to maintain adequate blood oxygenation. We were moments away from inserting a breathing tube down her throat, but several doses of morphine controlled her pain well enough for us to abandon placing Ella on the ventilator.

A CT scan of Ella's brain showed no damage to her skull or brain, but scanning down through her neck unfortunately revealed two fractures through the second of the seven cervical spine vertebrae. Bone fragments were not displaced, and there did not appear to be any threat to her spinal cord. However, her injuries presented us with a conundrum as we needed to affix a rigid, immobilization collar to her neck—something which would ordinarily have already been done well before she ever even made it into our hospital—but Ella's neck was so short and stout that there wasn't a collar available that would fit her and provide the protection she needed. Fortunately, as we do with all of our trauma patients, we presumed that she had broken her neck before our knowing the CT scan results and we had kept her immobilized from the shoulders on up by securing sandbags to either side of her head to prevent any right or left movement. But now knowing that Ella would need long-term immobilization, we needed to come up with a better plan.

CT scans through her chest revealed three broken ribs on her right side. Ribs three, four, and five were cracked, but her lung and vascular structures all seemed to be relatively uninjured. Hopefully, with the right amount of pain medication, we would be able to control Ella's pain well enough to keep her off the ventilator. We couldn't sedate her too much, since that might potentially slow her breathing to the point of causing her lungs to retain carbon dioxide. That would be a very precarious problem that could necessitate us putting her on the machine at any time, the inevitable result of which would require a tracheostomy since once we put her on the ventilator, we would likely not be able to get her off for several weeks.

A CT scan through her abdomen and pelvis showed no injury to her liver, spleen, gastrointestinal tract, or kidneys, but it did show in great detail the fractures to her pelvis. Her sacrum and both the left and right sides of her pelvis were fractured. Fortunately, nothing had displaced significantly. The force that broke her pelvis did, however, rupture a portion of Ella's bladder, but the rupture was small and was contained within the peritoneal lining of her pelvis. It would not require surgery, as no urine leaked into her abdomen proper.

Once we had obtained all of our diagnostic studies, I made of list of all of Ella's injuries and began to formulate a plan to address each of her problems. From head to toe, Ella had a broken neck, three broken ribs, a broken scapula, a broken arm, an extra-peritoneal bladder rupture, multiple pelvic fractures, and fractures to both bones of her right leg. She had lost a large amount of blood but all had been contained within the soft tissues of her muscles and pelvis. Three units of transfused blood and the IV fluids had stabilized her.

Her broken neck was a serious problem. I talked with our trauma spine surgeon as well as with our trauma orthopedist to formulate plans to get all of Ella's bony injuries stabilized as quickly as possible. We took Ella to the operating room where the anesthesiologist secured her airway with what we had hoped would only be a temporary breathing tube. Once safely anesthetized, we decided that Ella's neck injury was our first priority. Ordinarily, the spine surgeon might have been able to surgically fuse the fractured bone segments through a carefully placed incision down the back of her neck. But Ella was a diabetic, and her uncontrolled disease had resulted in her having a chronic yeast infection in the floppy, fatty structures of the skin from the base of her skull extending to the tops of her shoulders. Operating through skin infected with yeast was a disaster waiting to happen. The inevitable result would be a fungal infection deep within Ella's neck bones, which could easily cause her demise. We agreed that Ella needed a surgically placed halo brace.

A halo is a steel ring placed around the head, screwed into the skull with four pins drilled directly into the bony cortex. Attached to the metal ring was a series of rods placed parallel to Ella's neck, which were bolted to a large corset brace placed around her corpulent, upper chest. We rarely use halo braces any longer, but considering Ella's morbid obesity and the yeast infection of her neck, we had little alternative but to place the hugely cumbersome device and attempt to allow her fractures to heal spontaneously over six-to-eight weeks' time. Ella's large body limited her mobility even before her accident, and we knew that attaching the heavy contraption to her head and chest would make her a temporary invalid. But we had to do what was necessary, and after several hours of work fitting together pieces of orthopedic hardware, Ella's upper torso was rigidly fixated within a circumferential cage which surrounded her from her mid chest on up.

Following the meticulous application of the halo brace, we all felt comfortable enough to proceed with fixing Ella's arm, leg, and pelvic fractures. The orthopedic surgeon and his assistant spent the next four hours fixing all of her remaining fractures. Rods placed directly though Ella's right humerus and tibia provided rigid stabilization of the fractures. An anterior, external fixator device was then placed across her fractured pelvis, firmly attached to her skeleton via four pins drilled into the barely palpable, bony prominences of her iliac crest bones deeply hidden within her multiple layers of fat. When all procedures had been completed, Ella had titanium and carbon fiber hardware protruding in a most unnatural manner from her upper and lower body, all attached to cagelike structures resembling something from the Middle Ages.

One of my partners was on duty that evening in the trauma center and fortunately had the time to spend nearly all night at Ella's bedside continuing to resuscitate her with additional units of transfused blood and IV fluids. By the time the morning sun had risen, Ella's blood pressure had once again stabilized completely and we collectively decided to try to get her off the ventilator. It was a bold move, but knowing that we had only a limited window of opportunity to attempt extubation, we removed her breathing tube and hoped for the best. We were well aware of the likely possibility of having to emergently replace the breathing tube. Hoping to ward off any evil spirits, we kept all of the reintubation equipment nearby at Ella's bedside. Thankfully, Ella tolerated removal from the breathing machine very well, and she didn't require anything other than supplemental oxygen by way of a nasal cannula.

The odds were against Ella doing well. Any one of a number of terrible complications could develop at any time. I gathered Ella's family together and briefed everyone as to the stormy course all of us who were treating her had anticipated. I wanted to sound optimistic, but at the same time, I needed to paint a realistic picture of statistically what would likely occur over the next several weeks. Yes, Ella was stable, but she could easily develop pulmonary failure and needed to be placed back on the ventilator. She was at high risk of developing pneumonia, and she was at high risk of developing a deep vein thrombosis—a clot within any of her leg or pelvis veins, any one of which could break off and migrate into her chest, obstructing the blood flow to her heart or within her lungs. Ella

could develop one of any number of wound infections, and her obesity and diabetes could even precipitate a heart attack.

In a nutshell, Ella had a much greater chance of getting sicker than getting
better. I told them all that we would do everything possible to anticipate any
problems and we would even be placing a filter into her vena cava to catch any
clot that might be forming in the veins of her lower body. Her family understood everything I told them, and they were all very appreciative for what we
had done for Ella. They also appreciated my very candid and honest comments,
but they all stated repeatedly that Ella was a tough old lady who had defeated
problems before. They felt that she would somehow weather this storm as well.
I encouraged them to remain optimistic, but I also asked that they not be
surprised if any of us called them at any time with news of any complications.

Meanwhile, while Mrs. Morgan had been fighting for her life in our hospital, her husband had been having his own problems at the other facility. Despite Roger being stable throughout his emergency room workup, his blood
pressure started to drop. Apparently, he drifted into shock throughout the night
as he bled from an unrecognized injury, exacerbated by the fact that his blood
was incapable of forming clot due to the necessary blood thinner he had been
taking daily to prevent thrombus from forming on his artificial heart valve.
Doctors had been monitoring Roger's blood count at the other hospital throughout the night, which had slowly drifted down over the eighteen or so hours since
his admission. When nurses took Mr. Morgan's morning blood pressure, it measured a critically low seventy over forty. To complicate matters, his urine output
had trickled down to almost nothing by sunrise. Realizing that Mr. Morgan's
injuries were more severe than they had originally anticipated, they aggressively
transfused multiple units of red blood cells and plasma in order to restore Roger's
circulatory volume and thicken his pharmacologically thinned blood.

They also again reviewed the CT scans performed the previous day and
realized that what they had originally felt was an incidentally identified liver
tumor was more likely a contained hemorrhage within the large abdominal
organ. The bleeding from the tear in his liver had no reasonable chance of stopping as his ability to form clot had been impaired by his medications. At
some time in the middle of the night, his bleeding liver must have ruptured
and Roger began hemorrhaging into his abdomen. Mr. Morgan's situation had
changed from stable to critical, and he needed a higher level of trauma care
than could be provided to him at the other hospital. Just as with Mrs. Morgan

the day before, the doctors caring for Mr. Morgan asked that we also take our patient's husband in transfer. The helicopter was spun up and within an hour, Mr. Morgan was whisked away to our hospital, where we received him in our intensive care unit.

On arrival to our hospital, Roger looked very pale. His blood pressure was borderline low and he was clutching his chest. We quickly assessed Mr. Morgan from head to toe and reviewed the previous day's CT scans. I'm sure that in retrospect the other hospital's surgeons and radiologists would agree that there was no question that Roger's abnormal liver CT reflected a traumatic injury and was not an incidental tumor. But regardless, none of that was important once Roger was with us. Mr. Morgan was bleeding from a tear originating deep within his liver in an area that would be nearly inaccessible by any surgical approach. We needed to stop the ongoing hemorrhage and the best chances of saving our patient's life would be in the interventional radiology suite.

Interventional radiology is a subspecialty practiced by highly skilled radiologists who drain abscesses, deploy vascular devices, and plug bleeding vessels with tiny instruments and catheters passed into the body under fluoroscopic or CT imaging guidance. We contacted the interventional radiologist in-house that day and asked him to get his team ready for our patient. While preparing Roger for his procedure, we transfused additional units of blood, performed an electrocardiogram, and ran additional cardiac tests, which revealed that he was having a mild heart attack due to the physical strain of the ongoing, internal blood loss. We began infusing intravenous medication to protect Roger's heart from further damage, but we knew that none of it would make a bit of difference unless we could get the bleeding stopped.

Once on the interventional radiology table, the radiologist catheterized Mr. Morgan's right femoral artery, which is a similar procedure interventional cardiologists perform when catheterizing the heart. The radiologist slid a long, narrow catheter through Roger's right groin vessel up into his abdominal aorta. Using radio-opaque, injectable contrast to visualize the otherwise impossible-to-see vessels, the radiologist then maneuvered the catheter into the highest branch of Mr. Morgan's abdominal aorta—a four-to-five-millimeter diameter vessel called the celiac trunk. The celiac trunk has three primary divisions, and the branch coursing off to the right is the one which supplies the majority of the blood to the liver. After squirting an additional dose of contrast into the vessel, it was apparent that a branch of Roger's right hepatic artery was actively hemorrhaging, as intravascular dye leaked out of what could be mistaken for nothing other than an arterial injury. Snaking the long catheter a little farther into our patient's body, the interventional radiologist then deployed several, clot-forming, vascular coils from the tip of the long tube, plugging the hole in Mr. Morgan's bleeding liver artery.

With almost magical qualities, the clot-forming coils did what they were supposed to do. The bleeding stopped almost immediately, as verified by a final blast of the arterial contrast, which showed no leakage outside of the subsequently occluded vessel. The radiologist removed the several feet of narrow catheter tubing from Mr. Morgan's right groin and he turned the patient back over to me. We then took Mr. Morgan to the intensive care unit for further, critical care management, which included caring for Roger's mild heart attack.

When the nurses who cared for Mr. Morgan that evening learned of all that had happened to the Morgan couple, they couldn't help but feel very bad for Roger. All night long, Roger asked about his wife, feeling great remorse for all that Ella had just been through. He was sick over the thought of his wife's suffering, and he was terribly distraught over the possibility of Ella dying. Touched by the emotional heartache Mr. Morgan was experiencing over his wife's injuries, the ICU nurses began to repeatedly mutter in consolation, "Poor Roger; poor, poor Roger."

Over the following several days, Roger's cardiac condition worsened. His heart attack weakened his cardiac muscle, making it less able to circulate blood throughout his system, and causing fluid to back up into his lungs, which resulted in congestive heart failure. We placed an invasive catheter through the large vein below his collarbone and threaded the monitor through Roger's heart—through his right atrium, right ventricle, and his pulmonary artery—in order to obtain specific measurements of the volumes and pressures of the various parts of his heart and circulatory system. Using the values obtained on a continuous, ongoing basis by the invasive monitor, we adjusted potent, continuous, cardiac infusions and we adjusted the volumes of fluid we administered through the intravenous lines to keep Mr. Morgan's heart function optimized. We kept him from decompensating, and after a few days, Roger's condition stabilized.

But on about the third day, Roger took an abrupt turn for the worse. He could not breathe and we were forced to place him on a ventilator. Roger's blood pressure dropped and he was becoming septic—a condition where a source of infection was spreading throughout his circulatory system causing generalized organ failure. His belly was becoming distended, and a second CT scan of his abdomen suggested that decreased blood flow to Roger's large intestine had caused a portion of his bowel to necrose and die. He simultaneously began to bleed from his rectum, further suggesting that Roger had an area of dead bowel. We inserted an endoscope into Mr. Morgan's lower gastrointestinal tract where we identified large areas of dead, black intestine, and the unquestionable source of his rectal bleeding. Roger was again unstable, and his only chance of surviving his new problem was with an emergency operation. We talked with his family and we obtained consent to take Roger to the operating room to perform the necessary emergency, exploratory surgery.

In the OR, we found most of the left side of Roger's large intestine to be dead—a diagnosis we refer to as ischemic bowel, a condition which is often the result of poor blood flow through an area of diseased blood vessels, not uncommon in older patients with coronary artery disease. Roger's hemorrhagic shock secondary to his liver injury, compounded by the weak circulatory efforts of his diseased heart, certainly must have resulted in an area of decreased blood flow to the colon, resulting in the dead bowel. Dead bowel is a terrible problem, from which older patients often don't recover. Knowing that Roger had a wife and family who did not want him to die, we aggressively treated his condition by surgically removing all of Mr. Morgan's abnormal bowel. We brought out the remaining, healthy end of the right side of his intestine through his abdominal wall and we created a colostomy. We sealed off the lowest portion of Roger's large intestine, beyond the level of the dead bowel, with a surgical stapling device, creating an end intestinal segment, which could still evacuate its residual contents through his rectum.

After thoroughly washing out Roger's abdomen, we closed the dense layer of abdominal wall fascia but we left his large, skin wound open, packed only with saline-moistened gauze dressings. It is a technique surgeons often use to minimize postoperative wound infections in any patient who has had internal leakage of intestinal contents, or dead bowel. Roger was sick enough already. He did not need any additional sources of infection.

After surgery, we took Mr. Morgan back to the intensive care unit, still very, very sick, but with a renewed chance of surviving—something which could not have occurred without the emergency operation. The nurses caring for Roger were notably bothered by all that the man had already been through, and wondered just how much more his sickly, old body could take. With great professionalism and compassion, they meticulously attended to all of Roger's critical care needs, occasionally shaking their heads, and uttering the words, "Poor, poor Roger."

For the next three days, Roger slowly improved. The insult to his body from the generalized infection and the surgery seemed to be coming under control. His blood pressure and heart rate were again normalized, and he was no longer having fevers. He remained too sick and too weak, however, to be removed from the ventilator, but he was making progress.

On his third postoperative night, Roger went into full cardiac arrest. Without warning, his ventricle began to fibrillate and he lost his pulse. Nurses instinctively began cardiac compressions and the in-house, on-call trauma surgeon was notified and at the bedside within minutes. Blasts of electrical energy were delivered to Roger's chest, causing his body to jump with each high voltage shock, and numerous ampoules of epinephrine and other cardiac drugs were pushed into his frail blood vessels. After repeated shocks and nearly thirty minutes of CPR, someone suddenly felt a pulse in Roger's groin artery and his heart again began to beat in a normal, rhythmic fashion.

But the thirty minutes of cardiac arrest and extremely effective chest compressions had taken a significantly adverse toll on Roger. Many of Roger's ribs had been broken from the chest compressions—an expected occurrence if good CPR is performed for even a few minutes. A postresuscitation chest X-ray confirmed the fractures, and also revealed that one of Roger's lungs had collapsed as a result, necessitating a large diameter chest tube be inserted to fully reexpand the injured pulmonary tissue. Having no spontaneous heartbeat for a half hour often results in strokes, kidney failure, and damage to the heart muscle itself. Roger once again had a pulse, but his blood pressure was far from normal. Two different continuously infused medications were needed to keep his blood pressure at a level sufficient to maintain oxygenated, circulatory flow to Roger's organ systems. One of those medications was Levophed—a drug I typically used only in the most dire of situations.

The following morning, Roger was still alive, and like his previous brushes with death, he somehow seemed to tolerate the otherwise grave insult to his body. The intensive care unit nurses had managed to wean off the Levophed entirely, but Roger was still dependent on a fairly high dose of one of the other pressure-elevating medications. As we had predicted, Roger's kidneys failed, and it would only be a matter of days before he would begin requiring dialysis.

On that day, nearly everyone caring for Roger started repeating the words that were becoming rather familiar: "Poor, poor Roger."

A week passed and Roger again stabilized in the intensive care unit. Still very sick by all standards, he was off all medications required to keep his blood pressure in the normal range, but he was on countless other drugs. He was receiving several different antibiotics, each targeted to kill the different organisms cultured from his blood. He was also receiving numerous other agents to both treat as well as prevent other conditions associated with critical illness. He still required full ventilator support, as he remained too weak to take in a breath. All of his nutrition was provided via a tube passed through his nose and threaded into his stomach. Despite the tube feedings, Roger was still very malnourished. His body consumed more calories trying to heal than his gastrointestinal tract could absorb. His kidneys had shown no signs of recovery and he was receiving daily dialysis treatments to rid his body of the toxic byproducts he generated, as well as the excess water his urinary tract could not eliminate.

We changed Roger's abdominal dressings two times each day. One morning after I removed his abdominal wall packing, I spotted brown, feculent material in the lower aspect of his wound percolating up between the sutures holding his midline abdominal fascia together. He was leaking stool! It was a terrible sight for a surgeon to witness, as it could only mean that the staple line I had previously fired across his left-sided colonic stump had blown out and the residual feces contained within were leaking, undoubtedly now throughout his entire abdominal cavity. There was only one place where Roger again needed to be, and that was back in the operating room.

Redo operations are never as easy as first-time surgical procedures. His intestines had formed an inflammatory rind over everything, as if a sticky paste had been poured over his bowels. Like a pot of cooked noodles left in a bowl overnight, his intestines were all stuck together. I carefully peeled loops of bowel away from one another with my gloved fingers, taking great care not to injure any more of the delicate segments. After spending several hours meticulously freeing up the matted loops of intestine, I finally exposed Roger's left lower quadrant, where his colonic stump lay. As I had expected, his stump had completely blown out. I washed out his abdominal cavity with five liters of saline until the material I suctioned out ran clear. Knowing that his inflamed, thickened, colonic stump would never again hold a stapled closure, I sealed up the blown-out segment of large intestine with multiple, large, hand-sewn sutures. Once confident that his colon was again sealed shut, I rewashed his abdominal cavity an additional time and reclosed his abdominal wall fascia.

His postoperative complication was demoralizing and painful for me. Despite having done everything correctly at the original surgery, his staple line had failed. But as all surgeons should do, I second-guessed what I originally did and wondered if perhaps I had hand-sewn his colonic stump the first time he might not have had the setback. Despite knowing that I had done everything correctly from the very beginning, I still lamented Roger's complication. I, too, began to wonder just how much more Roger's frail body could take. And I, too, began saying "Poor, poor Roger."

For the next several weeks, we chased Roger's fevers. Infectious disease specialists changed Roger's antibiotics several times, and we performed CT scans of his abdomen every week, each time identifying a new collection of pus that had formed in a hidden corner of Roger's peritoneal cavity. Each time, the interventional radiologists drained the pus pockets with tubes and drains placed directly through Roger's abdominal wall, guided by CT imaging techniques to ensure accurate placement of the drainage catheters.

Finally accepting that Roger would not be able to be weaned from the ventilator, I performed a tracheostomy and a surgically placed feeding tube, which I sewed directly into Roger's stomach. Roger looked terrible. Drains, tubes, and lines of every diameter pierced his abdominal wall. The mucous membranes of the end of Roger's remaining colon billowed out through his colostomy site, and his midline wound remained open, covered only by the saline-moistened, gauze material we replaced in the mornings and evenings.

Meanwhile, Ella was making great progress. The lady who we all originally thought was the more seriously injured of the two was out of the intensive care unit and up on the general medical floor, eating and drinking by mouth, and getting around in a wheelchair pushed by nurse's assistants. She asked us about her husband daily and we kept her apprised of his overall status. After a while, she was finally well enough to be wheeled down to Roger's bedside for a brief visit. There she spent a half hour holding his weak hand, crying quietly as her spouse of nearly fifty years lay next to her, too weak to reciprocate the squeeze of the woman's hand. It was such a sad sight to witness the two, elderly car-crash victims in such a state of extreme disability. I couldn't help but wonder if they would ever again be able to spend any quality time together.

Ella left us the following day as she was transferred to an acute, inpatient rehabilitation center where she would spend the next month regaining her strength and independence so that she could again care for herself and resume her activities of daily living. Few people ever think twice about how they will get themselves into the shower each morning, how they will comb their hair and brush their teeth, and how they will get themselves on and off the toilet throughout the day. But nearly all of our severely injured trauma patients face these seemingly trivial challenges with great difficulty, and often require many weeks of reconditioning and relearning the basic tasks which—with only rare exception—they all previously took for granted. Ella would spend at least four hours every day at the rehab center practicing the essential skills necessary to again achieve independent living.

But Roger would not be so lucky to be able to yet graduate to the rehabilitation center. On the day that Ella left us, Roger was still breathing with the assistance of a machine. He hadn't even the strength to move himself within his bed. He certainly could neither feed himself nor manage his own basic hygiene needs. Despite having stabilized and being free of fever and infection, Roger still needed extensive nursing care on an almost continuous basis.

After additional time, however, Roger no longer required inpatient hospitalization in our trauma center, but he did need the fairly extensive services of a skilled nursing facility—basically, a maximal support nursing home, where nurses and doctors provide high-level chronic care for patients with long-term medical conditions. No one knew just how long Roger might spend at the skilled nursing facility, or whether or not he would ever even make it to the rehabilitation center. Some skilled nursing facility patients never become independent and eventually have to settle for traditional nursing-home living, never achieving the strength or endurance to participate in the level of physical therapy required of the acute, inpatient rehab facilities.

I couldn't wait for Roger to leave us. As harsh as it may sound, I began to dread rounding on Mr. Morgan day after day, seeing little to no progress, wondering if yet another, major complication or setback would become apparent to me, necessitating additional diagnostic workups, interventional treatments, or even surgical procedures. Seeing Roger, tediously reviewing the reams of data we collected on him every day, and examining him each morning sucked the life out of me. I feel guilty about this whenever I care for a patient like Roger, but I recognize it as a personal limitation of mine. I have never been a person who felt good about my patients' tiny improvements, but rather one who required more dramatic demonstrations of progress to give me satisfaction as a treating physician.

This is a phenomenon many surgeons share, and is especially true of trauma surgeons who thrive on taking patients who are dying in a dramatic fashion and exhaust their own energies to give their patients the chance to live. There is a reason why some physicians choose to pursue slower-paced specialties such as internal medicine, family practice, and administrative medicine. God bless all of them, because I surely couldn't do what they do for a living. But conversely, they couldn't do what I do, and they would never want the responsibilities associated with my job. Thankfully, there are avenues in the profession of medicine for all personality types. Roger needed a different set of doctors. The trauma surgeons had done all that they could.

Mr. Morgan transferred out of our trauma center into a skilled nursing facility several weeks after his wife left us. For two months, I heard nothing of how he had been progressing or otherwise. In some cases—as with Roger—no news was considered to be good news. But one afternoon while I was working in-house, I received a page from one of our emergency room physicians. Roger was back! He had apparently started bleeding from a small area on his abdominal wall. The doctors who attended to Roger at the skilled nursing facility didn't feel comfortable attempting to control the blood loss.

I went to see Roger in the emergency room, cringing at the very likely thought of having to readmit him to our service. When I entered Roger's room I was shocked at just how bad he looked. He was thinner than ever and he looked as if he had aged a decade since I last saw him. He lay on the emergency room cart looking pathetic and depressed, with no trace of hope or will to live left on his gaunt, beard-stubbled face. I had no problem controlling what I thought was fairly trivial bleeding—more like oozing—from the lowest part of Roger's abdominal wound with a few quick applications of a handheld, electrocautery probe. I tried to boost Roger's spirits by assuring him that his bleeding wasn't a problem, and I lied with the best of intentions when I told him how good he looked.

But Roger was no fool. He knew that he was dying a slow death. I knew it as well: Roger had slipped to the point of no return and would never again leave the confines of a health-care institution. Seeing Roger in such a miserable state ate away at me. He looked at me with his deeply set, weakly opened eyes and he moved his lips as if he desperately was trying to tell me something very important. Sadly, no words came out of Roger's mouth; he was too weak to even speak. I wondered if he was asking me to let him die—something that I could, of course, never actively facilitate.

I did consider if Roger would be better off in a hospice environment, where nurses could give him as much pain medication as needed to ease Roger's suffering, and let him die peacefully with compassion and dignity when it was his time to leave this world. But I knew from my previous dealings with Roger's family that hospice was something they would not be interested in. At that point, all I could do was hold Roger's hand firmly. I hoped that spending a few quiet moments with him with his hand in mine might give him at least some temporary peace to his tormented existence. The words I had heard so many times before when Roger was lying in our intensive care unit rang out in the quiet of my own thoughts: "Poor Roger; poor, poor Roger."

I transferred Roger back to the skilled nursing facility later that day and I hoped that his suffering would soon come to an end. About a week later, I heard the news of Roger's passing. One of the ward secretaries in our intensive care unit had become close to one of Roger's sons and she kept in contact with him fairly often. Nearly everyone had developed a relationship with the Morgan family, but unit secretary Karen had become closer than any of us to Roger and his children. Roger's son called Karen to courteously inform all of the nurses and doctors who had cared for his father that Mr. Morgan had quietly passed away in his sleep at the skilled nursing facility. The sad but anticipated news spread quickly throughout the intensive care unit, and the overall mood of the forty-four-bed critical care department was unusually somber that day. His suffering had finally ended, and poor, poor Roger was finally at peace.

26

The Final Chapter

It Has Been a Privilege

Losing a patient like Roger was a painful blow for me. If I was to dwell on his sad death, I might abandon my profession entirely. Roger was a case where all hope had been lost. Fortunately for me, though, I would encounter many more patients teetering on the brink of death, whose splendid recoveries would mitigate my sad and painful memories. Patients with successful outcomes always bring me great satisfaction and are my source of hope, allowing me to drive on and keep working at the trauma center.

Rachel McKay was one such source of hope. She was a bright, young, university senior of twenty-one years who had been home with her family over Thanksgiving break. After celebrating the holiday the evening prior, she journeyed out to the outlet malls with her mother to partake in her annual ritual of Black Friday shopping. Along with thousands of other early-morning shoppers, Rachel and her mom hoped to find a few exceptional Christmas special deals.

The outlet-mall parking lot was jammed with cars. Despite the fact that the sun had not yet even broken the horizon, every parking space on the vast asphalt perimeter of the shopping complex was occupied. Rachel drove around for about ten minutes before finding one open space, which she quickly claimed. Exiting her car, she noted dozens of other drivers weaving up and down the rows of parked cars looking for their little piece of empty lot. While walking toward the mall entrance, she was forced to jump out of the way of a car whose driver decided to quickly back out of a space without looking. Without so much as a wave or acknowledgement from the hurried driver, the exiting car sped off. The rest of what happened was nothing more than a blur for Rachel, as moments later she was on the ground, bleeding and unconscious.

As soon as the driver hastily abandoned his parking space, a second driver stepped on her accelerator pedal, eager to take the newly vacated spot. The driver barreled into the open space, not seeing that Rachel was in harm's way. The side view mirror of the speeding vehicle smacked into the back of Rachel's head, knocking her to the ground. The car's tires narrowly avoided running over Rachel as her head impacted the hard asphalt. Her mother heard what sounded like a coconut being cracked. Blood began pouring from Rachel's ear, and she lay lifeless on the ground in front of her.

Paramedics arrived less than five minutes later. By that time, Rachel had regained consciousness, but she had no recollection of the events that had just occurred. Rachel's head throbbed, and she was a bit stuporous. She was able to tell paramedics her name and address. She was able to follow all of their commands. But she seemed somewhat confused to her mother, who worried greatly about the bleeding that persistently oozed from Rachel's ear. A short while later, the lights on the ambulance were turning and the siren was blaring. Rachel was being taken to a local hospital for an emergency evaluation.

I received a call about an hour later from an Emergency Medicine physician thirty miles west of us, requesting that Rachel be transferred to our facility for a higher level of care. According to the transferring doctor, Rachel had been brought to their emergency room awake and alert, but her mental status was declining. He had performed a CT scan of Rachel's brain, which revealed a lens shaped collection of blood between the left side of her cerebral cortex and the skull. The epidural hematoma was compressing Rachel's brain, and the Emergency Medicine doctor was concerned that Rachel might die as the bleeding expanded inside her skull. With no neurosurgeon at the other hospital able to accommodate Rachel's immediate needs, my help was needed. I accepted Rachel without hesitation, and arranged for a helicopter to pick her up.

About twenty minutes later, the sound of rotors chopping through the early-morning air notified me that my patient had arrived. Having spent considerable time around helicopters as a military physician, I was keenly aware of the distinct sound of an approaching aircraft. Moments later, my trauma alert sounded and I knew with certainty that Rachel had arrived.

I arrived in the trauma room even before the flight crew had time to extricate Rachel from the chopper and bring her into the hospital. As she was being wheeled down the hall, I saw the petite girl's head wrapped in bloody gauze. She was restless and somewhat agitated. My senses told me that she was not well, and that she needed my attention as quickly as possible. As soon as Rachel was transferred onto the trauma room cart, I assessed her airway, breathing, circulation, and her mental status. Although her airway was patent and she was breathing well on her own, she would only open her eyes when I ground my knuckles into her breastbone. From my discussion with the transferring hospital's emergency room physician less than a half hour before, I knew that Rachel's mental status had declined significantly. So, to keep her airway protected, I told one of our emergency medicine physicians to insert an endotracheal tube and place Rachel on the ventilator. I knew that Rachel would only be getting worse, and intubation would eventually become an emergency requirement. I wanted the tube inserted under more controlled, less urgent circumstances.

I checked Rachel's pupils. Her right pupil constricted vigorously when I shined a flashlight into her eye, but her left pupil was sluggish. It was not behaving normally. I ordered an emergent dose of Mannitol to decrease any brain swelling. I then whisked her off to the CT scanner to repeat the study performed at the previous hospital. Having the luxury of being able to compare the recent scan with the one taken just thirty minutes prior, I saw that the epidural hematoma in Rachel's head had expanded to nearly twice its previous size. Rachel needed surgery, and she needed it as quickly as possible.

I alerted the operating room and I told them to prepare for an emergent craniotomy. I called the on-call neurosurgeon who then quickly jumped into his car to meet us. I ordered a few additional tests as I went looking for Rachel's mother. She would need a thorough briefing as we were about to open her daughter's skull to drain the expanding blood threatening Rachel's very existence. But I would have little time to go into great detail.

I found Mrs. McKay and explained everything as quickly yet thoroughly as time allowed. Rachel's mother nearly collapsed when I told her that Rachel had an epidural hematoma and would die if we didn't operate emergently. Her mother asked me if her daughter had suffered the same injury that had taken the life of Liam Neeson's wife eight months prior. In fact, it was the identical injury.

In March 2009, Natasha Richardson had suffered a brain injury while skiing in Canada. The actress suffered the injury remote from a tertiary care medical center, and there was no brain surgeon available to provide the emergent surgery needed. Ms. Richardson was helicopter-evacuated to another Canadian hospital, where she underwent emergency surgery. But it was too late. She was already brain dead. The expanding mass of blood had created so much pressure in Ms. Richardson's head that her brain became irreversibly compressed resulting in brain death. Her actor husband painfully authorized the doctors to remove his wife from life support, and the actress died shortly thereafter.

My patient's mother was devastated by the news I told her. She trembled as she signed the consent authorizing the neurosurgeon to open her daughter's skull and evacuate the expanding blood. I assured the woman that we would do everything possible to save her child. Moments later, we sped Rachel to the operating room.

I helped move Rachel onto the operating room table. The anesthesiologist administered intravenous drugs and inhalational gases to our patient ensuring that she was sleeping deeply. I placed Rachel's head into a set of tongs, which would hold her head securely in the perfect position while the neurosurgeon operated. I ran an electric razor over the young woman's scalp, clipping away all the hair covering the left side of her head. I then asked the nurses to begin painting antiseptic solution over the bare area of her cranium, and I left the room to scrub.

The neurosurgeon walked toward me as I kicked the panel in front of the scrub sink, which activated the water faucet. He told me that he reviewed the CT scans and would join me at the scrub sink just as soon as he made his presence known to the OR staff. Once back at the scrub sink with me, we discussed Rachel's physical findings. I then warned him that Rachel's mom had brought up Natasha Richardson's injury and her subsequent death. We agreed that we could only do what we could—and we proceeded into the operating room.

I don't always assist the neurosurgeons when they perform emergency brain surgery. The neurosurgeons are the experts in that area; they certainly don't need my help. But I periodically assist them in the OR to maintain my proficiency should I ever be tasked with having to emergently open a head should a neurosurgeon be unavailable. I can't imagine such a situation arising at my hospital, but I had been tasked with crazier situations at other hospitals, as well as when on deployment with the military.

We covered Rachel's head with special drapes fashioned specifically for brain surgery. The neurosurgeon then created the classic question mark–shaped incision used for most brain trauma operations. The large cut began just in front of her left ear and curved back just as the scalpel cleared the top of her auditory cartilage, extending several inches. The incision then curved up toward the top of her head, and then forward. By the time the single, curved wound had been created, it extended nearly fifteen inches. The entire wound, except for the part in front of Rachel's ear, was within the hair-bearing area. When her locks grew back, the scar would be nearly imperceptible.

Her scalp bled, as it always does—profusely at times. We quelled the pooling blood with numerous bursts from the electrocautery device. I placed removable plastic clips on the edges of the scalp wound, each one positioned immediately adjacent to the next, to further control the hemorrhage. Once all of the dozens of clips were secured, the neurosurgeon peeled Rachel's scalp wound from back to front, removing it from the underlying temporalis muscle, which one can feel bulge at the temple while chewing. We detached the muscle from its connections to the skull with additional blasts from the electrocautery and it, too, was peeled forward.

The white bone was all that kept us from Rachel's life-threatening blood clot. A jagged fracture line was visible through the center of the temporal bone—the thinnest portion of a person's skull. Undoubtedly, the blow to Rachel's head cracked the bone, which then tore the high-pressure middle meningeal artery lying just deep to it. The middle meningeal artery is anatomically positioned between the skull and the outer covering of the brain—the dura mater. When high pressure bleeding occurs within the space, the collection of blood is called an epidural hematoma. If a different source of bleeding resulted in blood to accumulate in the space deep to the dura mater, it would be called a subdural hematoma. Subdural bleeding is usually due to low-pressure, venous bleeding, but epidural bleeding is almost always due to high-pressure arterial bleeding. Epidural hematomas are notorious for causing rapid deterioration and death if not evacuated expeditiously.

We drilled four burr holes into Rachel's skull. Each one was placed several inches from the other. The neurosurgeon then took an oscillation saw with a right-angled blade and hooked it under the edge of one of the burr holes in Rachel's head. He powered up the saw and ran the cutting edge of the blade through the bone, connecting each of the holes. The result was a plate of skull completely detached from the rest of Rachel's cranium. We dissected the plate free from its underlying attachments, and we set it aside on the sterile back table of the operating room.

The culprit causing Rachel's potential demise was obvious. The three-inch, mulberry-shaped clot sat in a pool of fresh blood, which welled up from below. We picked away the thrombus exposing the pulsatile flow of the damaged middle meningeal artery. We found exactly what we were looking for. A few quick bursts from a bipolar, electrical coagulator seared the bleeding vessel, and the worst was over. We washed away the excess blood with a thorough application of saline solution and we evacuated the fluid with a suction tool. All that was left was to close Rachel back up and then move her to the intensive care unit.

We closed Rachel's wounds in the reverse manner as we had created them. We refitted the bony plate back into its defect and we secured it in place with miniature screws and plates after passing a few sutures through Rachel's dura mater and tiny holes were drilled into her skull plate. Those few sutures would prevent additional blood from forming in the epidural space during the postoperative period. After the final skull plate was secured, we flipped the temporalis muscle back into its normal position and we tacked it into place with heavy sutures. We then rotated the scalp back into its normal position, and after removing each of the plastic clips, we stapled the skin edges together. A thick, gauze, turbine dressing fitted tightly to Rachel's head and completed our work. Nearly three hours after starting the procedure, we transferred her still-anesthetized and intubated body back to the intensive care unit, and we waited for her to recover. I stayed at Rachel's bedside and composed a complete set of postoperative orders while the neurosurgeon briefed Mrs. McKay of the work we had just performed.

Rachel did extremely well following surgery. Within a few hours after leaving the operating room, she was wide awake and breathing through the tube without the assistance of the ventilator. A short while later, I removed the tube entirely and Rachel began speaking to her mother. The mom wept with tears of relief and joy. She thanked me and the neurosurgeon profusely. Mrs. McKay was so overcome with emotion that Rachel had to intervene and calm her mother's fears. Feeling confident that my patient was doing well, I left the girl and her mother to spend some quiet time together.

Rachel was eating by the following day, and she was up and walking on the

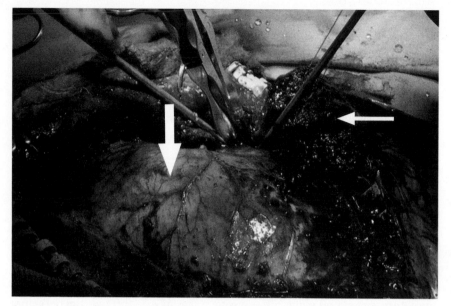

A surgeon's view of a craniotomy. The skull is open and the large, vertical arrow points to the dura mater covering the brain. The smaller, horizontal arrow points to a portion of the epidural hematoma clot peeled off the dura.

second postoperative day. She spent the next few days receiving assessments from the various rehabilitation specialists, including physical therapists, occupational therapists, and speech therapists. Speech therapists often help determine if any subtle, neurocognitive deficits have occurred as a result of brain trauma. If identified, traumatic brain injury rehabilitation is usually indicated. Our speech therapists performed several different brain-function assessment tests, but they could not identify any area of cognitive deficiency.

By the fifth postoperative day, Rachel was well enough to be discharged to home. She and her mother thanked us again for all that we did. They assured me that they would return to our trauma clinic within a few weeks so that we could again assess Rachel's postoperative progress.

Ten days later, Rachel and her mother returned to our clinic. She was doing great! She no longer had headaches, and she denied any nausea, dizziness, or subjective problems otherwise. She eagerly wanted to get back to school. She had been studying to be a financial manager, and she didn't want to miss any more of her classes. Finding no good reason to deny her desire, I authorized her to travel back to the university and get back to her studies.

A few weeks later, I received a small note from Rachel. She again thanked me for all that everyone on the team had done for her. She told me that her studies were going well, and that her professors had granted her extra time to take exams she had missed while convalescing. She said that she was happy to have met us, but assured me that she would no longer be taking advantage of the post-Thanksgiving, Black Friday events.

Rachel was one of my most memorable patients, and I am proud to have been able to help her. Rachel's success once again reminded me that quitting my job would never be an option.

When I reflect on all of the great experiences and opportunities that I have been blessed with, I conclude with certainty that I have been very fortunate. I have been enriched by a multitude of experiences afforded to me by patients, mentors, work associates, and everyday people who have made a favorable and lasting impact on my professional and personal development. I've had challenges and I've had some adversity, but I believe with conviction that my rewards have been more than plentiful.

I am grateful for having had the honor to serve my country. If I had not joined the military, I would never have chosen to go to El Paso, Texas, where I was selected sight unseen by my residency program director to train to become a surgeon. William Beaumont Army Medical Center and its surgical residency staff will forever be the precious gem that prepared and trained me better than any other surgery program could have. The military introduced me to countless interesting and noble people, many of whom my wife and I still remain in contact with. The military allowed me to experience living in many unusual and interesting places, within every time zone of the continental United States. I have traveled to no fewer than ten different countries on military orders and I have learned so much about the world outside of my homeland by way of my personal experiences.

Despite having served in war, the military has brought me peace. War has taught me to better appreciate all that is good, and has taught me that a bad day in a land free of fighting is probably better than a good one in a combat zone. I also recognize that my two-year period spent serving as a military general practitioner—during which I matured as a young doctor, enjoyed the thrill of parachuting and SCUBA diving, and when I was given ample time to relax my mind and body before completing my residency—was a blessing most physicians and surgeons today might have chosen in retrospect if they had been given the option.

Having been given the opportunity over the years to treat many severely injured patients with complex psychological and social lives has also been an ongoing education in and of itself. The complexity of my patients' injuries has provided me with a continuous source of opportunity to maintain my surgical skills to a high standard, and the diversity of their wounds has afforded me numerous endeavors while operating on every body part, cavity, and structure created by the Maker.

Whereas only trace amounts of my education while in medical school and during my postgraduate training taught me how to deal with the psychiatric and social aspects of illness and injury, my patients themselves have enlightened me plenty. My dealings over the years with the countless criminals, substance abusers, mentally disabled, and social derelicts who seem to have a high predilection for getting themselves injured have taught me how to best manage the complex intricacies of trauma care, which extend well beyond the traumatic wounds themselves.

It has been my distinct privilege to care for the thousands of patients who have entrusted their lives to me. I realize without any uncertainty that there are many people in this world who would love to have had the opportunity to do what I have been allowed to do: to provide care to those in their darkest hours of need, and to save some lives along the way. Indeed, I have been so very fortunate. Indeed, I have been so very blessed. God has been very kind to me. He has been my chief of trauma and the lead surgeon in the operating room, who has guided my hands and my mind during my most difficult cases. And although the very nature of my subspecialty has forced me to deal with more chaos, drama, pain, and suffering than I might ordinarily choose to experience, I wouldn't trade my past or my present for a more tame and predictable lifestyle—at least not at this point in my life. Doing anything less than that which I engage in on a daily basis would be to deny my calling to serve the critically injured, and to care for those who cannot care for themselves.